M000205629

Clinical Data Management

SECOND EDITION

Clinical Data Management

SECOND EDITION

Edited by

RICHARD K. RONDEL
University of Surrey, UK

SHEILA A. VARLEY
Quintiles (UK) Ltd. Berkshire, UK

COLIN F. WEBB
Amgen Ltd, Cambridge, UK

JOHN WILEY & SONS, LTD

Chichester · New York · Weinheim · Brisbane · Singapore · Toronto

First published 1993 (reprinted 1994; 1995, twice; 1996; 1998, twice), Second Edition published 2000

Copyright © 1993, 2000 by John Wiley & Sons Ltd,
Baffins Lane, Chichester,
West Sussex PO19 1UD, England

National   01243 779777
International (+44) 1243 779777
e-mail (for orders and customer service enquiries):
cs-books@wiley.co.uk
Visit our Home Page on http://www.wiley.co.uk
or http://www.wiley.com

Reprinted October 2002

All Rights Reserved. No part of this publication may be reproduced, stored in a retrieval system, or transmitted, in any form or by any means, electronic, mechanical, photocopying, recording, scanning, or otherwise, except under the terms of the Copyright, Designs and Patents Act 1988 or under the terms of a licence issued by the Copyright Licensing Agency, 90 Tottenham Court Road, London, W1P 9HE UK, without the permission in writing of the publisher.

Other Wiley Editorial Offices

John Wiley & Sons, Inc., 605 Third Avenue,
New York, NY 10158-0012, USA

WILEY-VCH Verlag GmbH, Pappelallee 3,
D-69469 Weinheim, Germany

Jacaranda Wiley Ltd, 33 Park Road, Milton,
Queensland 4064, Australia

John Wiley & Sons (Asia) Pte Ltd, 2 Clementi Loop #02-01,
Jin Xing Distripark, Singapore 129809

John Wiley & Sons (Canada) Ltd, 22 Worcester Road,
Rexdale, Ontario M9W 1L1, Canada

Library of Congress Cataloging-in-Publication Data

Clinical data management / edited by Richard K. Rondel, Sheila A. Varley,
  Colin F. Webb. — 2nd.
     p. cm.
  Includes bibliographical references and index.
  ISBN 0-471-98329-2 (cased)
  1. Medicine—Research—Data processing. I. Rondel. R. K.
  II. Varley, S. A.
  [DNLM: 1. Information Systems. 2. Automatic Data Processing.
  3. Data Collection. 4. Data Display. 5. Quality Control. W
  26.55.14 C641 1999]
  R853.D37C55 1999
  610′.285—dc21
  DNLM/DLC
  for Library of Congress   99-31926
                                                                  CIP

British Library Cataloguing in Publication Data

A catalogue record for this book is available from the British Library

ISBN 0-471-98329-2

Typeset in 10/12pt Cheltenham Book by Dorwyn Ltd, Rowlands Castle, Hants.

Contents

Contributors

Steve Arlington
PricewaterhouseCoopers, West London Office, Harman House, 1 George Street, Uxbridge, London UB1 1QQ, UK

Paul Athey
PricewaterhouseCoopers, West London Office, Harman House, 1 George Street, Uxbridge, London UB1 1QQ, UK

Moira Avey
2 Loughton Villas, Crowborough, East Sussex TN6 5UD, UK

Elliot G. Brown
EBC Ltd, 7 Woodfall Avenue, High Barnet, Herts EN5 2EZ, UK

Kenneth Buchholz
INC Research, Charlottesville, Virginia, USA

Heather Campbell
Covance Clinical & Periapproval Services Ltd, 7 Roxborough Way, Maidenhead, Berkshire S16 3UD, UK

John Carroll
PricewaterhouseCoopers, West London Office, Harman House, 1 George Street, Uxbridge, London UB1 1QQ, UK

Stuart W. Cummings
Merck Sharp & Dohme (Europe), Inc., Clos du Lynx 5, Lynx Binnenhof, Brussel 1200, Bruxelles, Belgium

Linda Heywood
Amgen Ltd, 240 Cambridge Science Park, Milton Road, Cambridge CB4 0WD, UK

Steve Hutson
Barnett International, Parexel, River Court, 50 Oxford Road, Denham, Middlesex, UB9 49L, UK

Ruth Lane
MDS Therapeutic Director, Glaxo Wellcome UK, Greenford Road, Greenford, Middlesex UB6 0HE, UK

Munish Mehra
M² Worldwide, 1401 Rockville Pike, Suite 300, Rockville, Maryland 20852, USA

Louise Palma
Berlex Laboratories Inc., 340 Changebridge Road, PO Box 1000, Montville, New Jersey 07045-1000, USA

Pankaj 'Panni' Patel
Manager, Contract Operations and Resource Management, SmithKline Beecham Pharmaceuticals, New Frontiers Science Park (South), Third Avenue, Harlow, Essex CM19 5AW, UK

Andreas M. Pleil
Pharmacia & Upjohn AB, Lindhagensgatan 133, S-112 87 Stockholm, Sweden

Richard K. Rondel
HPRU Medical Research Centre, University of Surrey, Egerton Road, Guildford, Surrey GU2 5XP, UK

Michael F. Ryan
460 Foothill Road, Bridgewater, New Jersey 08807, USA

Alistair Shearin
PricewaterhouseCoopers, West London Office, Harman House, 1 George Street, Uxbridge, London, UB1 1QQ, UK

Beverley Smith
Amgen, Inc., One Amgen Center Drive, Thousand Oaks, California 91320-1789, USA

John Sweatman
7 Fox Covert, Lightwater, Surrey GU18 5TU, UK

Chris Thomas
Covance Clinical & Periapproval Services Ltd, 7 Roxborough Way, Maidenhead, Berkshire S16 3UD, UK

Tom Tollenaere
T2 Data Consult BVBA, Willemstraat 28, B-3000 Leuven, Belgium

Sheila A. Varley
Customer Strategic Business Unit, Drug Development Services, Clinical Services Europe, Quintiles Ltd, Ringside, 79 High Street, Bracknell, Berkshire RG12 1DZ, UK

Emma Waterfield
Clinical Trials Research Ltd, 107/123 King Street, Maidenhead, Berkshire SL6 1DP, UK

Colin F. Webb
Amgen Ltd, 240 Cambridge Science Park, Milton Road, Cambridge CB4 4WD, UK

Jon Wood
Phoenix International UK, Mildmay House, St Edwards Court, London Road, Romford, Essex RM7 9QD, UK

Louise Wood
Epidemiology Unit, Post Licensing Division, Medicines Control Agency, Market Towers, 1 Nine Elms Lane, London SW8 5NQ, UK

Foreword

Clinical data management is a profession with increasing importance within pharmaceutical research and development. The diverse lineage of clinical data management coupled with a wide range of responsibilities makes a clear, clean definition of 'clinical data management' difficult at best. As complex and diverse as the profession is, it is a field in which the number of substantial publications is extremely small. The first edition of this book provided one of the very few in-depth resources for clinical data management professionals. This second edition continues in that tradition by expanding and updating that knowledgebase.

Authored by professionals on both sides of the Atlantic, this text is reflective of the current trends of global harmonisation of clinical research and development. With the global consolidation of the industry, it is critical to understand, appreciate and be able to work within the framework of global clinical development. This text should contribute to that understanding.

As the global clinical data management discipline continues to grow we can rightfully expect an increase in the amount of research and reference material, such as this book, available to those working in and around the pharmaceutical industry. This is good for all involved—authors, publishers and readers!

Paul R. Loughlin
Chairperson,
Association for Clinical Data Management (ACDM)

Dr Kenneth Buchholz
Chairman of the Board of Trustees
Society for Clinical Data Management

Preface

Clinical Data Management has come a long way in the last decade. It is now a firmly established discipline in its own right, and is becoming an area that people know about and can progress their careers within.

We feel that the next decade will see major changes with the advantage of electronic data capture. The clinical and data jobs/disciplines as we know them today will become one as companies use more and more sophisticated hardware and software to streamline and eliminate duplication from the clinical trial process. Gone will be the days of the Investigator giving the CRF to CRA, CRA giving the CRF to DM, DM giving the CRF to DE. DE enters it, gives CRF back to DM and so on.

The ever increasing computerisation of the worldwide healthcare system will mean a practically paperless environment when study protocols will specify what data points at which intervals need to be transmitted from the clinic to the company headquarters via electronic means.

The need will then be for strict computer validation to audit trail data edits, electronic querying of data and mechanisms to ensure the host database at the hospital site is updated correctly and not corrupted.

The industry is still contracting, with more and more mergers and aquisitions occurring daily. The world of Contract Research Organisations has started to follow, with CROs, often of considerable size, going through takeovers and mergers to supply the type and size of service that the new emerging pharmaceutical companies need. We are seeing the emergence of virtual pharmaceutical/biotechnology companies who have no intention of having their own clinical research staff, but who just buy in a drug and then rely on the service industry to take it to the market place.

We predict that the top pharma/CRO companies today will not be the players of tomorrow unless they now address the necessary structures and technology to move themselves into the New Tomorrow, and the true advent of electronic data capture.

RKR
SAV
CFW

1 Chapter Review

STUART W. CUMMINGS

Merck Sharpe & Dohme (Europe), Inc., Brussels, Belgium

INTRODUCTION

The breadth of topics covered in this second edition reflects the range of regulatory, technical and operational areas of clinical development which are all impacted by the need for sound and effective Clinical Data Management (CDM) practices. The many authors who have contributed to this book are able to draw on many years of practical experience from within the pharmaceutical industry and have themselves either initiated or implemented many of the ideas described in the chapters that follow.

ICH AND ITS IMPACT (Smith and Heywood)

Since the first edition of this book was published in 1994, the International Conference on Harmonisation (ICH) has had a significant impact on how clinical trials are conducted and has set new expectations regarding how sponsor companies and drug regulatory authorities will interact in the next millennium. The impetus for ICH stems from a common desire on the part of industry to reduce development costs, from a regulatory perspective to reduce approval times and from a public health viewpoint to make more economical use of human subjects in scientific research studies. In Chapter 2 of this new edition of *Clinical Data Management*, Smith and Heywood present a concise overview of the recent history and conclusions resulting from the four ICH conferences that took place between 1991 and 1997.

The authors begin their review by describing the ICH organisational structure and defining the stepwise process whereby guidelines are developed and approved. A chart is provided which displays the status of each guideline. Particular consideration is given to surveying the five ICH guidelines (E2A, E3, E6, E8 and E9) which include specific references to

Clinical Data Management. Second Edition. Edited by R.K. Rondel, S.A. Varley and C.F. Webb.
© 2000 John Wiley & Sons, Ltd

clinical data management. Procedural and system changes which may be needed to assure compliance with ICH are reviewed in depth and the need to assure appropriate training and education is emphasised. Key areas where pharmaceutical companies will have to devote considerable energy include system validation, harmonisation of adverse experience terminology and the reformatting of key tables and listings for reporting purposes. ICH also underlines the role and contribution of data management staff throughout the drug development process including design activities, generating CSR tables and listing and satisfying electronic submission requirements.

Reference is also made to other guidance which complements ICH but has been developed separately in different regions. This includes the EU GCP Directive and a number of FDA guidance documents focusing on the submission of electronic case record forms (CRFs) and data listings. The authors note that the involvement of regulatory agency staff in the development of ICH and other guidelines, particularly with regard to electronic submissions should ultimately facilitate the review process, reduce the review period and further encourage consistency across regulatory agencies.

ICH is already impacting how data management departments are structured, how data management tasks are executed and how data are exchanged between sponsors and regulatory authorities. Widespread adoption of ICH will confirm the common framework against which research working practices will be evaluated, new clinical data management systems implemented and training and education goals will be set. However, it will probably take several years before it will be possible to assess whether the goals of ICH have been reached.

CRF DESIGN (Avey)

Despite the recent emphasis on electronic data capture tools, 95% of clinical data are still captured on paper and considerable resources are still applied to achieving efficient design, production and distribution of CRFs. Good CRF design offers the opportunity to minimise data processing delays due to poor data quality or loss of data. However, CRF design alone cannot compensate for inadequacies which may be inherent in the protocol. Moreover, since study objectives differ between early phase clinical trials and confirmatory trials it is to be expected that data collection and hence how CRFs are designed will also vary. These observations, from Avey, form the basis for a detailed account of CRF design and implementation. The author proposes a life cycle model which considers how a CRF is used at each stage of its evolution, encompassing the perspective of the designer, the user (form filler), data entry staff and data reviewer.

Creating a time and event schedule (study flow chart) derived from the study protocol can be helpful in designing the CRF and clarifying where standards can be applied and is strongly recommended as a key preparatory step. The author gives examples of modules which may generally be regarded as 'standards' and offers guidance as to the types of changes to 'standards' that should be permitted or even mandated. The use of standards must be balanced with a degree of flexibility to accommodate diverse trials since, if standards are applied slavishly, modules become foreign to the form filler's environment and data quality will be jeopardised.

Advice is offered as to how to identify, construct and organise data items onto CRF pages, noting that accuracy and legibility can be affected by the availability and presentation of space for recording responses. CRF 'performance' can also be enhanced through the use of a 'positive thinking bias' by presenting optional responses ranked by relevance and importance. Amongst alternatives for responding to multiple choice questions 'tick marks' are favoured in preference to other indicators. Readers are also cautioned that, when presenting an ordered categorical list, the positioning of response boxes relative to the question text can influence the response. Design features that help to minimise ambiguity (e.g., 'should' could mean may or must, and avoiding of double negatives) are also discussed. The order, format and physical characteristics of CRF pages can all influence how they are completed. There is also some discussion regarding various CRF production features, for example the use of different types and weights of paper, use of colour, margins, shading, fonts, insertion of additional pages, and so on.

CRF design impacts all stages of the clinical trial process. CRFs designed to facilitate data recording must also recognise how and where data will be entered and subsequently reviewed. A life cycle analysis to evaluate competing needs among different partners in the CRF process at different timepoints can help to achieve a balanced solution.

DATA CAPTURE (Waterfield)

For more than a decade, there has been a drive towards using electronic data capture tools in the belief that these technologies could be developed at reasonable cost, would reduce processing time and enhance data quality. It has also been recognised that facilitating data capture through technology solutions alone would not be sufficient and that changes in work processes and in job roles would also have to occur if such solutions were to be successful. However, the scalability of such solutions has often been questioned not only in terms of development and support costs but in terms of the computing architecture necessary to sustain such solutions globally. Technology and cost constraints have limited the widespread adoption of new approaches to data capture. Most major and medium-sized pharmaceutical companies have experimented with RDE solutions but few companies have embraced this approach as their primary data capture solution. In this chapter, Waterfield first examines how attitudes towards data capture have evolved in recent years and then reviews a number of different remote data entry (RDE) technologies.

The author stresses that data entry systems must be designed from the perspective of the person keying the data. For example, the data entry screen and data entry guidelines may be more or less complex depending on the skill set and medical background of the person keying the data. Understanding how a user will interact with the data entry screens determines the extent of edit check functionality built into the system and in particular the extent to which autoencoding may be used. Data capture requirements also change as one graduates from a centralised approach using 'heads down' data entry staff to one where data entry is distributed on a global scale and where the data entry would be carried out by clerical staff, study monitors or investigators.

Data capture is not just limited to processing of CRF data and Waterfield next considers various design concepts and issues surrounding the capture of data from external sources as well as considering the pros and cons of alternative data capture technologies that can be used, for example, fax-based systems, optical character recognition (OCR) and image character recognition (ICR) systems.

There is a good discussion on the rationale and some of the design issues concerned with the development and implementation of RDE technology. The potential benefits of using RDE must be assessed against the development and the support costs associated with global ambitions to achieve early access to study data. Successful RDE systems must be flexible and be based on careful protocol selection. Factors which influence the choice of data capture tools include cost, maintenance, security and regulatory compliance.

To date, only the larger pharmaceutical companies have been willing to invest heavily in new electronic data capture technologies and modify their work processes. With the advent of the next generation of data capture tools, embracing Web-based solutions and the prospect of controlled access to medical records, companies of all sizes will have to introduce electronic data capture technologies if they are to remain competitive. However, most companies may expect to live with a mixed data entry approach for the foreseeable future and should remain vigilant to the issues involved in scalability and user support as data entry becomes even more decentralised.

PLANNING AND IMPLEMENTATION (Thomas)

Dependent on the trial in question, up to 40% of the total resource spent in drug development can be attributed to tasks related to data management. This large cost can be mitigated if, in particular, projects teams elect to integrate data management early in the planning phase and involve data managers as key members of design and implementation teams. In this chapter, Thomas reviews the key steps associated with the planning and execution of a clinical trial system, emphasising not only the process involved but also the data management products delivered at each stage of the process.

Planning starts with a basic understanding of the business needs, a clear definition of objectives, a budget proposal, a summary of the assumptions and constraints that may affect both development and implementation and a notion of timeline. Only once the timeline has been established can those tasks and key milestones which fall on the critical path be identified. An early product resulting from the planning process is a list of feasible solutions supported by a statement of the manpower and materials required to support each solution together with a framework against which alternatives can be evaluated. The evaluation should include scope (single vs multiple protocols), deliverables (study database, statistical report, clinical study report), customer focus (internal, external), data sources and data flow (CRFs, laboratory data), ownership (processes and tasks) and constraints (budget, skills, time).

From the data management perspective, the project plan defines process flows against which specific data management and study tracking solutions can be developed. If a new technology is to be introduced then the impact of change on existing work processes and job roles must be taken into consideration before confirming the final solution. The planning phase must also consider such items as data validation, reconciliation of adverse experience (AE) data, SOP development and training, dictionary management and how the liaison with CROs will be handled, if applicable.

Throughout the project, timelines, budget, process efficiency and product quality as stated in the project plan are under constant review. In this regard, it is important to report on metrics representing performance, quality and resource utilisation to determine if the study is being conducted according to plan or if certain processes are not in control. Responses to processes which are found not to be in control may include renegotiation of tasks and priorities, shifting resources, providing incentives and possibly changing work processes.

DATA VALIDATION (Patel)

GCP and regulatory reporting requirements emphasise the importance of validation of systems, process and data. Since the quality of trials depends on the acceptability of data and results, all trial participants have a role to play in ensuring this success and in sharing the responsibility for continuous data validation. However, data recorded on CRFs do not always represent data held in source documents and even if data are correctly recorded on CRFs they may not always be correctly represented on the clinical database, and study reports may not always reflect the contents of the database. Whereas electronic data capture solutions and automated query and review tools have, to some extent, reduced the time and effort required to review and correct data at different stages, data validation still commands considerable resources to ensure success. Resources to support validation efforts can be reduced through careful definition and execution of data review and audit plans and by encouraging a continuous data validation process throughout the study.

In this chapter, Patel considers data validation as a stepwise process starting at the investigator site and ending only when the final clinical study report is published. The roles of the investigator and study monitor in assuring that source document verification (SDV), data entry and subsequent data review steps are conducted in accordance with GCP are discussed. Data validation during data entry is accomplished by executing edit checks against the data being entered. The number and complexity of edit checks will be dependent on the underlying data management process and the job roles of those involved.

Steps that can be taken to enhance data quality before the study starts are discussed in some detail. In particular, the role of SOPs found in regulations and in company policies can be helpful in establishing the environment and setting expectations regarding how data will be processed and validated. Parallel development of the protocol and CRF, development of clear data handling guidelines, timely training and support of investigator and field staff can all lead to increased data quality. Headquarters staff too can benefit from a clear understanding of the data management guidelines in an effort to reduce the number of review questions raised and presumably to increase the proportion of questions raised that are relevant and lead to database changes. There is also mention of how validation should be carried out for data from external sources (e.g., laboratory data).

In conclusion, Patel notes that the introduction of new technologies will have a significant impact on data validation. As automated processes for data capture and review become standard practice, it is expected that there will be a shift from data validation late in the process towards early validation of the systems and procedures that govern the clinical data management process.

QUALITY ASSURANCE AND CLINICAL DATA MANAGEMENT
(Campbell and Sweatman)

Definitions of quality assurance (QA) and quality control (QC) can be found in guidance issued by the FDA and in ICH GCP. In general, this guidance refers not just to data but also to the systems procedures and validation steps which give assurance that data have been processed correctly and that the CSR is a true representation of the trial that took place. Although audit findings cannot give 100% assurance with regard to all aspects of a trial, they should accurately reflect what has happened. Moreover, QA should not just be viewed as a confirmation step to ensure compliance with regulations and procedures but as an opportunity to positively influence decision making across all phases of development before problems arise.

In the opening sections of the chapter, Campbell and Sweatman quote the definitions of QA and QC and related terms as defined in ICH GCP and take care to distinguish between these two terms, which are frequently confused. One key distinction is that QC is carried out by all staff throughout the trial whereas QA is an independent audit activity.

There follows a review of how audit practices have evolved in recent years, characterised by a shift away from site audits and the late involvement of QA staff to an earlier and more continuous effort focusing on processes and procedures starting at the protocol review stage and continuing throughout the lifetime of a study. The early involvement of QA staff also positions this group to play a more proactive role as the trial progresses, including selection of investigator sites, setting the data review strategy and the training of site and other study personnel. The benefits of early and interim audits are also described.

From a data management perspective, audit activities focus on five key areas—study documentation, completion of CRFs, emphasis on key variables, content and format of table and listings, and the CSR. Advice is offered as to how groups supporting these various activities can prepare for both internal and external regulatory audits. Guidance is also given in terms of how compliance can be achieved and measured although some caution is suggested against over-interpretation of error metrics unless the structure behind their meaning is clear.

Future audit activities are expected to be greatly influenced by the impact of technology changes—particularly the expansion of electronic data capture systems and regulatory acceptance of electronic signatures, for example, by FDA. QA will also have an expanded role to play in ensuring harmonisation of submissions. The contribution of QA is dependent on the quality and expertise of the staff performing this role. Criteria for selection and recruitment of audit staff are mentioned, emphasising both external as well as internal training opportunities. In conclusion, the authors suggest that the time may be right to introduce a formal QA qualification in response to the increasing role, contribution and size of QA departments.

PERFORMANCE MEASURES (Wood)

Measurement of performance is necessary to demonstrate successful project management and to identify opportunities for continuous improvement. Yet measurement of clinical development processes, and in particular data management activities, has proved to be notoriously difficult. Part of this difficulty concerns the fact that drug development timelines tend to be driven less by an underlying process but rather by setting target dates and subsequently adding resources or adjusting priorities to ensure that targets are met. Nevertheless, organisations that can generate meaningful measures against which performance can be judged and future targets set should be more successful in achieving continuous improvement than those which do not.

In his review of the challenges and opportunities that impact our ability to measure performance, Wood highlights three key dimensions where measurement is desirable—productivity, quality and cycle time—noting that aggregation of data across protocols may be difficult or inappropriate since protocols have varying characteristics and operate under different processes.

The key to successful measurement, Wood suggests, is defining a framework or process flow from which processing units (e.g., a complete CRF) can be defined, and against which measures (e.g., CRF visit date to CRF reviewed) can be determined. Successful measurement involves gathering input and buy-in from all team members since only by understanding how measures relate to each other can a true appreciation of the process flow be understood.

The use of metrics data for reporting or diagnostic purposes should reflect the underlying work process (e.g., it should be possible to distinguish between queries raised by field monitors and in-house staff). Such metrics, however, may be subject to misinterpretation and the author cautions against inappropriate use and the need for relevant subanalyses to ensure that performance is correctly evaluated. Wood also stresses the importance of being able to capture resource data although getting staff to record time spent per task will rarely by successful.

CDM still represents about 30–40% of total effort and expenditure in drug development. Measurement of current and assessment of future practice should identify improvement opportunities leading to reduced cycle times and accelerated data clean up and reporting practices. Although we can measure CDM performance, this is not always done or applied consistently. As a consequence it is difficult to assess the real economic and material benefits of change. Interest at lower levels can only be successful if project teams buy-in to a methodology and measures of common interest. In conclusion, Wood suggests that network-based technologies will continue to significantly impact current performance and the standards that we use. However, without metrics the effect of change is likely to be at best inaccurate or at worst it will lead to missed opportunities for further improvement.

DATA PRESENTATION (Mehra)

In designing a clinical trial, most attention is given to those activities concerned with the trial set up, for example, CRF design, data capture system specifications and data handling guidelines. Less attention is paid to how data will be presented and reported. This is surprising when one realises that it is the report and the way data are presented to regulatory agencies that will determine whether approval is granted or not. Although some effort is generally made to include reporting needs at the study design stage, for example through the adoption of data analysis and data management plans, most data presentation needs can only be finalised well after the trial has started. To add to this confusion some companies have found that the common formats defined by ICH have caused considerable rework and some uncertainty, in determining how data will be presented in clinical study reports.

In his analysis of how data should be displayed to meet regulatory requirements, Mehra considers two uses of data presentations. Firstly, to assist in the review and screening of data leading to clean files for analysis, and secondly, for the purpose of permitting reviewers to accept or reject a hypothesis under test on the basis of data presented in a submission document. He points out the difficulty in designing clinical database systems that are optimal for data capture, data retrieval and data

presentation and notes that in most cases data capture needs are favoured. This practice may become even more widespread as data entry
becomes more decentralised. Database designers have traditionally
focused on structures which are optimal for storage and can allow transformations for other purposes—the so called third normal form.
However, for database presentations, non-normalised databases are
preferred.

Another issue which designers and programmers alike have to face is
that different reviewers may require different presentations of the data. To
facilitate this debate, Mehra proposes certain rules governing data presentations. He notes that displays of raw data, for example by CRF form type
or by patient across forms, may not necessarily be optimal for screening
purposes. This task is better accomplished through summary table displays (graphs, figures, plots, as well as data listings). Such listings are also
used for validation purposes and frequently use distribution statistics to
highlight abnormal values or trends of interest.

The author next presents a characterisation of different data types and
reviews how presentation needs differ between continuous and categorical variables and between visit datapoints and those that are patient oriented. Another issue covered is that of combining data across different
protocols where, for example, different units, variable names or methods
of data collection may have been used.

In conclusion the author stresses the importance of displaying data not
just for review and validation but also for interpretation of results. Data
displays demand the skills of both data management and statistical programmers and should ideally be amenable to statistical modelling and
analysis.

CODING OF DATA (Brown and Wood)

Brown and Wood dedicate this chapter to the late Dr Sue Wood, formerly
of the MCA, whose work is widely recognised as being a driving force in
the harmonisation of the use of medical terminology now reflected in the
work of the MedDRA and ICH M1 working parties. Brown and Wood both
work at the MCA and it is therefore appropriate that they also present
the benefits that coding brings from the perspective of a regulatory
authority.

The authors begin their review by assessing the need for coding
systems, particularly those linked with medical terminology, in response
to the need to manage large volumes of text data at a time when
computing technology was not well designed to meet this need. Coding of
data not only provides an opportunity for storing data more concisely and

consistently but also greatly facilitates the summarisation and reporting of text data. The irony that today's computing technology solutions are well able to handle large text databases is not lost.

Coding systems which permit the aggregation of data help sponsors to meet legal obligations and aid in the identification of signals to detect rare adverse experiences. In particular the use of recognised coding systems effectively eliminates the risk that different processors could obtain different results based on determining their own rules for aggregating verbatim terms.

The authors next review the history and characteristics of a number of the commercial dictionaries which have been embraced both by industry and by drug regulatory agencies. Particular attention is given to the origin of MedDRA which dates back to 1993, with further work culminating in the acceptance of MedDRA as a new international standard endorsed by ICH. There follows a concise overview of the structure, use and maintenance of MedDRA, highlighting the expected advantages in comparison with existing commercial and indeed some in-house coding schemes. In certain instances, MedDRA can be regarded as being more complex than existing systems and will require a more in-depth knowledge of dictionary structures and a possible need to adjust MedDRA output for presentation purposes. The authors note that over time MedDRA will become the gold standard for pharmacovigilance and expedited reporting. However, its acceptance by industry and industry support organisations is more likely to be driven through its adoption by regulatory authorities.

In closing, the reader is reminded why the creation and acceptance of a single medical terminology having the support of ICH will provide long-term benefits both to sponsors and to agencies. As a consequence expectations are high that data quality, electronic interchange of data and hence speed of development, review and approval of drug applications and pharmacovigilance will all improve for the public good.

DATABASE DESIGN ISSUES FOR CENTRAL LABORATORIES
(Tollenaere)

Guidelines regarding laboratory data systems are briefly mentioned in EC GCP requirements and again in GMP whereas GLP advice is more directed towards animal experimentation. In this chapter, Tollenaere considers the special case of database structures for the management of clinical laboratory data. He begins by pointing out that, in general, the rules for normalising data do not necessarily apply to laboratory data, in part due to regulations and in part to particular requirements which characterise laboratory data processing.

By way of example, the author explores the structures, advantages and disadvantages of normalised datasets, pointing out the particular difficulties caused by erroneous or inconsistent laboratory data. Normalised datasets minimise storage needs, avoid duplication of data and can easily be updated. However, they have the disadvantage that data retrieval and interrogation is somewhat more complex and may require sophisticated programming techniques. This point is illustrated by examining the impact of just one erroneous laboratory value. Conversely, storing data in a denormalised form and selecting the right key can result in correct output. A clean database can often be normalised for delivery to a sponsor although the effort in creating it has not followed non-normalised rules.

Next, a set of principles for managing laboratory data are described including the need to be able to store inconsistent data. Again by example, the difficulties resulting from one or more erroneous identification field are explored in detail.

Another issue affecting the processing laboratory of data concerns the need to process unscheduled or unexpected laboratory results. In practice, when repeat test results occur two choices are available to resolve this situation—either programs are written to selectively add new values or the database is designed with placeholders in such a way that any number of results can be accommodated. Tollenaere emphasises the need for a 'good correction system' to ensure an adequate audit trail and offers two alternatives—one where all changed values are held and another which retains only the original and most recently changed record. He advocates that the former method offers greater advantages.

In conclusion, the author reminds the reader that understanding the prerequisites of managing laboratory data and careful consideration of database design issues can greatly improve the speed and efficiency with which the data can be processed and reported. This statement is all the more striking when one appreciates the greatest processing in any trial concerns the processing of laboratory data.

COMPUTER SYSTEMS (Palma)

Increased computer literacy, advances in technology and a desire to accelerate drug development and approval has encouraged both industry and regulatory authorities to invest in new database structures and state-of-the-art computing infrastructure. In this chapter, Palma presents an overview of current thinking in clinical systems design and focuses on the growth and potential of a number of commercial clinical data management systems available.

A necessary first step in defining a new clinical data management system is to conduct a present state analysis and establish criteria which will allow the organisation to put forward clearly defined objectives and to define a process whereby the selection and evaluation of candidate products can be conducted. Objectives should be multidisciplinary and incorporated into a requirements statement from which standards, strategy and functionality and the potential for integration with other (internal and external) systems can be derived. The author leads us through a stepwise process and provides guidance for determining technical and operational specifications and for conducting acceptance testing. User acceptance test plans should mention the need to perform 'gap analysis', a determination of how feedback will be incorporated, a transition strategy and specify how training will be given.

The features of three of the more popular commercial systems (Clintrial 4, DLB, Oracle Clinical) are discussed in detail. The author comments that many commercial database systems have been upgraded to include document management needs, provide links to CROs and accommodate data from external sources.

A product review is also provided of commercial workflow systems and associated technology solutions designed to allow the receipt and tracking of data from different sources. In general these systems are based on varying combinations of fax, scanning and image applications, some of which are able to integrate CRF data directly into a clinical database. A useful table contrasting these different options is provided.

Palma concludes that if data management systems are to be fully effective, they must be integrated with workflow and document management systems and with data from other sources. Such systems require the necessary time to plan, develop and implement and require attention to training needs.

SYSTEMS VALIDATION (Hutson)

Historically, data management systems and data managers place greater emphasis on data validation rather than systems validation. Only within the past five years has this emphasis been reversed, driven in part by greater reliance on computer systems and technology to replace manual tasks and partly by regulatory guidance which now requires systems validation to be demonstrated. Companies must have in place both internal validation steps as well as a procedure for responding to external regulatory inspections. Regulatory guidance is primarily contained in the EC GCP guidelines and in ICH E6. In this chapter, Hutson reviews the current validation environment governing clinical systems, including rationale for developing a validation policy, and a description of what regulatory auditors may request.

From a regulatory perspective, organisations should develop SOPs, policy statements and record meeting materials and minutes in such a way that inspectors can easily and quickly determine how compliance has been achieved. A useful reference in this regard is the joint PSI/ACDM guideline on Computer Validation published in 1997. It is not, however, sufficient to have SOPs in place for each protocol or system component. Rather organisations need to demonstrate that they have developed and indeed implemented a validation policy covering roles, personnel, training, and organisation and implementation of QA programs.

Retrospective validation generally applies to older systems which predate the more recent guidance referenced above. In such cases, it is a question of 'filling the gaps'. Retrospective validation begins by establishing an inventory of systems components and configurations, documentation, and a historical perspective on system use. Since not everything can be included, a risk assessment must be conducted taking into account resource availability and timeframe. In extreme circumstances, it may even be necessary to take the system out of commission for a short time. The key steps involved consist of planning, validation, reporting deficiencies, correcting defects and revalidating the system.

Prospective validation is an inherent part of systems development methodology and is commonly presented within the context of a Systems Development Life Cycle (SDLC) model. The classic SDLC approach is illustrated in the text and provides a useful distinction between validation and verification. Testing provides evidence that inputs and outputs are processed correctly and particular mention is made of the need for integration and stress testing to ensure scalability.

The chapter includes a case history concerning the steps taken by a development team in validating a Phase II/III clinical database. The discussion details the data characteristics, the use of software packages, and highlights the complexity of validation in a multidisciplinary setting. The author identifies tips to aid in this process, including reference to sponsor SOPs, a clear definition of scope, and a component analysis with an assessment of risk for each component.

Hutson concludes by echoing a theme repeated elsewhere in the book that as we have moved to integrated CDM systems, so the emphasis has shifted from data to systems validation. Such systems are complex, must meet regulatory requirements and strike a balance with good business practice. As a consequence, systems should be more reliable, development costs and implementation costs will be reduced and overall product and process quality enhanced.

RE-ENGINEERING (Arlington, Athey, Carroll and Shearin)

Innovation in basic research and development, health care reform, competition, globalisation of research practices, new regulations and demands to demonstrate economic benefit have led pharmaceutical companies to re-engineering current practices. However, the expectation that re-engineering would result in candidate nomination to launch within five to seven years has still to be proven. In this chapter, Arlington et al. describe how re-engineering methodologies have been embraced by industry and propose that much improvement can be obtained by eliminating non-value-added tasks, partly through harnessing technology solutions but also by changing the process used to perform data management. Their discussion, although general, contains specific and informative references to re-engineering of CDM practices.

Arlington et al. point out that success is not just a case of change in practice but is also reflected in the ambition within the organisation. Experience with both success and failure has led to rules designed to 'get it right' the first time and the bulk of the chapter is concerned with expanding on this advice. Criteria for the success and failure of re-engineering efforts are discussed, citing figures that 40% fail and only 33% claim success.

Barriers to successful re-engineering efforts include the culture of the organisation, management style, skills, technology systems—the last of which may be difficult to change quickly. Change also requires the commitment of cross-functional resources and a mechanism to prioritise and develop change. Success factors include the ability to demonstrate quick wins, assessing feasibility of implementation during development, not implementing novel solutions too quickly, continuous communication to stakeholders and a clear understanding of barriers to development and acceptance of proposed solutions.

Strategies designed to ensure success include an early analysis of performance gaps, building consensus, following a structured approach based on agreed priorities and a broad agreement on goals and criteria for evaluating success. The actual solution development may need to extend into other disciplines, suggesting the formation of multidisciplinary development teams, and workshops to handle the human and behavioural aspects of change are advised, emphasising the respective AS-IS versus the TO-BE process models. Once development is complete the organisation must move quickly from a go-decision to implementation to maintain momentum and here the choice is to go for a gradual roll out or a 'big bang' approach.

In concluding this discussion, Arlington et al. underscore the power of re-engineering if applied correctly and again remind the reader of the high rate of failure arguably due to failure to set and follow rules and the failure of those responsible for implementation to willingly embrace solutions.

WORKING WITH CROs (Buchholz)

In the face of increased internal and regulatory pressures, organisations are not always able to grow resources to meet demands posed by increased workload and greater complexity of data systems and the introduction of change. There are two choices—either to reduce or reprioritise the workload or to invest in additional resources, primarily relying on Contract Research Organisations who provide either stand alone or full service support. Under the CRO option there is an increasing preference on the part of companies to form preferred partnerships with CROs, resulting in greater flexibility and increased efficiency. On the other hand, enlisting the help of different CROs can spread the risk should a CRO fail. In this chapter, Buchholz describes how CROs have emerged to become fully integrated service partners or in some cases are able to bring a product through full development to registration. Their growth continues to be fuelled by mergers and acquisitions.

There are many reasons why a company may engage a CRO and why maintaining such relationships in the long term makes both scientific and economic sense. A CRO may be employed not only to meet a resource shortfall or a lack of in-house technical or therapeutic expertise but can also help to train and develop staff on new systems or to release staff for other priority work.

Buchholz explores the range of factors involved in selecting a CRO, commenting that this process can be helped if companies have CRO management services in place which can pre-qualify CROs, thus limiting the time taken to research and evaluate tenders. It is increasingly important that sponsors develop negotiating expertise. The author cautions that price alone should not be the sole determinant for selecting a CRO, mentioning that size, geographic spread, financial viability, staff stability, references from clients and audit results should all be considered. The chapter offers clear guidance on how to enhance the sponsor's ability to recover data on communication to ensure success.

The sponsor is ultimately responsible for the terms and conditions defined in the contract with the CRO. The purpose of the contract is to set expectations and list the extent of documentation, timelines, quality, billing, reporting and other deliverables that will control the activity. Where possible, statements as to how the quality of the data and process steps will be measured should be included. The merits of fixed price contracts versus those based on time and materials are also discussed.

Nor does Buchholz ignore the human component in ensuring a success-ful outcome. He stresses the need for a communication plan and argues this must be a two-way communication to the point where, under certain conditions, CRO staff could be invited to participate as a member of the project team in preference to appointing a person from within the sponsor organisation.

In conclusion, there is a discussion on alternative indirect ways of work-ing with CROs which builds on greater use of computing networks to permit database access and e-mail between sponsors, clients and sites. The pros and cons of permitting direct database access with the inherent security problems are discussed as well as the longstanding issues of integration of CRO work with company systems and procedures.

DATA MANAGEMENT IN EPIDEMIOLOGY AND PHARMACOECONOMICS (Ryan)

Partly in response to regulatory reporting requirements as defined in pharmacovigilance and partly in response to a desire on the part of com-panies and research institutions to evaluate large databases to test new hypotheses, the disciplines of epidemiology and pharmacoeconomics have become established as key areas supporting drug development and delivery. As a consequence, clinical data managers have had to become familiar with a range of different types of data, sources of data, analysis and reporting needs. In this chapter, Ryan introduces the reader to the key concepts which underlie both epidemiological and pharmaco-economic research and considers the particular data needs that pertain to both areas.

Epidemiology has evolved through the need to better understand long-term drug safety and to examine drug effects in large diverse populations and is primarily concerned with assessing populations at risk, tracing the natural history of disease, determining clinical endpoints, defining disease incidence and supporting health economists. Pharmacoeconomics is a discipline which is concerned with determining the economic benefit of drug therapy, especially in support of reimbursement arguments. A range of different types of health economic studies is presented which vary in their objectives, endpoints and outcomes.

Regarding data management in epidemiological and pharmacoeconomic studies, Ryan comments on how unreliable secondary data can be, given that they come from multiple sources and that they are usually neither complete nor consistent and contain unknown bias. This is particularly true for safety data which can come from spontaneous reports, health authorities and drug companies. Some degree of harmonisation has been achieved through the CIOMS process although most countries still operate independently. In the US public and private databases are generally accessible while in Europe, access is much more restricted. In circumstances where existing databases are insufficient, prospective studies may be conducted and have been used to advantage where, for example, a sponsor may wish to demonstrate a competitive advantage because of a superior safety profile. Data managers, for their part, need to understand the strengths and weaknesses of various study designs of this type.

In conclusion, Ryan considers the distinction between experimental designs exhibiting scientific rigour and non-experimental (observational) studies—both of which are widely used in epidemiological and similar studies. Observational studies which do not employ randomisation techniques and are not designed with a predetermined selection of therapy are of major importance in characterising disease and treatment relationships. He provides examples of different experimental designs used in pharmacoepidemiology studies, observing that the same principles apply as for economic studies.

FUTURE REVISITED (Lane)

Ruth Lane, in her chapter on the future of clinical data management, makes the point that despite much promise the new technologies have not radically improved the process or reduced the paper mountain. Pressure within the industry is to reduce costs and data management, which accounts for 6% of clinical development costs, is no different from other functions. Adopting more effective methods of managing clinical data could enhance the speed with which the drug is developed and commercialised, increasing competitive advantage.

It is now acknowledged that clinical data are a key corporate asset. The trend in the industry has been to use data capture tools to ensure that high-quality data are now available early for review and rapid decision-making. Although the regulatory agencies are often considered the primary customers of the information and it is recognised that a speedy response to questions has commercial benefits, increasingly the customer-base is widening. Patients and the numerous advocacy groups are becoming powerful and increasingly more knowledgeable, especially with the advent of the Internet.

The data management function is very much involved in building a knowledge base which may need to serve the company for the lifetime of the product (15–20 years) with its attendant problems as technology changes and advances.

As far as the data management function is concerned in the future, its boundaries with statistics and clinical will probably become more blurred, as the structure of organisations is flattened and teams are empowered.

The expected progress and impact by new technology has not so far materialised. However, the Internet is permeating the world at an unprecedented speed which will inevitably impact clinical data management, potentially making the transfer of patient data electronically from investigator sites plus improving communication between clinics, laboratory and sponsor. Potentially the Internet and other data capture alternatives to the keyboard, for example, optical mark reading, optical character and voice recognition, could make the biggest impact in the future, but we have said this before—time will tell.

2 The International Conference on Harmonisation and its Impact

BEVERLEY SMITH[1] and LINDA HEYWOOD[2]

[1]*Amgen Inc., California, USA*
[2]*Amgen Ltd, Cambridge, UK*

OVERVIEW

Since the publication of the first edition of this book in 1993, the regulatory scene governing medicinal product development has been very active. The initiatives of the International Conference on Harmonisation of Technical Requirements for Registration of Pharmaceuticals for Human Use (ICH) have produced lively debate and interpretation of regulatory expectations and a number of written scientific and technical standards (guidelines) for medicinal product development and registration. Since its inception, the ICH process has produced over 50 technical documents (Appendix 1), several of which have been formally adopted by regulatory bodies and their requirements implemented by industry. During the second ICH meeting in 1993, Kessler (from the US Food and Drug Administration) gave a keynote address where the *vision* of a single universal new drug registration package was speculated. The concept of a Common Technical Document for submitting medicinal product applications was discussed during the fourth ICH meeting in 1997, and development of this technical standard commenced during 1998. Kessler's *vision* now seems more of a reality despite the language, cultural and medical practice differences between geographical regions.

One ICH document which specifically references data handling obligations of the Sponsor is the ICH Harmonised Tripartite Guideline for Good Clinical Practice. This guideline defines standards and expectations which encompass the conduct, performance, monitoring, auditing, recording, analyses and reporting of clinical research. The guideline will have a significant impact on clinical data management practices as sponsor companies and clinical investigating sites work towards compliance with the requirements. The adoption of this guideline in Europe, Japan and America re-enforces the cultural diversity, as further language modifications and interpretive clarifications to the already agreed document were made in each region prior to adoption.

Clinical Data Management. Second Edition. Edited by R.K. Rondel, S.A. Varley and C.F. Webb.
© 2000 John Wiley & Sons, Ltd

Several of the ICH technical documents define standards, procedures and requirements relating to clinical data management practices. Information repositories sited on the Internet now provide a rapid method of retrieving the latest information to enable industry to keep abreast of the developing documents. In addition to this, training courses are widely advertised to industry offering the latest updates to the ICH documents and guidance on their interpretation and practical implementation.

Before discussing the impact of the current ICH guidelines on clinical data management, the history of the ICH initiative will be presented.

HISTORY OF ICH

The ICH initiative started in November 1991 in Brussels. The purpose of this initiative was to bring together regulatory agencies and experts from the pharmaceutical industry of the three largest markets (Europe, Japan and the United States of America) in an effort to harmonise regulatory requirements for the registration of new human therapeutics. If harmonisation could be achieved without compromising the quality, efficacy and safety of medicinal products, then much of the repeat testing required to register a product in the three regions would be reduced or eliminated. This lofty goal would also result in reduced times to medicinal product approval, more economical use of human, animal and material resources, and would potentially reduce the costs of medicinal product development. Patent protection time was also an issue for small companies without financial stability and where the costs of researching and developing biotechnology derived drugs outweighed any potential financial gain. Ways of increasing patent protection times were subsequently investigated. The ICH initiatives excluded medical devices and were targeted to harmonising technical requirements for medicinal product development (from pre-clinical through clinical requirements) and defining new standards for biotechnological products. In summary, the aims of the ICH process are to:

- Unify the registration requirements for new medicinal products
- Accelerate medicinal product licensing times
- Reduce medicinal product development costs
- Increase patent protection times

ICH Conferences

ICH conferences are widely advertised in advance and are held every two years. They are attended by the ICH committee members, observers from regulatory agencies and interested parties from academia and industry. Four ICH conferences have been held to date:

ICH 1: November 1991, Brussels
ICH 2: October 1993, Orlando   Phase 1 of the ICH process
ICH 3: November 1995, Yokohama
ICH 4: July 1997, Brussels

ICH 4 was intended to mark the end of the first phase of ICH activities. These activities concentrated on ensuring that the scientific research and testing required to approve and market new medicinal products only needed to be carried out once to satisfy regional registration requirements. Finalisation of all the technical documents should be completed before ICH 5 which is scheduled to take place in San Diego, California, during November 2000.

Organisation of ICH

The ICH organisation involves representatives from three principal regions the European Union, Japan and the United States of America, with the assistance of observers from the World Health Organisation (WHO), the European Free Trade Association (EFTA) and the Canadian Health Protection Branch. There are six co-sponsors of the ICH process, two from each of the following geographical regions:

Europe
> The Commission of the European Communities (CEC)
> The European Federation of Pharmaceutical Industries Association
>   (EFPIA)

Japan
> The Ministry of Health and Welfare (MHW)
> Japan Pharmaceutical Manufacturers Association (JPMA)

USA
> Food and Drug Administration (FDA)
> Pharmaceutical Research and Manufacturers Association (PhRMA)

Secretariat

The International Federation of Pharmaceutical Manufacturers Associations (IFPMA) provides the ICH Secretariat. The Secretariat coordinates meetings of the Steering Committee and the Expert Working Groups. It also organises the biennial conferences, including coordinating all the documentation and speakers required for the meetings.

Steering Committee

The ICH Steering Committee oversees the conference organisation. Each co-sponsor has two seats on the Steering Committee and the IFPMA has two seats, resulting in a total of 14 seats. The committee is chaired by one of the regulatory agencies and the chair is rotated to match the region of the location of the meeting. Observers also participate in the meetings but they are non-voting members of the Steering Committee. The Steering Committee is responsible for selecting topics for harmonisation. A representative from each of the six sponsors is responsible to act as ICH coordinator with the Secretariat to ensure that all ICH documents are distributed to the relevant personnel within their area of responsibility.

Expert Working Groups

The Expert Working Groups (EWGs) consist of joint regulatory and industry representatives nominated by the six ICH co-sponsors. Several EWGs are appointed to advise the steering committee on topics for the harmonisation process. These topics are grouped under four areas:

1.   Quality
2.   Efficacy
3.   Safety
4.   Multidisciplinary (Cross-topics)

Topics identified for technical harmonisation pass through five administrative steps (Figure 2.1). The time taken for documents to pass through all five steps is highly variable and has taken up to four years for some topics. The time taken is usually related to the complexity of the topic and the difficulty in reaching consensus on all issues. Step 5 of the ICH process tends to differ in each ICH region because the guidelines are adopted and implemented by different mechanisms, as follows:

Europe	Japan	United States
Issued as guidelines by the CPMP. Member states of the EU transpose and implement guidelines into local requirements. This may include revision of local regulations.	Issued as law by the Ministry of Health and Welfare (MHW), with implementation dates set in the future.	Issued as guidelines under 21 Code of Federal Regulations Part 10, and printed in full in the Federal Register (FR). Later consideration may be given to revising the regulations, if necessary.

The Future of ICH

Having harmonised the technical requirements for demonstrating the quality, efficacy and safety of a new medicinal product in phase one of the

STEP 1

> Preliminary discussion of topic by EWG. Consensus draft guideline produced and forwarded to the Steering Committee.

STEP 2

> Steering Committee approves the draft and issues it for comment to regulatory agencies in Europe, Japan, USA and other interested parties.
> Distributed via pharmaceutical representative bodies or published in the guideline section of the regulatory authority's publications.

STEP 3

> Review comments are collated by the regulatory agencies. The EWG incorporate these comments to a revised draft of the guideline.
> EWG review and sign off the revised guideline and forward it to the Steering Committee.

STEP 4

> Guideline is endorsed by the Steering Committee.
> Recommended for adoption to the regulatory agencies in Europe, Japan and USA.

STEP 5

> The process ends when the guideline is formally adopted by the three regulatory agencies.
> The guideline is incorporated to domestic regulations, or other administrative measures are taken to implement the guideline according to local procedures.

Figure 2.1 ICH administrative steps

ICH initiative, the second phase of harmonisation activities was initiated during ICH 4. The following terms of reference were revised to ensure the ICH momentum was sustained:

- Maintenance of the forum for dialogue between regulatory authorities and the pharmaceutical industry on the differences in technical requirements for product registration in the ICH regions, in order to ensure the timely introduction of medicinal products
- Monitoring, revising and updating the technical requirements with a view to achieving greater mutual acceptance

- Avoiding divergent future requirements by proactively selecting topics for harmonisation as a result of therapeutic advances, and the development of new technologies for the production of medicinal products
- Adopting new or improved technical approaches which permit a more economical use of human, animal or material resources without compromising safety
- Maintaining the momentum already established in the ICH process by facilitating the dissemination of guidelines and encouraging the implementation and integration of common standards

The second phase of ICH (post-ICH 4) will continue its commitment to international harmonisation and countries such as Australia, Canada and South Africa will be included. The real focus of the second phase will be on the development of a Common Technical Document for submissions. Harmonisation of the format and content of product application documents is intended to save time and resource for companies who submit applications across more than one region. Work commenced on this initiative in February 1998, and the final objective of reaching consensus on a Common Technical Document is to be completed by the three EWGs for Quality, Safety and Efficacy in time for discussion at ICH 5.

ICH 5 plans to primarily review the requirements of the Common Technical Document and the scope, format and specifications for an electronic Common Technical Document. Other topics to be reviewed include post-marketing safety surveillance and electronic reporting of adverse drug reactions; new technologies and other challenges, and globalisation of the ICH achievements. In March 1999, the *Medical Dictionary for Drug Regulatory Affairs* (MedRA) was launched. Progress in its implementation will be studied at this meeting.

The impact of specific ICH guidelines on clinical data management activities will now be discussed.

ICH GUIDELINES AND CLINICAL DATA MANAGEMENT

Of the several technical guidelines developed through ICH, Table 2.1 lists 15 ICH topics which contain elements relating to clinical data management practices. Their ICH reference number and current status in each ICH region are also provided. Two ICH guidelines—General Considerations for Clinical Trials (E8) and the Guideline on Statistical Principles for Clinical Trials (E9)—mention these topics specifically because of their inter-relatedness and relevance to clinical research. When the status 'effective' is reached in each region, the implications for industry are that the guidelines should be complied with and represent current best practice. Not all of the topics are final documents but the reader should be familiar with their current status and contents.

Table 2.1 ICH topics affecting clinical data management

Area	Topic	Reference (Europe, US & Japan)	Status
E1	The Extent of Population Exposure to Assess Clinical Safety	CPMP/ICH/375/95 60 FR11270 YAKUSHIN No. 592	Effective 1 June 95 Effective 1 March 95 Effective 24 May 95
E2A	Definitions and Standards for Expedited Reporting	CPMP/ICH/377/95 60 FR 11284 YAKUSHIN No. 227	Effective 1 June 95 Effective 1 March 95 Effective 20 March 95
E2B	Data Elements for Transmission of ADR Reports	CPMP/ICH/287/95 63 FR 2396 YAKUSHIN	Effective March 98 Effective 15 January 98 Not yet published
E2C	Periodic Safety Update Reports (for Marketed Drugs)	CPMP/ICH/288/95 62 FR 27470 YAKUSHIN No. 432	Effective 18 June 97 Effective 19 May 97 Effective 27 March 97
E3	Structure and Content of Clinical Reports	CPMP/ICH/137/95 61 FR 37320 YAKUSHIN No. 335	Effective July 96 Effective 17 July 96 Effective 1 May 96
E4	Dose-Response Information to Support Drug Registration	CPMP/ICH/378/95 59 FR 55972 YAKUSHIN No. 494	Effective 1 November 94 Effective 9 November 94 Effective 25 July 94
E5	Ethnic Factors in the Acceptability of Foreign Clinical Data	CPMP/ICH/289/95 63 FR 31790 YAKUSHIN No. 739	Effective September 98 Effective September 98 Effective August 98
E6	Good Clinical Practice: Consolidated Guideline	CPMP/ICH/135/95 62 FR 25692 YAKUSHIN No. 430 (Ministerial Ordinance No 28)	Effective 17 January 97 Effective 9 May 97 Effective 27 March 97
E7	Studies in Support of Special Populations: Geriatrics	CPMP/ICH/379/95 59 FR 39398 YAKUSHIN No. 104	Effective March 94 Effective 2 August 94 Effective 2 December 93
E8	General Considerations for Clinical Trials	CPMP/ICH/291/96 62 FR 66113 YAKUSHIN No. 380	Effective March 98 Effective 17 December 97 Effective August 98
E9	Statistical Considerations in the Design of Clinical Trials	CPMP/ICH/363/96 63 FR 49583 YAKUSHIN No. 1047	Effective March 98 Effective 16 September 98 Effective November 98
E10	Choice of Control Groups in Clinical Trials	Under development	Step 3 July 99
E11	Clinical Investigation of Medicinal Products in Children	Under development	Step 1 adopted as a new topic September 98
M1	International Medical Terminology	MedDRA v 2.0 issued	Step 5 reached July 97
M3	Timing of Pre-clinical Studies in Relation to Clinical Trials	CPMP/ICH/286/95 62 FR 62922 YAKUSHIN No. 1019	Effective September 97 Effective 25 November 97 Effective November 98

E = Efficacy, M = Multidisciplinary

Five of the above ICH documents will now be discussed in further detail as these are thought to most affect clinical data management in terms of the roles, responsibilities and procedures of clinical data management groups.

General Considerations for Clinical Trials (E8)

Readers who are unfamiliar with the ICH requirements for clinical trials can use this document for orientation purposes. It presents an overview of the ICH clinical and safety documents, and is intended to:

(A)   Describe internationally accepted principles and practices in the conduct of clinical trials and overall strategy for new medicinal products.
(B)   Facilitate the evaluation and acceptance of foreign clinical trial data by promoting a common understanding of general principles, approaches and the definition of relevant terms.

In Section 2 of this document, the general principles state that clinical data should be reviewed by competent clinicians and other experts to assess their implications for the safety of trial subjects. The emphasis on sponsor company research staff being qualified through education, training and experience to perform tasks is a recurrent theme in several ICH guidelines and will be discussed again later.

Data management staff are routinely involved in the design and review of study protocols and tools for data capture. This guideline outlines several considerations related to planning the objectives, design, conduct, analysis and reporting of clinical trials. Points to consider include:

1.   Clearly stated objectives of the study.
2.   Appropriate design of the study (e.g. parallel group, cross-over, dose escalation etc.), appropriate comparators, primary and secondary endpoints, methods to monitor adverse events, follow-up of patients who stop treatment prematurely.
3.   Appropriate selection of subjects.
4.   Appropriate selection of a control group.
5.   Number of subjects—based on magnitude of treatment effect, disease being investigated, study objectives, endpoint criteria, number of trial sites.
6.   Planned efficacy and safety variables—prospectively defined.
7.   Methods to minimise bias—randomisation, blinding, compliance checks.
8.   Conduct of the study—according to the ICH guideline on Good Clinical Practice and adherence to protocol, protocol amendments, timely adverse event reporting.

9. Analysis—according to a specified analysis plan for the protocol appropriate to its design, deviations from the plan indicated, procedures and rules for early stopping described, appropriate collection and tabulation of safety data.
10. Reporting—adequate documentation according to the ICH guideline on Structure and Content of Clinical Study Reports.

The initial provision of a well-designed protocol to data management groups will determine the subsequent design of case record forms for data capture. The quality of the protocol will also impact other plans written to support a study, for example, plans for any database design, clinical data management, statistical analysis, monitoring, clinical logistics and audit. During protocol development, clinical data management groups should discuss data requirements and data flow processes to ensure the optimum tools, methods and resources are assigned to manage the tasks.

Good Clinical Practice Consolidated Guideline (E6)

This guideline became effective during 1997 in all of the ICH regions and represents a significant step forward in terms of harmonisation. It is anticipated that sponsor and investigator compliance with this guideline will provide public assurance that the rights, well-being and confidentiality of the trial subjects are protected and that the trial data are credible. The guideline has become the superseding document to the former European Community Good Clinical Practice Guideline (EC GCPs, effective since July 1991). During its development, the US FDA guidance documents for Informed Consent and Institutional Review Boards were revised for consistency with the guideline. In Japan, revisions were made to the pharmaceutical drug laws to enable requirements of GCP to be met. Source document verification, sponsor access to subject medical files and sponsor audits of clinical investigators should become accepted practices in Japan, although a significant change from current practice. Sponsor companies operating in Japan will need to hire and train staff and develop standard operating procedures to enable compliance with the guideline.

This guideline includes an initial glossary of terms with harmonised definitions for: adverse drug reaction; adverse event, audit trail, blinding/masking, case report form (CRF), essential documents, interim and final study report, quality assurance, quality control, randomisation, serious adverse event, source data, source documents, standard operating procedures and subject identification codes. These harmonised definitions should be used in all documentation generated by the sponsor during the conduct of a clinical trial.

Appendix 1 of the document provides the minimum information that should be included in an Investigators' Brochure. It also lists the Essential Documents for the Conduct of a Clinical Trial and their desired location with regard to the Investigator/Institution or Sponsor and Contract Research Organisation. This list represents the essential documents to be collected and archived to meet the ICH recommended archiving timeframes and to ensure study data and any study management issues can be reconfigured. The list will provide archive directions to clinical data management groups routinely responsible for CRF tracking, CRF correction documentation (queries forms), CRF signature sheets, laboratory normal ranges and certification/accreditation, adverse event reporting documents and relevant communications (letters, memos, telephone reports).

Consistent with the topic on General Considerations for Clinical Trials (E8), the Principles section of this guideline also requires the use of appropriately trained staff. Three statements are applicable to personnel working in the clinical data management field:

Section 2. 8   Each individual involved in conducting a clinical trial should be qualified by education, training, and experience to perform his or her respective tasks.

Section 2.10   All clinical trial information should be recorded, handled and stored in a way that allows its accurate reporting, interpretation and verification.

Section 2.13   Systems with procedures that assure the quality of every aspect of the trial should be implemented.

The implications of these three principles can be interpreted by sponsor companies to ensure the following are met:

- Staff should maintain job descriptions, training records and evaluations of competency
- Systems (computerised or non-computerised) that handle clinical trial information should be validated, include audit trails, maintain the trial blinding, include security systems and version control. See Section 5.5 of the document for more details
- Archiving and disaster recovery procedures should be in place
- All aspects of the clinical data management process should be described in procedures that are monitored by quality control activities (to ensure that the data are reliable and have been processed correctly) and are periodically subject to quality assurance activities

Another important aspect needed to support clinical data management activities is the provision of validated databases. Section 5.5.3 of the document includes the requirement that all electronic aspects used in the management of clinical trial data should be validated. Without the confidence that data entered manually, scanned-in or transferred electronically has occurred reliably, then further activities to address the accuracy and completeness of the database are futile. This becomes even more important as companies increase the use of modem data transfers from central analytical laboratories, Phase I houses, contract research organisations and remote data entry.

This expectation to evaluate the validation process and documentation prior to selection of a contract research organisation (central laboratory or other service) has created additional resource needs in many pharmaceutical companies. A team of specialists is now employed to visit and evaluate not only the suitability of the vendor or process but also the reliability of the computer systems used. The skills of the clinical data manager in these assessments should be routinely co-opted. Clinical data management plans and standard operating procedures require revision to incorporate new data handling technology, process changes and ICH requirements.

'Validation' workshops and courses for computer system validation are widely advertised to the pharmaceutical industry, but care should be employed when selecting a suitable course for training purposes. Many of these courses are designed for the industrial environments governed by the current Good Manufacturing Practice (cGMPs) regulations. These regulations are far more stringent in their validation expectations than might be expected for computer systems operating to GCP standards. Use the following as a guide:

Can data being entered onto the database be recreated from source data? If the answer is NO, then cGMP expectations apply.

A new requirement which will be beneficial to most data management and clinical research groups is the requirement in Section 6.4.9, that the protocol define in advance what fields included in the CRF will be considered source data. This is in cases where there are no prior written or electronic records of data (e.g., required data for a protocol test/assessment is not routine hospital practice). In order to determine these data, communication between sponsor clinical groups, investigating staff and data management groups during the design phase of the study should occur. Identification of source data up front should also increase the quality of the fields designed to be used for source data collection, and hopefully reduce the number of queries when cleaning data.

Definitions and Standards for Expedited Reporting (E2A)

This guideline falls under the broad topic of Clinical Safety Data Management and is associated with topics E2B, E2C and M1. These guidelines provide standard definitions, an international medical terminology (via the *Medical Dictionary for Drug Regulatory Affairs*—MedDRA) and standard data elements for reporting medical information. Timeframes for reporting safety information to regulatory authorities, both for investigational product and marketed product, have been recommended. The harmonised definition of a serious adverse event is:

> A serious adverse event (experience) or reaction is any untoward medical occurrence that at any dose: results in death, is life-threatening, requires inpatient hospitalisation, results in persistent or significant disability/incapacity, or is a congenital anomaly/birth defect.

This new definition will have to be incorporated to sponsor study protocols. Investigating staff will need to be trained in the reporting of such events to sponsor companies within a specified timeframe (usually 24 hours). This will then enable the following regulatory reporting timeframes to be met: 7 calendar days (for fatal or life-threatening unexpected adverse drug reactions) and 15 calendar days (for serious, unexpected adverse drug reactions that are not fatal or life-threatening). The change from a working day timeframe to a more rigorous calendar day timeframe presents new challenges to clinical safety data management groups in terms of re-engineering their processes to further expedite data receipt, tracking, data entry, review, querying and reporting.

Appropriate quality control (manual/electronic checks) should be employed during data cleaning to ensure all serious adverse events have been reported. For companies that maintain separate systems/databases for clinical trial adverse event handling and serious adverse event handling, this guideline has not removed the need for database reconciliation. Sponsor databases will have to be upgraded to ensure the specified reports can be derived containing the required data elements for transmission to regulatory authorities.

Unfortunately, the ICH definitions and reporting timeframes are not currently reflected in local country regulations. Until all three ICH regions harmonise their own local requirements to those of the ICH guideline, additional resources will be required to monitor and ensure that the appropriate information is reported to the designated regulatory agency in the correct timeframe.

Guideline on the Content and Structure of Clinical Study Reports (E3)

This guideline is intended to facilitate the compilation of a single worldwide core clinical study report acceptable to all regulatory authorities. By developing a report that is complete, unambiguous and organised, it is hoped that the review of such reports by regulatory agencies will be made easier. In the US this guideline replaces the existing Guideline for the Format and Content of the Clinical and Statistical Sections of the New Drug Applications.

This guideline will also require sponsor companies to update their standard operating procedures, statistical report templates and clinical report templates in order to meet the ICH standard.

Key tables and data listings described in this guideline (Section 16: Appendices) are required to be made available to regulatory authorities upon request, and therefore will have to be prepared concurrent with the final report development. It is probable that further software development will be performed in order to generate the standard tables if the generic code is not already written or cannot be adapted. Specific examples of table format are also suggested. This is a useful document for staff members responsible for preparing tables or listings for inclusion to study reports. The tables address both efficacy and safety evaluations and include the following:

- Disposition of Subjects
- Demographic Data
- Discontinued Subjects
- Dosing Compliance and/or Drug Concentration Data
- Randomization Scheme and Codes
- Protocol Deviations
- Subjects Excluded from the Efficacy Analysis
- Individual Response Data
- Adverse Events by Subject
- Deaths, Other Serious Adverse Events, and Other Significant Events
- Individual Laboratory Measurements by Subject
- Abnormal Laboratory Values by Subject

An area that has been a topic of lengthy discussions between the clinical research staff, data management staff and the statisticians is the prospective definition of protocol deviations that must be captured for review. Section 10.2 of this guideline defines the protocol deviations that must be captured and collated for discussion in the final study report.

Rationale for not including certain tables will almost certainly be a discussion point among staff. Such strict defining of data may, however, induce sponsor companies to consider more carefully what data must be collected during a study and to be more efficient in their collection and handling.

Statistical Considerations in the Design of Clinical Trials (E9)

This extensive guideline was written in order to harmonise the principles of statistical methodology applied to clinical trials for marketing applications submitted in the ICH regions. The guideline focuses on statistical principles as opposed to statistical procedures and methods, and consists of the following detailed sections:

- Considerations for Overall Clinical Development
- Study Design Considerations
- Study Conduct
- Data Analysis Considerations
- Evaluation of Safety and Tolerability
- Reporting

Many data management groups adopted the suggestions of this guideline before it reached step 5 of the ICH process. Several sections are worthy of discussion here:

Section 2.1.1   'ensuring that common standards are adopted for a number of features of the trials such as dictionaries of medical terms, definition and timing of the main measurements, handling of protocol deviations.'

The role of Clinical Data Management in achieving this expectation is obvious. The majority of groups are either solely or partly responsible for the choice of medical and concomitant medication dictionaries. Version control of the dictionaries is an important issue if the development time of the investigational product is lengthy. Additions to the dictionaries to cope with new terms must be performed with care particularly if final study reports for earlier trials have already been completed. With the advent of MedRA in March 1999 the choice of dictionaries should be simplified. MedRA is designed to support the classification, retrieval, presentation and communication of medical information.

Section 2.1.2   'Confirmatory trials are intended to provide firm evidence in support of claims and adherence to their planned design and procedures is particularly important; unavoidable changes should be explained and documented, and their effect examined.'

Protocol amendments that necessitate a change in the design of the CRF, subject diaries, study worksheets and the clinical trial database need to be controlled. This means that extensive up-front research must be performed and wherever possible standardisation determined and agreed upon before project initiation. Investigator site processes for data generation and capture are usually assessed by clinical staff, with the exclusion of data management staff. It would be preferable to include data management staff in site pre-evaluation activities so that data management plans are written with consideration to the investigating sites' data management processes.

Where changes to the protocol procedures are unavoidable then documented explanations or version control on documents (such as protocol amendments and revised case report forms) must be made to enable simple reconfiguration of the changes at a later date. This point is even more critical when clinical database line listings are provided to regulatory agencies, such as the FDA, for verification purposes.

Section 3.6   'Whatever data capture instrument is used, the form and content of the information collected should be in full accordance with the protocol and should be established in advance of the conduct of the clinical trial. . . . Missing values should be distinguishable from the value zero or characteristic absent.'

Whenever the electronic transfer of information occurs to the sponsor it is important that the data transmitted match the requirements of the protocol. This is particularly applicable to laboratory data where a standard panel of tests is routinely performed for the subject. Data must be selected and validated prior to transmission to match those parameters required by the protocol.

The coding of comments such as not done, not available, not applicable or the value of zero should be defined in advance. Clinical data management can input effectively when preparing study guides used with case report forms or user guides for electronic transfers. The computing specialists or data management personnel need to decide who will be responsible for the codes.

Section 5.2.1   'There are a limited number of circumstances that might lead to excluding randomised subjects from the full analysis set, including the failure to satisfy major entry criteria (eligibility violations), the failure to take at least one dose of study medication, and the lack of any data post-randomisation. . . . violations of the protocol that occur after randomisation may have an impact on the data and conclusions, particularly if their occurrence is related to treatment assignment.'

Most data management groups are responsible for developing methods for identifying and coding protocol violations. The classification of protocol deviations must be defined in advance in the clinical data management plan. As stated earlier the ICH guideline E3 gives more guidance on what protocol deviations must be discussed in the final study report. The information collected on this topic is a powerful study management tool and should be shared with the study team on a regular basis.

Section 5.3   'Missing values represent a potential source of bias in a clinical trial. Hence, every effort should be undertaken to fulfill all

the requirements of the protocol concerning the collection
and management of data.'

This point emphasises the importance of data coding conventions, the
monitoring of protocol deviations and the importance of raising data queries to the site (rather than assuming data are missing) when it is not
clear if the data were generated or not.

NEW RULES/GUIDELINES SUPPORTING ICH CONCEPTS

New rules and guidelines that support the ICH concepts, but are not formally part of the ICH process, are emerging from the US FDA and the
European Commission (Table 2.2). They are of interest to clinical data
management groups as they provide specific instructions to companies
seeking compliance with the ICH requirements.
    Discussion of these seven documents and their consideration by spon-
sor clinical data management groups will follow.

Directive of the European Parliament and of the Council of the EU

This definitive proposal for the first ever EC Directive on Clinical Trials
forms part of a legislative framework being developed in Europe which will
eventually mandate for ICH GCP being followed. The directive also aims to
make legal the GCP inspections performed by regulatory authorities in
order to verify Sponsor/CRO/Investigator compliance. This move has been
taken in Europe because the requirements set down in ICH GCP guidelines
are not binding. The message for sponsor companies is that ICH GCP will
have to be followed and all parties conducting trials will now be open to
inspection. The draft Directive reinforces ethical principles already harmonised between Member States and also proposes some new standards.
In summary, 10 provisions are laid down relating to:

- Protection of Trial Subjects
- Ethics Committee Opinion
- Commencement of a Clinical Trial
- Conduct of a Clinical Trial
- Exchange of Information
- Manufacture and Import of Investigational Medicinal Products
- Labelling
- Compliance with Good Clinical Practice
- Notification of Adverse Events
- Notification of Adverse Reactions

Table 2.2 Emerging new rules and guidelines

Directive of the European Parliament and of the Council of the EU	Status
On the approximation of the laws, regulations and administrative provisions of the Member States relating to the implementation of good clinical practice in the conduct of clinical trials on medical products for human use	Draft version September 1997 Redrafted November 1998 Planned for adoption in 2000 Implementation by Member States thereafter

FDA Final Rule	
Electronic Records: Electronic Signatures	Issued under 21 CFR Part 11, effective 20 August 1997 Enforcement Policy 64 FR 39146 effective 21 July 1999

FDA Guidance Documents	
Computerized Systems Used in Clinical Trials	Final guidance April 1999
Providing Regulatory Submissions in Electronic Format—General Considerations	Final guidance January 1999
Providing Regulatory Submissions in Electronic Format—NDAs	Draft April 1998
Electronic Submissions of a Biologic License Application (BLA) or Product License Application (PLA)/Establishment License Application (ELA) to the Center for Biologics Research and Evaluation	Draft May 1998
Electronic Submissions of Case Report Forms (CRFs), Case Report Tabulations (CRTs) and Data to the Center for Biologics Research and Evaluation	Draft May 1998

FDA Guidance Documents

The FDA-derived documents relate to the proposal from the agency to move from paper regulatory submissions to electronic submissions in stages. These documents will help facilitate the transition. Since these topics represent rapidly growing areas, the FDA acknowledge that the guidance will need to be updated periodically.

Concurrent with the development of the final rule on Electronic Records, the FDA established a docket on electronic submissions in which it notifies sponsors when it is ready to accept specific types of submission. Details can be obtained from http://www.fda.gov/ohrms/dockets/ dockets/92s0251/92s0251.htm. Technical guidance on how to make the submission according to the receiving unit's capabilities is provided within the guidance documents prepared by the Centers for Drug and Biologic Research and Evaluation, listed above. The FDA's goal is to establish an approach for submitting electronic applications that create minimal work and reduced costs for sponsors and reviewers, as well as encouraging consistency in information transfer requirements across the agency.

Electronic Records; Electronic Signatures

This new rule makes it possible for sponsors to submit applications or parts of applications in electronic-only form without requesting a specific waiver from the FDA. The need for the new rule was forced since regulations were originally written for the 'paper world' which did not anticipate the impact that information technology would have on business operations. Industry subsequently requested changes to provide electronic records and electronic signatures to the agency in lieu of paper records. FDA has acknowledged that the agency must function on the same technological plane as the industry it regulates. The document describes the agencies' expectations for electronic systems and electronic signatures. The FDA will consider:

Electronic records   ≡   Paper records
Electronic signatures   ≡   Hand-written signatures

as long as the company intent to use electronic signatures has been submitted to the FDA, and the provisions in the rule are complied with.

The rule has definitions for: biometrics, closed and open systems, digital signature, electronic record, electronic signature, and handwritten signature. For electronic records the controls for closed and open systems are specified. Expectations include appropriate validation of the systems used; inclusion of an audit trail; appropriate security systems; authorised access; implementation of quality control; users are appropriately trained; users have access to written policies and procedures governing the use of the system, revision and change control procedures are in place. Sponsors who take advantage of this practice will have to consider its application to remote data entry systems and electronic transfer of data supporting a clinical trial.

All of these requirements support those listed in the ICH GCP guideline (Section 5.5). What is new are several requirements for the electronic signature, which include:

- The signed electronic record must include the printed name of the signer; the date and time the signature was executed and what the signature represents, e.g., review, approval, responsibility or authorship

- Before an electronic signature is permitted to be used, the company must verify the identity of the individual and upon request from the agency be able to provide additional certification or testimony that the electronic signature is equivalent to the handwritten version

An important area for consideration is the Investigator's signature required on CRFs and data queries. Any remote data entry system must have the capabilities to fulfil the first bullet point and appropriate security measures will need to be available to ensure that only the Investigator can electronically sign documents or data fields. In addition to CRFs, other potential applications for the use of electronic signatures include laboratory notebooks and standard operating procedures. Clinical data management should commonly be being included in defining company information technology strategy, as IT is continually mapped to new business processes.

The Enforcement Policy emphasises that sponsor companies must take steps to ensure that legacy systems still in use, and used to provide data to the agency, comply with the requirements of the rule. The FDA recognises that the validation activities required to retrofit existing systems are likely to take longer than prospectively implementing a compliant (or new) system. Therefore, an expectation has been set that the sponsor company will create a timetable for modifying legacy systems and monitor the validation progress. This timetable and progress will be subject to review during an FDA inspection. In addition to clinical trial databases, Data Management Departments have other electronic systems (and applications) at their disposal to facilitate data handling. Each one of these systems must therefore be evaluated for compliance with the rule, and a documented decision made as to whether or not to retrofit or replace the system.

Computerised Systems Used in Clinical Trials

This document details the FDA's current thinking on the use of computer systems in clinical trials. It defines in much more detail than Section 5.5 of the ICH GCP document what is expected with regard computer system validation. The current document includes the following sections:

- Introduction, Definitions, General Principles
- Standard Operating Procedures
- Data Entry (Electronic signatures, Audit trails, Date/time stamps)
- System Features (Facilitating the collection of quality data, Facilitating the inspection and review of data, Retrieval of data, Reconstruction of study)

- Security (Physical security, Logical security)
- System Dependability (Systems documentation, Software validation, Change control)
- System Controls (Software version control, Contingency plans, Back-up and recovery of electronic records)
- Training of Personnel (Qualifications, Training, Documentation)
- Records Inspection
- Certification of Electronic Systems

We expect the contents of this guideline to be incorporated into company standard operating procedures and checklists for the evaluation of CROs and IT providers.

Providing Regulatory Submissions in Electronic Format—General Considerations

Representatives from the Biologics and Drugs divisions of the FDA drafted this guidance document. It covers the general issues common to all types of electronic regulatory submissions and points to consider. The document is divided into the following sections:

- Background of FDA guidance documents
- File formats for documents
- File formats for datasets
- Procedures for sending electronic submissions
- Type of media that may be used and how to prepare them
- FDA processes and contact information

It is hoped that this standard policy will facilitate the handling and continued access to all electronic archival submissions.

Sponsor companies have long been required to meet regulatory defined archiving timeframes for clinical trial data used in licence applications. The advancements in computer technology and imaging have forced the creation of specialist groups in companies to support records management system development and business contingency (disaster recovery) planning. Sponsor companies must continue to ensure that electronic data are recoverable and reconfigurable when exported to regulatory agencies, as well as preserving the data in an appropriate long-term storage environment. Data management staff responsible for preparing line-listings or images of case report forms should use this guideline as an introduction to the FDA's requirements. Detailed information is available from the Drugs and Biologics Division and will be discussed below.

Providing Regulatory Submissions in Electronic Format—NDAs

This document is intended to reduce the need to consult the Center for Drug Evaluation and Research for details on submitting the archival copy of the New Drug Application (NDA), including amendments or supplements, in an electronic format. The document covers the following information:

- Definition of the sections to be included in the archival copy
- Use of fonts, page orientation, paper size and margins
- Sources of electronic documents and datasets
- File naming conventions
- Hyperlinking requirements
- Security

Of special interest to data management staff are Item 11 Case Report Form Tabulations (CRTs) and Item 12 Case Report Forms (CRFs). Patient profiles and domain profiles may be provided as part of the submission. Patient profiles are defined as all study data collected for an individual patient organised by time. Domain profiles are defined as patient line listings and consist of all data collected for a single CRF domain from one study. Patient profiles should be provided as Adobe PDF files and domain profiles may be provided by either Adobe PDF or SAS transport files. The reviewing division should be contacted to determine the preferred method for domain files.

The reviewing agency also requires that an annotated blank CRF be provided that maps each blank on the CRF to the corresponding element in the database. This document is usually prepared by the data management staff as part of the development of the clinical trial database. Any updates to the design of the CRF or database should be reflected in this document; the author must also remember to include the date when an element changed.

Electronic Submissions of a Biologic Licence Application (BLA) or Product Licence Application (PLA)/Establishment Licence Application (ELA) to the Center for Biologics Research and Evaluation

This guidance document covers the same details as the one prepared by the Center for Drug Evaluation and Research. Data management staff responsible for preparing information for NDAs, BLAs and PLAs should familiarise themselves with all documents.

Electronic Submission of Case Report Forms (CRFs) Case Report Tabulations (CRTs) and Data to the Center of Biologics Evaluation and Research

This document describes the specific features that are recommended for electronically imaged CRFs and electronically searchable submissions which include:

- An index/table of comments
- Ability to read and print each page exactly as it would have been printed in the paper submission
- Ability to create hypertext linking and bookmarks
- Accessibility on any computer platform
- A format commonly available which requires minimal training
- Ability to search for a character string or multiple character strings
- Ability to select and save a subset
- Ability to print selected CRFs
- Ability to view the audit trail for selected CRFs

Electronically imaged CRT files are recommended to contain similar elements to the above. Electronically functional CRTs (electronic data) are extensively specified and all data sets should be provided as SAS transport files. The FDA also recommend the use of Adobe Portable Document Format (PDF) and Adobe Acrobat tools for computer/image output, the creation of specified indexing fields and ASCII output printing. Such technical recommendations published by regulatory agencies will impact the sponsor selection of computer platforms, hardware and software purchases, database development methodology, regulatory publishing style guides and staff training.

The documents discussed demonstrate that regulatory agencies involved in the ICH process are incorporating the good ideas into their local practices. Industry needs to remain vigilant and keep abreast of this and future developments. Comments in favour of the documents should be forwarded to the agencies as well as concerns when the practices recommended appear to be departing from the ICH principles.

CONCLUSIONS

The importance of the ICH effort cannot be overstated. A framework for global medicinal product development now exists and with an established mechanism to continue this process. There is now a common language presented in the various ICH documents which include harmonised requirements applicable to data management staff and their activities. The challenges ahead for regulatory bodies and industry are to ensure that consistent application of the ICH recommendations occurs. This is not an easy task, as pharmaceutical companies working internationally and attempting harmonisation efforts with standard operating procedures can attest. We must all strive to overcome cultural and nationalistic barriers between regions and agree to implement 'best practice', no matter where it originates.

Three main themes recur within the ICH documents which impact data management groups and must be considered in all activities:

1. Have written work procedures.
2. Train new and existing staff appropriately to perform their designated tasks.
3. Implement computer-related system validation.

In addition, the concept of approved software and database vendors (required in the pharmaceutical manufacturing environment and the defence industry), will become more common in clinical trial application selection. Contract research organisations providing data management services now have a major stake in contributing to regulatory licence applications. Therefore, expectations of what sponsor companies will be looking for during CRO evaluation and selection and subsequent audits must be pre-defined.

The next phase of the ICH process will include monitoring the implementation of the guidelines. Europe is in the process of establishing Member State Inspectorates to facilitate this goal. In the United States it is not yet established whether the Compliance Divisions will incorporate ICH requirements into their inspection process. It is more likely that this will occur as the Federal regulations are amended to match those of ICH.

It will be interesting to look back in five to ten years' time and evaluate whether or not the ICH efforts have resulted in medicinal products reaching the marketplace sooner and at reduced costs. The concept of a paperless drug development program and one regulatory dossier for all regions of the world may also be a reality by then. The ICH initiatives continue to be a challenge, but commitment and persistence by regions has demonstrated that problems can be surmounted.

E-MAIL ADDRESSES

http://www.ifpma.org/ich1.html
http://www.fda.gov.cder/guidance.htm
http://dg3.eudra.org/eudralex/vol-3/home.htm

Appendix 1: List of ICH Topics and Guidelines

Safety Topics

	Carcinogenicity Studies	
S1A	Guideline on the Need for Carcinogenicity Studies of Pharmaceuticals	Step 5
S1B	Testing for Carcinogenicity in Pharmaceuticals	Step 5
S1C	Dose Selection for Carcinogenicity Studies in Pharmaceuticals (S1CR—revised version)	Step 5
	Genotoxicity Studies	
S2A	Genotoxicity: Specific Aspects of Regulatory Tests	Step 5
S2B	Genotoxicity: Standard Battery Tests	Step 5
	Toxicokinetics and Pharmacokinetics	
S3A	Toxicokinetics: Guidance on the Assessment of Systemic Exposure in Toxicity Studies	Step 5
S3B	Pharmacokinetics: Guidance for Repeated Dose Tissue Distribution Studies	Step 5
S4	Single Dose Toxicity Tests	Step 5
S4A	Duration of Chronic Toxicity Testing in Animals (Rodent and Non-Rodent)	Step 4
	Reproductive Toxicology	
S5A	Detection of Toxicity to Reproduction for Medicinal Products	Step 5
S5B	Reproductive Toxicology: Male Fertility Studies	Step 5
	Biotechnological Products	
S6	Safety Studies for Biotechnological Products	Step 5
	Pharmacology Studies	
S7	Safety Pharmacology Studies	Step 1

Efficacy Topics

	Efficacy	
E1	The Extent of Population Exposure to Assess Clinical Safety	Step 5
	Clinical Safety Data Management	
E2A	Definitions and Standards for Expedited Reporting	Step 5
E2B	Data Elements for Transmission of ADR Reports	Step 5
E2C	Periodic Safety Update Reports for Marketed Drugs	Step 5
	Clinical Study Reports	
E3	Structure and Content of Clinical Study Reports	Step 5
	Dose Response Studies	
E4	Dose Response Information to Support Drug Registration	Step 5
	Ethnic Factors	
E5	Ethnic Factors in the Acceptability of Foreign Clinical Data	Step 5
	Good Clinical Practice	
E6	Good Clinical Practice: Consolidated Guideline	Step 5
E6A	Addendum on Investigator's Brochure	Step 5
E6B	Addendum on Essential Documents	Step 5
	Clinical Trials in Special Populations	
E7	Clinical Trials in Special Populations: Geriatrics	Step 5
	Clinical Trial Design	
E8	General Considerations for Clinical Trials	Step 5
E9	Statistical Considerations in the Design of Clinical Trials	Step 5
E10	Choice of Control Group in Clinical Trials	Step 3
E11	Clinical Investigation of Medicinal Products in Children	Step 1
E12	**Guidelines for Clinical Evaluation by Therapautic Category**	
E12A	Clinical Evaluation of Drugs by Therapeutic Categories: Antihypertensives	Step 1

Quality Topics

	Stability Testing	
Q1A	Stability Testing of New Drugs and Products	Step 5
Q1B	Photostability Testing	Step 5
Q1C	Stability Testing for New Dosage Forms	Step 5
	Validation of Analytical Procedures	
Q2A	Text on Validations of Analytical Procedures	Step 5
Q2B	Methodology	Step 5
	Impurity Testing	
Q3A	Impurities in New Drug Substances	Step 5
Q3B	Impurities in New Drug Products	Step 5
Q3C	Impurities: Residual Solvents	Step 5
Q4	**Pharmacopoeial Harmonisation**	
	Quality of Biotechnological Products	
Q5A	Viral Safety Evaluation	Step 5
Q5B	Genetic Stability	Step 5
Q5C	Stability of Products	Step 5
Q5D	Cell Substrates	Step 5
	Specifications for New Drug Substances and Products	
Q6A	Chemical Substances	Step 3
Q6B	Biotechnological Substances	Step 4
	GMP for Pharmaceutical Ingredients	
G7A	Good Manufacturing Practices for Active Pharmaceutical Ingredients	Step 1

Multidisciplinary Topics

	Regulatory Communications	
M1	Medical Terminology	Step 5
M2	Electronic Standards for Transfer of Regulatory Information (ESTRI)	Step 4
	Joint Safety/Efficacy	
M3	Timing of Pre-Clinical Studies in Relation to Clinical Trials	Step 5
	New Topic	
M4	Common Technical Document	Step 1 (1998)

3 Case Report Form Design

MOURA AVEY

Crowborough, East Sussex, UK

INTRODUCTION

Someone wisely said 'if we take care in the beginning, the end will take care of itself'.

This is true for the creation of both the protocol and the Case Report Form (CRF), which illustrates it, at the beginning of the clinical trial. If we take care in getting these two 'right' the remainder of the process, up to and including the Final Study Report, will take care of itself.

Whatever medium is used for the CRF, paper, electronic or combinations of both, the CRF is only as good as the protocol. As a translation/illustration of the protocol the CRF can never be better than the protocol or compensate for its inadequacies or oversights. Ultimately, the Final Study Report, which is the product of sophisticated computer programs and a statistical analysis, is only as good as the data collected in the CRF.

The whole process from defining the data to be collected, collecting, checking, analysing and presenting it, is resource intensive, utilising sophisticated technology and employing highly skilled professionals. Unexpected delays can occur at any of these stages, which is costly. The process does not need the additional cost burdens and delays due to poor data quality or loss of data. Minimising these are within our control at the start with the protocol and CRF design.

FUNCTION OF THE CRF

The CRF is the tool we use to collect pre-defined data from a Subject in a clinical trial. The ICH Guidelines for Good Clinical Practice define the CRF as:

> A printed, optical or electronic document designed to record all of the protocol required information to be reported to the Sponsor on each trial Subject.

Clinical Data Management. Second Edition. Edited by R.K. Rondel, S.A. Varley and C.F. Webb.
© 2000 John Wiley & Sons, Ltd

Although considerable advances have been made in the study and production of electronic CRFs, the majority of trial data are collected on paper CRFs and the current review focuses on these, where the CRF refers to the total collection of pages for each Subject.

THE LIFE HISTORY OF THE CRF

The CRF must be robust in content and material. The Life History Table, Table 3.1, illustrates the uses made of the CRF, and by whom, and the emphasis of use which impacts on the design. The Users can be categorised as individuals concerned with the data collected on the forms—Form Fillers and Readers, and those concerned with pages or whole CRFs—Handlers.

Each User has created a process through which the CRF will pass. Ignore any User at your peril and delays will result. It takes less resource to incorporate their needs, within reason, in the design stage, than to amend the CRF during printing, or after distribution, or to expect Users to muddle through producing possible errors and/or delays.

STAGE 1: PROTOCOL

As the precursor to the CRF, review of the protocol before it is final provides the designer with an overview of the clinical trial, and the opportunity to assess its impact on the CRF design. Personal experience has shown that holding discussions focused on the CRF during the writing of the protocol produces a better final version and fewer protocol amendments.

Phases

The protocol defines the objectives of the study. Broadly speaking, these are concerned with safety and efficacy; the degree of emphasis for each is dependent on the phase of the clinical trial programme. Reviewing the protocol from this angle indicates the size of the task and where to focus energies for the design of the CRF.

In general, early phase studies collect data over a short period of time, such as a large number of safety measurements and intense monitoring of the drug's behaviour for a population selected by tightly defined exclusions, at a single site.

By Phase III the sheer numbers of Subjects, studied for a longer period of time, using subjective questionnaires/opinions, more specific safety, efficacy and population details at many centres, add to the complexity of the CRF.

Table 3.1 Life history of the CRF

Stage	How the CRF is used	Form User/ Contributor	Form use emphasis
1. PROTOCOL Precursor of CRF	• Content, and question structure, are generated by the protocol • Specific forms designed during draft protocol stage help highlight strengths and weaknesses of the protocol • Pilot new designs and changes • Review draft forms against protocol	• CRF designer • Medical staff • Monitors • Data scientist • Statistician • Pharmacokineticist • Investigator • Nurse	Reader Form Filler (testing)
2. CREATE CRF Design Master Copy	• Review data items against the protocol • Check for correct questions, flow and response format • Circulate drafts for input from reviewers • Finalise designs that have been piloted	• CRF designer • Medical staff • Monitors • Data scientist • Statistician • Pharmacokineticist • Health economist • Investigator • Nurse • Consultant/expert • Word processing • Laboatory staff • Pharmacist	Reader Form Filler (reviewing)
3. PRODUCE CRF Print and quality check CRFs	• Ensure Printer is able to recognise: 1. Order of pages 2. Copying instructions 3. Links between components 4. All components 5. Language requirements • Send electronic or paper version to Printer	• CRF designer • Printers • Assembly staff • Distributors	Handler
4. DISTRIBUTE CRF CRFs packed and shipped to sites	• Recognise all stationery components of clinical trial • Match CRF with other trial documentation, labels, diary cards, etc. • Track distribution of CRFs • Ensure correct number of CRFs are sent to sites	• Distributors • Couriers • Warehouse and stores staff • Recipients	Handler

(*continued over*)

Stage	How the CRF is used	Form User/ Contributor	Form use emphasis
5. COMPLETE THE CRF Record data in CRF	• Respond to questions • Complete by hand • Interpret/transcribe diary card data • Insert additional pages • Attach traces/expert reports • Subject's questionnaires are completed, views are requested • Source documentation verification by monitors • Signed off when complete	• Investigator • Nurse • Subject/Guardian • Technician • Consultant • Monitors • Pharmacists • Pharmacokineticist • Contract house staff	Form Filler
6. RETRIEVE CRFs Completed CRFs transferred to site of data entry	• Check for completeness of each CRF • Check that all CRF pages are accounted for • Track progress of retrieval • Bring part of CRF back (batch retrieval) or whole CRF • Transport CRFs • CRF pages may be photocopied or faxed	• Data scientists • Administrators • Monitors • Investigator • Nurse • Couriers • Distributors	Handler

Despite the number of Subjects per trial increasing in Phase IV, the data collected per CRF will be reduced to specific safety, efficacy and subjective data.

Movement from one phase to another is not always clear-cut from the CRF point of view, so it is important to question when data can be reduced. Sometimes a study is modelled on a previous one and data remain in the trial because their continuing usefulness was not questioned.

Time and Event Schedule

The best review of the protocol is achieved by constructing a Schedule of Events against Time from the protocol text. The benefits of the exercise are:

(i)   To highlight the Reviewer's interpretation of the protocol which may differ from the Author's.

(ii)   To check for omissions/discrepancies of the proposed study events.

(iii) To highlight potential logistic problems for the CRF if numerous sources provide data for each Subject.

(iv)   To generate a list of specific questions based on the following checklist:

- What data need to be collected if a Subject does not meet entry criteria?
- What standard data collection modules can be used? need modifying? are missing?
- What existing forms can be used?
- What new forms are needed?
- How is dosing/compliance being measured?
- What population-specific data are needed?
- Which data are needed for safety monitoring? efficacy?
- What happens if the Subject does not complete the study at any time point after enrolment?

Protocol Review Meetings and Version Control

It is a very good draft protocol that can provide answers to all the above. However, depending on the number of 'unknowns' contained in the protocol, a meeting with as many different Users of the protocol as possible allows various interpretations of the protocol to be voiced and the protocol can be changed to avoid different interpretations by future Readers. This is beneficial to the CRF designer by reducing the risk of various interpretations of the protocol being prompted later in response to a carefully drafted and detailed CRF.

Delays can be avoided when new forms have been identified, by drafting them and issuing them to the relevant Form Fillers for piloting in existing clinics or using data from medical records, during protocol development.

The protocol is subject to change. It is important that the CRF bears the appropriate identifier of the protocol version to prevent CRFs being reviewed against an incorrect version, for example, the draft protocol version, final version, or protocol amendment version.

A 'near to final' good draft of the protocol is suitable for the drafting and reviewing of the CRF in the next stage.

STAGE 2: CRF DESIGN

Introduction

The CRF is a very specialised form. More forms are generated as our life becomes increasingly computer dependent. All forms collect data, but the use of the data varies, for example, applications, purchases and so on, which in turn influences the look of the form. Forms are composed of structured questions by someone else, demanding answers from us in a way that is foreign to our thinking and constraining to our freedom of expression of information. We are apathetic, possibly because we cannot interact with a form to, for example, clarify a meaning, request more space, provide an answer which has not been anticipated, or request a clean page if we make a mistake. Small wonder that for most, completing a form is a daunting task, and complex CRFs get a cool reception.

Over the past 30 years or so, students of typography, ergonomics and occupational psychology have examined in depth the use of written language, presentation and various media in an attempt to measure the factors that facilitate reading, comprehension and action—known as Human Factors. If these are understood, then we can incorporate those that motivate the Form Filler to provide better quality data into the structure of the CRF.

The application of the findings to Clinical Trial forms was reviewed by Wright and Haybittle when they proposed three aspects for consideration[1]:

1. **CONTENT**—do you need to collect it?
2. **PRESENTATION**—are you asking the question correctly?
3. **METHODOLOGY**—what design alternatives are available to avoid/minimise problems that Users have with the forms?

CONTENT—Do you need to collect it?

The protocol identifies the data to be collected during the trial to achieve the study objectives and meet regulatory requirements.

1. Date, phase and identification of the trial.
2. Identification of the Subject.
3. Age, sex, height, weight and ethnic group of the Subject.
4. Particular characteristics of the Subject (smoking, dietary, pregnancy, previous treatment etc.).
5. Diagnosis, indication for which the product is administered in accordance with the protocol.
6. Adherence to inclusion/exclusion criteria.
7. Duration of disease, time to last breakout, etc.
8. Dose, dosage schedule, administration of medical product, compliance record.
9. Duration of treatment.
10. Duration of observational period.
11. Concomitant use of other medicines and non-medicinal interventions/therapy.

12. Dietary regimens.
13. Recording of efficacy parameters met, date and time.
14. Recording Adverse Events, type, duration, intensity consequence and measures taken.
15. Reasons for withdrawal, breaking code.

Some study designs will legitimately omit a few of the above, for example, dietary regimens, breaking code, but the majority will be included.

Precision

As each data item is critically reviewed, its precision of collection will be considered for inclusion. The precision is dependent upon one or a combination of the following:

1. The study objectives defined by the statistical hypothesis.
2. The nature of the data item itself, e.g., administrative, historical, etc.
3. The precision of the scientific technology and accepted medical practices.
4. Human nature/culture.

What are the cleanest and most relevant data you can hope to collect in the given circumstances?

To improve the quality of collecting the data, ensure the following:

- Key dates and times used in the analysis will be prominently placed
- Durations and all derived data will be calculated by the computer from the raw data. Derived data will be collected when the sponsor needs to know that the investigator chose a clinical regime of care for the Subject as a consequence of the derived value, e.g., intensive-care situations
- Objective measurements are the data of choice, e.g., enzyme test results, height etc.
- With multivariable information provided in X-rays, ECGs, Scans, etc., target the relevant factors, resorting to simplifications such as asking if the factor of interest is present or absent
- Standard 'definitions' exist when asking if a result is normal or abnormal

Age

The datum, Age, can be used to illustrate the influence of culture. The Western world collects date of birth, leaving the computer to calculate age, but some countries do not follow our Gregorian calendar. A person's 'date of birth' may be defined by a significant event, or in terms of the lunar or early Gregorian calendars.

In these countries the datum needs to be reviewed against the following options:

- Dispense with age altogether
- Collect the 'date of birth' in the indigenous format and apply a conversion factor
  or
- Collect an estimate of age provided by another method

PRESENTATION—Are you asking the question correctly?

It is essential to reverse the thinking process and anticipate the response before asking the question. The types of responses are:

1. **Open**—including text, number, alpha numeric.
2. **Closed**—including binary and multiple choice.
3. **Combination**—of the open and closed response.
4. **Analogue scales**—alternative rating response.

Open—'The actual answer cannot be predicted so an allocated area is provided for the written response.'

Space. The main concern is to allow sufficient space for the answer. Handwriting is unique to the individual but measurements/numbers/alphanumerical identifiers of known magnitude can be allocated at least 0.5 cm width per character.

Dates and times. Dates and times are examples of open numerical responses. Duration is calculated from dates and times and data processing benefits from knowing that the format of the recorded date is compatible with the database, hence the adoption of a line with separators (allowing 0.5 cm per digit) and descriptors immediately underneath. It is best to use the format familiar to the Form Filler because the more the Form Filler manipulates the data, the more prone they are to error.

Dates. Various indigenous formats exist, that is:

- dd/mm/yy in most of Europe and parts of Canada
- mm/dd/yy in the USA and parts of Canada
- yy/mm/dd in Scandinavia

But with the advent of the millennium and for future multinational studies, the format of dd/mmm/yyyy is encouraged, using the first three letters of the month and 4 digits for the year, for example 01 Jan 2000.

Time. In CRFs, Clock Time is standardly collected using the 24-hour clock or military time, instead of the domestic format of a.m. or p.m. With reference to the 24-hour clock, two formats exist depending on the culture and the Sponsor's database; they are:

1. 00:01—24:00 (midnight).
2. 00:00 (midnight)—23:59.

Note that midnight straddles two dates, existing at the end of the day or the beginning of the next. The Form Filler needs to know which convention to use, but decorators alone do not guarantee against mistakes. On one occasion 00:00 was mistakenly interpreted to indicate that the clock time was not noted and therefore missing.

Clock time is only of value if it can be directly linked with a date. It is a good practice to ensure initially that date and time are collected together, despite appearing repetitive to the Form Filler, until testing and review identifies which dates can be removed without jeopardising the data.

Signatures. Signatures are a special form of the open text response and although signatures can be influenced, a personal survey suggests that 90% of signatures will be accommodated by a minimum space of 3.0 cm × 6.0 cm.

Character separators └─┴─┴─┴─┘ *or* ▢▢▢▢ . Separators, for example combs or boxes, are used allegedly to encourage legible writing. Separators actually constrain reading in several ways. A Reader recognises a word by its shape. Segmenting and unnatural spacing will change the word's shape, and reduce legibility further. Forced to write disjointedly, the Form Filler hesitates and even the most familiar material, such as one's own address, is prone to error. Corrections in delineated areas are difficult to decipher and the separating marks themselves can be mistaken for components of alphanumerics.

Using character separators for recording actual measurements, such as pressures, rates, lengths and so on, can influence the precision of the answer by anticipating its magnitude but this must be reviewed against capturing the unit of measurement with which the Form Filler is familiar, if different: for example feet/inches vs cm. Software can convert this datum into the preferred unit for analysis with fewer errors.

Unlike identifiers and measurements, text fields, for example comments, drug names and so on, cannot be anticipated, so delineation is not feasible. Some believe that separators will prevent the Form Filler from writing more than the space allowed on the database. If information needs to be reduced, it is better to understand the full text in the CRF and abbreviate it for the database, than to receive illegible contractions from Form Fillers.

Comment fields collect reasons for using Concomitant Medications and blood products, or reasons for dose modifications, but with some thought many reasons can be put into categories and used to construct multiple choice lists. Avoid comment fields, but some like those related to Adverse Experiences, death and clinically significant lab results will be required.

Studies of the use of character separators show that a 7-hour working day (without separators) increases to an 8-hour day (with separators)[2].

Closed—'The content of the answer is predicted, and a list of options can be provided, but the range is limited.'

The advantages to the Form Filler are that the list of answers clarifies the meaning of the question and it is simple to make a choice. For data processing, it focuses the response with the desired precision, making it automatically compatible for computer analysis, and forms of electronic data capture.

Selection methods. The selection method is important. The printed list can be annotated to show the correct choice by circling, underlining, ticking/ checking ($\sqrt{}$) the correct answer, or deleting the incorrect options. When studying time and accuracy of completion, Wright discovered that the $\sqrt{}$ box was the quickest for the Form Filler[2]. It is also easily read by data entry (Readers) and readily adapted to electronic capture, unlike underlining or circling the correct answers.

Example: If the answer 'Yes' is required it can be indicated by—

(a) circling   (Yes)/No
(b) underlining   <u>Yes</u>/No
(c) deleting   Yes/~~No~~
(d) ticking/checking a box   Yes ☑ No ☐

'D' is the preferred format.

Deletion. Deleting the inapplicable response is prone to error. Firstly it takes more time to complete than responding with the correct answer. It is easier for a Form Filler to search and identify a match than to find mismatches. There are some cultures where crossing through a response indicates the correct choice. There is a chance that these Form Fillers could misread the English deletion instructions and instinctively record a match, with the result that data processing will enter the unmarked choice, when the opposite is true.

√ *Boxes.* The majority of closed response formats in the CRF will be √ boxes, with codes and matrices being offered as alternatives in special circumstances.

Response order. Human Factors Studies describe a 'positive thinking bias', that is people looking for something to agree with (Yes) first before disagreeing (No), the natural order of the binary response. If Yes/No is expanded to include the unknown category, Yes/No/Unknown is more instinctive than No/Yes/Unknown. The inclusion of the unknown is frequently debated, because without it the question may remain unanswered or a guess, yet its inclusion is viewed as a means to opt out of making a committed response. The decision to use UNKNOWN is driven by the analysis plan and the precision of the data.

Option order. Order a multiple choice list to prevent the correct item being overlooked. There are advantages if the most likely options occur early in the list. When grading performance, the list is best ordered from good to worse.

Sorting numerical answers by categories requires particular attention (Figure 3.1). The answer—15—can be represented in either 'greater than or equal to' ($\geq$) or 'less than or equal to' ($\leq$) scales. Note some arrangements give rise to error when the Form Filler records the first option that matches. Figures 3.1(a) and (c) will be recorded correctly, by selecting the first choice that matches. In Figure 3.1(b), theoretically the second and third options are correct, as are the first two in Figure 3.1(d). The Form Filler will probably mark the first correct choice and may or may not read further to notice the error. Bearing in mind the 'positive thinking bias' of preferring values that are greater than or equal to, the most appropriate format is Figure 3.1(a).

How many episodes did you experience last week?

	√ one		√ one		√ one		√ one
(a)	≥ 30 ☐	(b)	None ☐	(c)	None ☐	(d)	≤ 30 ☐
	≥ 20 ☐		≥ 1 ☐		1 ☐		≤ 20 ☐
	≥ 10 ☐		≥ 10 ☐		≤ 10 ☐		≤ 10 ☐
	≥ 1 ☐		≥ 20 ☐		≤ 20 ☐		1 ☐
	None ☐		≥ 30 ☐		≤ 30 ☐		None ☐

Figure 3.1 Option order

Position of √ boxes. The position of the √ boxes can affect the accuracy of the data. Wright noted that the quickest response was achieved when the text and boxes were both right aligned[2]—Figure 3.2(a). The next easiest layout has the text left aligned, followed immediately by the answer boxes, Figure 3.2(b). Data entry benefits most when boxes are aligned right, whether or not the text is aligned left or right, Figure 3.2(a) and (c). Note that the accuracy of recording reduces as the boxes move away from the text. Avoid positioning the boxes before the response, Figure 3.2(d), forcing the Form Filler to read the answer and return to the start to mark it. Errors may arise from forgetting what has been read or marking the line below, as a result of the right to left movement when reading.

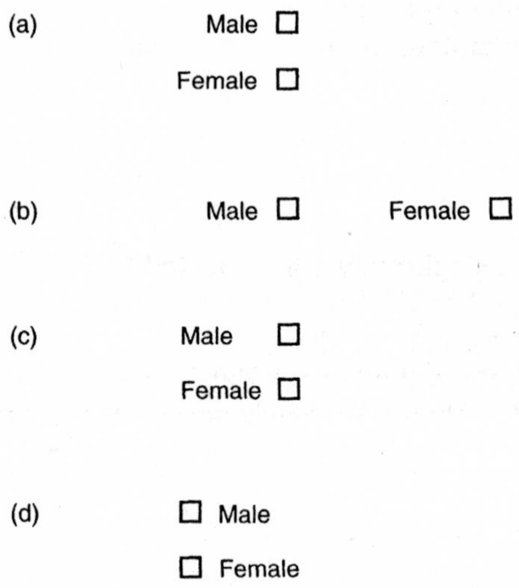

(a)   Male ☐

                       Female ☐

(b)   Male ☐   Female ☐

(c)   Male   ☐

                       Female ☐

(d)   ☐ Male

                       ☐ Female

Figure 3.2   Position of √ boxes

√ Box code descriptors. If printing the database code near the √ box to help data entry, consider these drawbacks:

- The position and size of the codes must not be obscured by the response mark
- There is a danger that the page will look busy and uninviting to complete, especially matrices
- Codes printed on the CRF become redundant if changed when building the database and difficult for data entry to ignore. Alternatively, design the data entry screens to mirror the CRF page, with codes programmed and linked in the background

Example:

(a) Mild [✓]   Moderate [2]   Severe [3] ⎤ Code obscured by

(b) Mild [✓¹]   Moderate [²]   Severe [³] ⎦ response mark

(c) Mild [✓] 1   Moderate [ ] 2   Severe [ ] 3   Page will be too busy

(d) Mild [✓]₁   Moderate [ ]₂   Severe [ ]₃   Best option if codes are

printed

Matrices. √ boxes for multiple choice can be organised as a matrix and although somewhat complex in structure, it is compact.

People tend to complete matrices by working along rows, that is from left to right, rather than down columns. The matrix limits the space for column and row headings. Abbreviations and links to footnotes are unsuitable because of the potential for ambiguities and transcription errors. Design the table to accommodate the longest headings, employing space, type size and type face effectively.

When more than a single answer is expected from a multiple choice list, a matrix of Yes/No or Yes/No/Unknown responses by each option, Figure 3.3(a), is preferred to a '√ all that apply', Figure 3.3(b). By requiring a response for each option, the Form Filler is encouraged to read and judge the alternatives rather than mistakenly accepting the first relevant answer in the list.

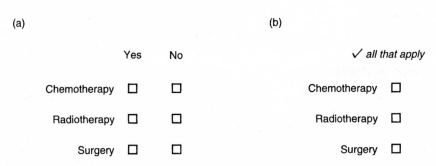

Which of the following treatments were given?

(a)   (b)

                    Yes   No   ✓ all that apply

Chemotherapy □   □   Chemotherapy □

Radiotherapy □   □   Radiotherapy □

Surgery □   □   Surgery □

Figure 3.3 Matrices

Recording codes. Although coding choices is easier for data input (Readers), the Form Filler's workload is increased with having to read and select the correct answer, memorise the associated code and transcribe it correctly to the appropriate position in the CRF.

There is a tendency to use codes to economise on space, but with an inevitable increase in complexity to the question.

As either the option text or the number of response options increases, the √ box approach becomes unwieldy and the coded response offers an alternative. Many medical conditions/descriptions are graded/coded within the medical vocabulary, and are appropriate to use although the Form Filler still has to transcribe the code to the correct position in the CRF.

To map and/or measure disease symptoms, anatomical diagrams/pictures of scans and so on can be overlaid with a coded grid, or divided into zones which are coded, for reference. An alternative to pictorial data is advised because they are difficult to set up, monitor and validate.

Combination—'Extends the range of the closed format by the addition of an open format.'

Other, specify. As the last item in a multiple choice list the open text response of 'Other, specify' introduces a disruptive element in the middle of a numerical database providing tables for analysis. Notice that the open text does not lend itself to mix easily with √ boxes arranged in a matrix.

'Other, specify' is included when all the possible options are not known. If the analysis is concerned only with the known options listed, the response 'None of the above' is better than 'Other, specify', while still inferring that other options exist. Note that both responses are last in the list to ensure all the anticipated options are considered first, that is by process of elimination.

In early phase studies of new indications, technologies and so on, this may be justification enough to include 'Other, specify' so that later studies will contain more 'known' possibilities in the list.

Analogue scales—'Alternative rating response'

Visual analogue scales (usually horizontal lines of 10 cm length) are used to measure an individual's perception of improvement, feelings and so on. Labels defining the range are put at either end of the line and the Subject is asked to mark the line at a position which best represents their own situation. The data are analysed using the distance measured to the mark on the line from one of the ends.

They are difficult to set up, monitor and validate, so it is important to:

- Provide clear instructions for marking the line (including an illustration if possible)
- Ensure the line is exactly 10 cm in length on return from the printers

Quality of Life (QOF)/Validated instruments. Before reproducing (QOF) instruments measuring subjective responses, check the copyright and validation properties:

- Copyright—this protects the intellectual property of the tool and, even if the layout is different, permission from the holder is required. When permission is obtained, a statement to that effect is included at the end of each copy produced
- Validated instrument—this is protected by using the instrument in the same manner in which it was originally tested, i.e., translation text, structure, order and instructions remain unchanged

Wording

Carefully word the written questions and instructions to complete the form correctly because the Form Filler:

- Cannot interact with the CRF to obtain clarification
- May be unfamiliar with the current English vernacular

Ambiguity. To minimise ambiguities:

- Avoid using words that have more than one meaning. Example: 'Should' can be replaced by 'may' (implying choice and giving permission to choose) or 'must' (removing choice and implying enforcement). Choose the most appropriate word
- Use a single word to replace unnecessary phrases; e.g., replace 'in the event of . . .' with the word 'if'
- Use connecting words, e.g., 'the'. Connecting words in speech are dropped successfully because the voice implies the meaning, but when connecting words are omitted from print, ambiguity results
- Avoid the double negative—use positively worded questions and statements. Apart from being difficult for English Readers, some languages interpret the double negative as emphasising the negative
  Example:
  Do *not* enrol the patient if the above criteria are *not* met.
  Preferred:
  Enrol the patient if the answers to *all* the above questions are YES.
- Avoid the passive voice. Use the active voice, linking actions with individuals, so that responsibilities for actions and lines of communication are clear to the Form Filler.
  Example:
  Permission for the next level of dosing can be obtained when these laboratory details are provided.

Preferred:
Send these laboratory details to the Monitor by fax (Number) or 'phone (Number). The Monitor will then inform you if this patient can proceed to the next level of dosing.
- Break down compound questions into a series of single idea questions. Use binary responses as filters, instructing the Form Filler to go to another question in the CRF, if needs be.

Example:
10. Is the patient female of childbearing potential and employing adequate contraceptive protection?

Preferred:
For male patients, continue with question 12. For female patients, answer the next two questions, then continue with question 12:
10. Is the patient of childbearing potential? Yes ☐ No ☐
If No, continue with question 12
11. If Yes, is the patient employing adequate contraceptive protection? Yes ☐ No ☐
- Avoid leading questions—Subjects may feel intimidated in a professional environment and try to please the investigator. For example, asking if any Adverse Experiences occurred can be better presented as—'Are there any other changes in health to report?'

Diary Cards

Design these with the CRFs so that it's obvious how the two link together, especially if data from the diary card will be reviewed and transcribed into the CRF. Depending on the indication, some diary card users may be very experienced and disciplined while others are less so, requiring that the diary cards be tested.

Use the appropriate terminology for Subjects to understand, that is:

(i)   Medical synonyms—e.g., 'skin redness' for erythema or 'dead skin' for necrotic skin.
(ii) Request domestic time using a.m. or p.m. instead of the 24-hour clock, e.g., 3:00 p.m. instead of 15:00.
(iii) Request concomitant medication doses in terms of—number of sprays, capsules . . . instead of total dose in mgs/ml, mgs, etc.
(iv) Structure as days and weeks instead of dates for daily routines.

Weekly Diary Card Example
In this example, leave the day column for the Investigator's staff to complete so the week starts with the correct day and date, for example

DAY	Did an attack occur today?	If yes, what time did the attack start?			How long did the attack last?		What were you doing when the attack started? e.g. walking uphill, climbing stairs, etc.	Medication taken?	
								GTN	ISMN
								No. of sprays	No. of tablets
EXAMPLE	Yes/No	1	3:00	am/pm	5	minutes	Cutting the grass	0	1
Wednesday 05 Aug 1998 dd/mmm/yyyy 1	Yes/No	1		am/pm		minutes			
		2		am/pm		minutes			
		3		am/pm		minutes			
Thursday 2	Yes/No	1		am/pm		minutes			
		2		am/pm		minutes			
		3		am/pm		minutes			

Medical staff to complete **dates** and record **drug names** when issuing

Wednesday 5th August 1998. They can complete the rest of the days, Thurs, Fri . . ., on the card, but the date is not needed after day 1. The medication boxes are also left blank for the Investigator's staff to complete for each Subject. Provide an example of completion of one row for the Subject to refer to which the staff can use to explain how the card will work. Consider issuing the Week 2 card as well, in case the Subject cannot return to the clinic on the correct day.

Data recorded on folds will not be legible for data processing or imaging. Avoid duplication of information between diary card and CRF, and between consecutive diary cards.

METHODOLOGY—how to minimise/avoid problems Users have?

The resultant House Style (choice of print layout and design of a published work) will be based on those factors (type size, type face, case, line length, spacing and graphics) which enhance readability and understanding and promote the desired use of the form.

Human Factors studies showed that legibility is best using:

Type size: 8–12 point
Type face: e.g., Times Roman, Helvetica, Ariel, Univers
Case: mixed; text all set in upper case impedes reading by 13–20%
Line length: 40–70 characters; avoid very short and very long lines

Spacing: less space shows items that are related, more space sepa-
                 rates unrelated ones; spacing between words is less than
                 between lines

Sentences or long phrases set in upper case (capitals) hinder reading by
13–20%. As mentioned previously, readers recognise the shape of the
word, produced by mixed case. Capitals result in rectangular or square
block shapes which are less distinctive. Capitals can be reserved for overall headings and not used for emphasis or important statements—see
Emphasis and Headings below.

House Style

Various combinations of these five factors are incorporated so the Form
Filler can easily recognise and comprehend areas designated for example
to specific activities. These conventions become familiar so the Form
Filler can concentrate fully on the response content. The additional benefits of an accepted House Style which can be used in any CRFs generated
by the Sponsor are:

- Easy recognition of the Sponsor's material and methods by all Users
- House Style does not need to be discussed in the CRF Review Meetings

Margins: Ensure top or left-hand space will accommodate binding without
interfering with text. Right-hand space will be sufficient to compensate for
paper shift during photocopying; make bottom space adequate so information is not lost when photocopying.

Pagination: Use Arabic numerals (1, 2, 3 etc.) and position number on the page
where it is easily seen by all handlers and does not get cut-off when copying.

Identifiers: Position printed, repeated information near the bound edge
margin if infrequently referred to, for example study number, drug name,
version, and so on. Production, dispatch, tracking during retrieval, submission and archive, rely on identifiers and page numbers to locate and
retrieve completed CRFs.

Use the right-hand top for information frequently referred to or recorded,
such as Subject number or initials.

Headings: Use a hierarchy in the same case, left justified descending in size to
denote main, then subordinate. Emboldened page headings of 14 point in size
and larger benefit from double spacing between words to improve legibility.

Question text: For the questions that make up the main body of the CRF,
whether open, closed or matrix formats, use one of the above type faces in

CRF A₄ page Housestyle Example

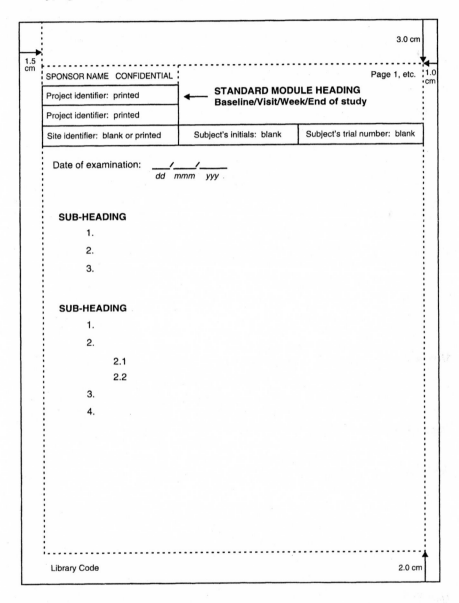

10 pt, mixed case, using 40–70 characters per line. Use a larger point size for elderly readers.

Emphasis: Embolden a single word or sentence without changing type size, type face or case from the convention being used.

Units: Units immediately follow the measurement or open response using the same size as text, and mixed case as is appropriate for any standard abbreviations. Ensure type face distinguishes I (international), from 1 (litre), number 1 and/(per).

Flow: Make the route through the questions obvious. Number the sections or questions using Arabic numerals (1, 2, 3, etc.). Use binary questions to filter and direct, but too many jumps become tedious. Look at the overall effect of space.

Use space to separate different ideas, and allow enough space for correcting entries to ICH requirements.

Well-ordered structured CRF's make communication easy between Users and facilitate recording, data entry, database set up, analysing, writing the final Study Report, and Approval.

Instructions: Devise a unique convention for each type of instruction to be used throughout the CRF. Choose a type face and size which is different to question text and keep instructions near the response, in sequence with events or on facing page for reference. Avoid footnotes, they won't be read properly and confuse flow.

1. Instructing the Form Filler how to respond—e.g., √ box, if Yes, complete AE section, etc.
2. Instructing the Form Filler to leave designated areas blank for other Users to use, e.g., data processing use, administration use only.
3. Instructing the Form Filler what to do when information is not available, or is incomplete; the procedure has not been done; there is more relevant information to record or items/pages to insert.

    Most of these directions can be incorporated into Guidelines for completing the CRF, occurring once near the front of the CRF in a way that is attractive and makes compelling reading.

    Providing an Investigator Comment Log in each CRF has discouraged investigators from writing relevant but unsought comments freely in margins, etc.
4. Instructing the Form Filler what to do next—CRF's can abbreviate protocols, in the form of single statements, numbered or bulleted lists, or the Time and Event Schedule. There needs to be a balance between too many instructions, which the Form Filler will skip, or too few, when the Form Filler becomes frustrated with the lack of guidance.

Open response format: Allow at least 0.5 cm per character response. Use a line for a single number or word and space for free text. Make date and time easily recognised using small descriptors (8 pt) to help completion.

Closed response format: Create a 0.5 cm^2 box, with lines that are not thick and align with text as previously discussed; if printing codes, use 8 point unobtrusively, near boxes, possibly in another typeface style.

Tables: Use very thick lines sparingly to separate unrelated items, and mixed case for table headings with no abbreviations, unless units. Order items (headings) to follow the order of the procedure where possible. Limit the size of each cell to the expected response. Keep the page in a portrait orientation and if the table continues onto two pages, look for the natural break in the procedure rather than attempt an even split. Avoid mixing landscape with portrait which is unwieldy for all Users.

Shading: Employed in tables that are repeatedly used in a CRF, to indicate that a certain response is not needed at that moment. Shading does not prevent information being recorded in that space though. The following alternatives are preferred:

1. If the cell at the end of a list is not needed, remove it rather than shade, and reinsert the cell when required.

Example:

Blood pressure systolic/diastolic mm Hg	Pulse beats/min	Weight kg	For baseline and end of study, e.g. week 12 visits
/			

Blood pressure systolic/diastolic mm Hg	Pulse beats/min	For weeks 2,4,8 visits, etc.
/		

2. If a whole column or row is not required in a matrix, remove it from the CRF and reinsert it when needed.

Example:

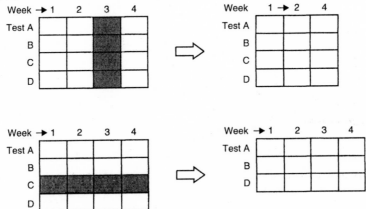

3. Finally, if there is no alternative to shading, especially if the cell is
   isolated in the middle of a column or row, then choose a shade or
   hatching that the Form Filler can recognise, but is of an intensity that
   doesn't cause problems for photocopiers, faxes and scanners.

Example:

Week →	1	2	3	4	5
Test A					
B			▓		▓
C					
D					

STAGE 3: PRODUCTION

A meeting with printers, to discuss a mock-up of the final CRF documents,
is the best way to communicate the details to production operators and
handlers.

The Mock-up CRF

General information that accompanies the mock-up will state:

- How the CRF will be finished?
  1. Drilling? Crimping? Pads?
  2. Folder? Ring binder? Covers?
- Numbers of CRFs required and when?
- Assembly instructions, order of pages
- Size, type, weight, colour, numbers, matt/shiny, thickness, etc. of all
  materials
- Position and orientation of print on materials
- Materials?
  1. Paper
  2. Inks
  3. Card
  4. Tab dividers
  5. Front sheets
  6. Acetates or laminates
  7. Attachment, insert stationery—wallets, folders, envelopes
  8. Labels
  9. Business reply cards?

Mark pages that require different materials, special printing, folding or
binding on the mock-up.

Colour

Coloured inks, paper and/or selected areas of a page can be used to show differences, similarities, for emphasis, make attractive, and make user-friendly.

Black ink on a white background is the benchmark against which usefulness of the colours of ink and backgrounds are compared. The subjective nature of colour necessitates a trial and error process, which is costly. Colour can be wasted on elderly or colour-deficient populations, by hindering readability.

We perceive colour differently, with changes in ink intensity, lighting types and levels, paper surfaces and sizes. The reprinting and reproducibility of colour has to be monitored carefully. Combinations of colour can negate other positive effects set up in the black on white master. For example, black ink is not legible on certain background colours, so to avoid difficulties use pastel colours. Spacing effects may be reduced or lost with the introduction of colour.

Reversing out (having white sections on a coloured background) has been used successfully, but is costly.

Keep to black on white, and only introduce colour, for example, as a background (tab dividers, NCR paper, etc.). Bear in mind that photocopying and scanning certain colours result in machine contrast adjustments which take ages and can obliterate the image.

Paper

Different coloured sets of NCR can be used to distinguish the original copy for data processing, the Investigator copy and if needed, a local company copy. The separating pressure card can be a flapover attached to a pad or a removable insert in a binder.

Check that the weight, shading used and colour of the paper can withstand photocopying or imaging techniques which may be used during production, retrieval, data entry, submission and archiving.

Pagination

Devise a system that allows for inserting additional pages in a logical fashion that Form Fillers, data handlers and printers can understand, and tracking systems can use, to identify all components for each Subject.

Administration

Ensure estimates of the number of CRFs, diary cards and so on allow for potential loss or damage and quality check the first CRF or card prepared.

If handling any translations, print the language name in full unobtrusively in a margin for the printer and Users' benefit.

STANDARD MODULES

Standard modules are developed to collect the same data across all trials and may be a whole page, part of or more than one page. The main benefits from using them are savings in time and effort by leading to:

- The development of standard procedures, such as data entry
- The complementary standard database module
- The basis for libraries of modules (both CRF and database) freeing up individuals to concentrate on the Science of the trial.

The following modules are commonly found to have similar CONTENT across the industry:

INCLUSION/EXCLUSION
DEMOGRAPHY
VITAL SIGNS
PHYSICAL EXAMINATION
MEDICAL HISTORY
CONCURRENT CONDITIONS
HAEMATOLOGY
CLINICAL CHEMISTRY
URINALYSIS
PLASMA SAMPLING SCHEDULE
CONCOMITANT MEDICATION
ADVERSE EVENTS
BREAKING BLIND
END OF STUDY DETAILS
INVESTIGATOR COMMENT LOG
INVESTIGATOR SIGN OFF

Standards will be designed to collect **all** the relevant data, allowing for some to be deleted from study to study. The standards will be adhered to unless an aspect is redundant, or the information will be collected differently. Some standard modules are not needed in every study, for example urinalysis, plasma samples for pharmacokinetics, breaking blind, and so on.

Deviations

Some situations will require a change to a standard. It is easier if items are removed, not added. Some examples are given below.

Demography

Date of birth may not be the appropriate way to measure Age. Sex for sex-linked diseases may be pre-coded on the CRF and hard coded on the database.

Vital signs

In clinical trials of babies, height will be replaced by length. In adult trials, height will only be collected once. In critical care, pulse will be replaced by a heart rate monitor reading. Respiratory rate will not be used in every study.

Physical exam

This is a general body system check. Omit the body system under study from the standard. Information will most likely be captured in more detail in a baseline indication module.

Lab data

Not all data will be collected in every trial—some tests can be removed.

There is the danger that if an organisation uses standards slavishly, the module may become foreign to a Form Filler's environment and will jeopardise the quality of the data recorded. Another problem which can arise consequently is requesting data more than once.

Data Duplication

Duplicated data is resource intensive for monitoring, data editing and entry. The Investigator does not expect to be asked for the same information more than once, with the result that the answers may be different through forgetfulness, or thinking another aspect is being questioned.
   Some situations commonly seen and to avoid are:

1.   Collecting age as well as date of birth.
2.   Putting a date in the header of a running log page that collects dates of events/medication changes, etc.
3.   Repeating data collected in a running log on separate visit pages, e.g., medication record.
4.   Asking for the date and reason for the patient stopping the trial early both on Visit pages and on the End of Study summary.
5.   Putting a date in the header of a laboratory page as well as asking for the date of sample/specimen.
6.   Asking for the same information in a diary card and a CRF.

Library

Standard modules may be organised centrally for all trials, and/or organised into therapeutic/indication areas with the agreed deviations to the modules. Within the therapeutic areas, there may be a subdivision for the population—such as paediatric, geriatric, immunosuppressed and so on.

REVIEWING THE CRF

The review team will represent the:

- Investigator
- Medical monitor
- Clinical monitor
- Data monitor
- Statistician
- Forms designer
- Database administrator
- Statistical programmer

Scanning and reading techniques are unique to individuals and dependent on the time allowed, so people need help to focus their attentions productively. Some reviews will require meetings, in the initial or problematic stages.

Initially supply one copy of each unique module which will occur in the CRF and, for each datum, standard module, ask:

1. Do you need to collect it?
2. What will you do with it?
3. Are you asking for it correctly?

Once each module has been agreed, expand the CRF fully and review:

- Cross-referencing of dates, data, instructions, etc.
- House style and layouts
- Consistency of grading and precision
- Baseline with following comparative data
- The need for deviations

Avoid or minimise:

- Duplicate data
- Pictorial data
- Comments

SUMMARY

These discussions have shown how the CRF is involved with, influences, or is influenced by, the stages of the clinical trial process. Ways to reduce the time and cost of the clinical trial which impact the CRF have been reviewed.

The competing/complementing demands made on the CRF by Form Fillers, Readers and Handlers have been highlighted and it is acknowledged that a CRF document could never meet all their needs.

However, no system is better than the quality of the information it handles. The User who can provide quality data is the Form Filler. That the Form Filler faces a daunting task has been recognised and to facilitate the achievement of quality the watchword is SIMPLE. Keep questions, words, layouts, identifiers, instructions . . . SIMPLE.

Guide the Form Filler through the forms using SIMPLE instinctive patterns of completion which are repeated to reinforce the learning process. In this way the Form Filler's memory load will be light so there is time and energy left to invest in answering the questions correctly.

REFERENCES

1. Wright, P. and Haybittle, J. (1986) Designing clinical trials forms to collect the right data. In H. Glenny and P. Nelmes (eds), *Handbook of Clinical Drug Research*, ACRPI; Blackwell Scientific, Oxford, pp. 247–270.
2. Wright, P. (1980) Strategy and tactics in the design of forms. *Visible Language*, **14**, 2, 151–193.

4 Data Capture

EMMA WATERFIELD

Clinical Trials Research Ltd, Maidenhead, Berks, UK

INTRODUCTION

The term 'data capture' refers to the accumulation of clinical data onto a database in a consistent, logical fashion so that it can be retrieved and searched. The content of the database should be an exact representation of the Investigator's observations at the clinical trial site, and capture of data must not obstruct this. For the purposes of this chapter, the term does not include the identification or interpretation of data errors or inconsistencies, except where this procedure is directly linked with the data capture step.

All companies, whether pharmaceutical/biotechnology organisations or Contract Research Organisations (CROs), will have similar objectives in mind when appraising the effectiveness of different data capture strategies. There is a universal need to submit data faster to regulatory authorities and also to submit to a larger number of authorities based in many more countries than was the case in the past. In addition, the volume of data collected in clinical trials has escalated, due both to the numbers of trials conducted and their increasing complexity and to increasing demands to prove drug safety. The chosen systems must therefore achieve the required balance between data quality and reduced drug cycle development time at the lowest overall cost.

Those involved in Clinical Data Management (CDM) are likely to experience an increasing pressure to review their data capture practices in an attempt to resolve this quality/speed/cost dilemma. By reviewing and understanding each data capture option, a considered judgement may be made as to which is most suitable for the individual organisation. Different solutions are likely to emerge depending on the individual factors involved.

This chapter explores the different types of data capture available to clinical data management, including the more established manual methods of data entry and newer electronic data capture technologies,

Clinical Data Management. Second Edition. Edited by R.K. Rondel, S.A. Varley and C.F. Webb.
© 2000 John Wiley & Sons, Ltd

the factors influencing choice of data capture method and some future prospects.

BACKGROUND

Historically, data capture methods have been restricted by available technology. The speed of computer systems, together with limited memory capability, restricted the numbers of users who could operate the system, the quantity of data and the complexity of programming possible. Reliability was also often a problem. Improvements to both hardware and software have developed to such an extent that technology is now rarely the limiting factor. Data capture will be considered firstly from this historical perspective, moving on to the newer technologies which in some cases completely bypass the methods utilised in the past.

TRADITIONAL DATA CAPTURE METHODS

Single/Double Data Entry

Traditionally, data capture has meant manual entry of data by trained specialist data entry operators who input data from a paper case record form (CRF) onto a central database via pre-set data entry screens, using a conventional keyboard. Data entry might occur only once (single entry) or successively (double entry), the latter with input by a second, separate data entry operator. Double entry aims to increase accuracy by highlighting the differences between the two operators' versions of the data. Reconciliation between the two entries may be achieved by either of two methods. On-line data point to data point verification by the second, more experienced data entry operator calls for a judgement to be made between the two conflicting entries, or flagging of the discrepancy for further investigation by CDM staff. An alternative is to run a report after double data entry which compares the two entries and indicates the inconsistencies. Subsequent comparison of the non-matching variables must then be accomplished by CDM staff before the data are transferred to the production area of the database. This represents an additional, time-consuming step in the data entry process.

The usual rationale for applying double data entry is that the increase in accuracy outweighs the additional expense and associated time delay in twice entering the data onto the system. One approach to maximise efficiency might be to employ single entry for text fields (which are notoriously difficult to enter accurately and are often subject to a later listings review by CDM staff), with double entry for non-text fields. In addition, by assessing the relative importance of different fields of the CRF to the final analysis, certain items of non-critical data might also be entered only once.

Legibility of text is likely to be a significant problem for the data entry operator. In general, operators are asked to identically reproduce the CRF page content onto the database, making no assumptions about the data that they see in front of them. In most cases, it is advantageous to use a flagging system, whereby illegible text is indicated by a keyed symbol which can later be reviewed by more medically aware CDM staff, thus reducing input time by the data entry operator and avoiding duplication of effort.

Data Entry Screen Design

Design of data entry screens is an important factor in determining the speed at which data can be entered. In general, the more similar the screen looks to the original CRF page, the easier it will be for an inexperienced data entry operator to enter the correct data in the appropriate field. However, experienced data entry operators often key very quickly, barely glancing at the data entry screen. If standard sets of CRF page templates are used to design the CRF, standard screen templates can be produced to minimise design effort for each individual study. Since similar pages are often repeated throughout the CRF, for example vital signs recorded at every visit, use of a single screen template for all such occurrences is often employed as a strategy. There is an additional benefit in maintaining a library of CRF page templates and matching data entry screen templates, since data entry operators will become familiar with the standard layout and require less study-specific training. A simple layout with individual data fields progressively one under the other is probably more effective when trained data entry operators are to perform the keying, as opposed to data fields placed randomly on the page. Obviously, ordering data entry screens in the same sequence that they occur in the CRF book also facilitates the entry of data.

It is often advantageous to program an 'index' table into the database which contains the unique patient identifiers, namely the protocol number, centre number and patient number. The index table can then be linked with all other tables in the database, allowing automatic population of these variables as each subsequent screen is accessed, thus simultaneously conserving data entry time and maintaining accuracy in key variables. A further benefit of such an index is that entry of duplicate records can be avoided.

Another consideration when designing data entry screens should be consistent formatting of analogous fields such as dates, which should preferably be entered in the same format throughout the database, for example always dd/mmm/yy in a single field or dd, mm, yy in three separate fields. The latter format may aid recording of partial dates, since a month and a year can be captured, even if the day is unknown. Attention should also be paid to the field attributes, (alphanumeric, integer, floating decimal, etc.) so that these are kept as consistent as possible across like fields, particularly where tables may later require merging, for example with an autoencoder program or imported Central Laboratory results, or be prepared for data transfer.

Restricting the input of data to a limited nomenclature can be achieved by the use of codelists. This reduces the possibility of error by the data entry operators, since only a finite number of keyed responses will be permitted, e.g. 'Y' or 'N' for 'yes' and 'no' respectively. Entry of any value other than those specified in the codelist would then be notified to the data entry operator, so that the correct value could be instated. As mentioned previously, ability to enter flags highlighting illegible or missing data can be a valuable facility, and should be designed to allow data entry operators to operate them using as few keystrokes as possible.

The draft data entry screens must be validated before use, both by the programmer who designed them and by the end user, preferably using test patient data. This provides assurance that the data typed into the screens is equal to that stored on the database, and assists creation of a user guide. A database listing of the test patient data should be checked against the original to confirm that the data are identical. All documentation of such validation should be signed, dated and retained in order to comply with GCP/ICH guidelines.

Centralised vs Local Data Entry

Data entry occurring in one central location is still standard practice for most companies. However, there is a time delay in mailing/couriering the paper CRFs to the central site from what may increasingly be multiple worldwide locations, as companies adopt globalisation policies. One solution would be to have entry occur at the Investigator sites or at several local office sites but this brings with it certain disadvantages:

- Entry staff less experienced with entry of data
- Requirement to maintain systems in remote locations and provide servicing and technical support
- Unlikely to be resource for second entry, therefore increased chance of errors
- Expense of initial outlay and ongoing support of data transfer mechanisms back to central site
- Compatibility of systems

By performing a company's entire requirement for data entry at a single central site, factors such as systems support, maintenance, stability and security can be more easily monitored and achieved. Trained dedicated staff are likely to be available on an ongoing basis to maximise the efficiency of the process. However, the nature of clinical research is such that flow of data in-house is unlikely ever to be at a constant rate, rather the organisation may at times experience a glut of data requiring urgent entry onto the database, whilst at other times it may be subject to periods of very low volumes of data requiring entry. An organisation may therefore find it practical to staff its data entry department with a baseline level of dedicated staff and supplement this with temporary staff as and when required. The use of temporary staff may not be an ideal solution to the problem of fluctuating data entry resource needs since the issues of training, quality standards and security must be considered.

An alternative solution to the challenge of retrieving paper CRFs from distant sites to either a central location or multiple local offices in the shortest possible timeframe is to use facsimile (fax) technology. This technology will be examined separately later in the chapter.

INCORPORATING DATA FROM AN EXTERNAL DATABASE

Manually entered paper CRFs may still be the norm in most companies engaging in CDM, however, many have embraced the opportunity to link with external databases to simplify the transfer of large volumes of specific data to their own database; for example, laboratory results from a Central Laboratory or blood pressure measurements direct from a monitor connected to a patient. Files of data can be downloaded onto disk, tape or via modem link and uploaded directly into the sponsor database, thus bypassing the need for a manual entry step. This is particularly advantageous in the case of laboratory data since before the availability of Central Laboratory data, entry proved very time consuming, especially when many different normal and alert ranges, units and repeat values had to be recorded.

Precautions must be taken to ensure that data integrity and security are maintained when data are transferred electronically. Either of two approaches may be selected: (i) ensuring that the two databases are compatible, or (ii) that suitable conversion programs are generated. Both systems must also be validated, common variables (e.g., protocol number, study number, centre number, subject number and initials, visit identifier) must be reconciled, and a procedure put in place for highlighting and resolving inconsistencies.

FAX-BASED DATA CAPTURE

Use of fax technology has accelerated throughout all industries in recent years. The potential benefits to CDM in speeding up the process by which clinical data can be gathered and tracked from diverse international sites and captured onto a centralised database have been quickly recognised, such that there are now a number of commercially available software packages designed specifically for use in CDM. The fact that the process can be relatively easily integrated into current working practices means that the idea of faxed CRF pages is more readily acceptable to those wary of, for example, remote data entry, since it represents a stepping stone between traditional paper-based data capture and full electronic data capture, requiring just a re-engineering of the paper CRF process.

Many sites will already have access to a fax machine, but if necessary, equipment can be provided at a relatively low cost and offering a high degree of resolution in terms of print quality. Maintenance and servicing costs must, however, also be considered. Provision of a (pre-programmed) free-phone number enables a user-friendly route to a central fax server, and training requirements are minimal. Transmission of data to the sponsor is less of a security concern using fax-based technology. Consideration must be given to the problem of tracking and reconciling duplicates of CRF pages of the type that are often updated periodically during the trial, for example adverse event pages or concomitant medication pages, which may have ongoing entries.

AUTOMATED DATA ACQUISITION FROM OPTICAL IMAGES

The drive to speed up the process by which clinical data are captured onto a centralised database has seen the development of more sophisticated scanning technology. When scanned, each mark on the original CRF page is viewed as a matrix of tiny dots which are stored electronically in the system so that an image can be assessed on a VDU screen rather than printed as a hard paper copy. The improvement over fax technology is that images can be recognised and stored in such a way that the information can later be deciphered. The step by which the optical image is interpreted onto the electronic database is known as automated data acquisition. Automated data acquisition can be subdivided into the following:

Optical Mark Recognition (OMR)

Where marks made on the CRF page in pre-determined areas are deciphered as meaningful data and converted to electronic values, e.g., yes/no check boxes on inclusion or exclusion criteria pages. Barcodes also rely on this technology.

| Optical Character Recognition (OCR) | Where the system can recognise numbers and characters. This is usually facilitated by restricting handwritten entry of individual digits or letters to specific boxes/areas. |
| Intelligent Character Recognition (ICR) | A type of OCR system which has the ability to 'guess' at unrecognised symbols, retain a 'memory' of those previously encountered, and apply rules of association to enable interpretation. |

Optical mark recognition can reach a very high level of accuracy if responses are restricted to check boxes. Optical character recognition as yet cannot match the levels of precision of OMR, but numerals recorded in boxes can be distinguished with a high degree of accuracy and short strings of characters such as patient initials are also fairly well identified. Accuracy levels for free handwritten text entries are poor, however. The degree of accuracy of data collected is obviously critical if subsequent automatic validation is to be performed effectively.

In order to make the transition to automated data acquisition, steps can be taken to modify familiar CDM procedures used for CRF design, database set-up and data entry screen design, thereby improving the likelihood of achieving an effective system. The designer will have to consider the ability of the scanning technology to comprehend the data, in addition to the more conventional requirements such as ease of data entry. It will be of paramount importance to maximise the ability to distinguish between marked and unmarked check boxes, and to identify the best methods of restricting handwriting in order to optimise accuracy of recognition. Another important technical requirement is the correct alignment of the image, which must be very precise in order for recognition to be performed. This can be facilitated by incorporation of location markers into the CRF page design.

Paper CRFs are collected from the trial site and either scanned at a regional office or central location, or faxed by the site directly to the main scanning point. Pre-printed study and page identifiers on the paper CRF are recognised by OCR and then subject and visit details can be used to uniquely catalogue the image and enable it to be tracked. A data entry reviewer can then check the data visually by on-screen comparison of image and data entry screen, and enter any unrecognised free text. Range and sense checks, including coding dictionaries and translation, can be programmed and the output reviewed by CDM staff, who annotate the screen with any queries before returning the image to the site for resolution. Queries annotated onto the CRF page tend to be more easily understood by site staff than traditional paper-based query reports. The process allows CDM to have earlier access to the data than is possible conventionally, and simplifies tracking and query management procedures. Storage of CRF images also greatly facilitates archiving obligations. Scanning data capture methods are effective for studies with numerous sites recruiting small numbers of patients, and for studies with complex data, which are more difficult to manage with the remote data entry process outlined below.

REMOTE DATA ENTRY (RDE)

Remote data entry means data capture at the point at which it is generated. If electronic transfer of the data to the sponsor's system occurs regularly, the data can be accessed and reviewed much more quickly than has been possible using traditional data capture methods. Crucially, the data can be validated as they are entered, by on-screen prompting, thus minimising errors early on in the process. The incentives for introducing remote data entry are therefore improved data quality, speed and flexibility of access to data, automatic avoidance of simple errors and early notification of error trends, which are all factors that can expedite time to database closure. Implementation of an RDE system is, however, very expensive. The following are likely to be significant costs:

- Purchase of a proprietary RDE package or design of an in-house RDE system
- Purchase of new hardware in-house
- Purchase of new hardware, e.g., PCs, laptops, palmtops, for remote sites and their delivery
- Communications charges and associated validation
- Training (both in-house and at site), support, e.g., helpdesk
- System maintenance and support
- Security of data transmission, integrity and access
- Compatibility with existing systems and data
- Re-engineering of processes and promotion in-house

Before investment in such a system, consideration must have been given both to the potential users of the system, and to the study requirements. Users will include Investigators, site staff, monitors, CDM, IS and potentially third parties such as a CRO or Central laboratory. Since a key element of the system is its integrated validation, all edit checks must be programmed in parallel with development of the electronic CRF (e-CRF). This makes it imperative that *all* members of the project team are involved in determination of the extent of data validation. Design of the screens must be from the perspective of the Investigator or site staff entering data, making use of the e-CRF as simple as possible, for example by logical sequencing of pages, on-screen prompts for missing or inconsistent data and skipping of irrelevant fields. There must be sufficient flexibility in the entry screens and edit checks to allow for data not available at the time of entry, which could also necessitate some checks being run separately in-house after transfer of data from the remote site.

The Investigator or designated site staff access the password-protected e-CRF on either a PC or laptop provided by the sponsor. By supplying a laptop, the sponsor can be certain that there is sufficient memory capacity and that the edit checks have been correctly loaded. Technical support of the trial may also be less complicated if all sites are using standardised equipment. Alternatively, use of a site-based PC would be cheaper and the software could be loaded and encrypted relatively easily. Data are entered onto the e-CRF directly from source documents which is aided by on-screen help messages and alerts such as range check outliers, protocol violation warnings or coding mismatches. The data are then downloaded at the end of each session to the sponsor's remote server via a modem link installed at the site. The sponsor, CRA or CRO can then immediately gain access to the data. Read-only, or read-edit restrictions can be placed as required to regulate access. Data management staff may initially be given read-only access to the data, and place electronic queries for any inconsistencies identified by their review, by either a pre-determined flag or using a query template. Once the Investigator has resolved the query to the CRA's satisfaction, the CRA can 'lock' the record, visit or patient data so that the Investigator no longer has edit access. This system has the advantage that the 'history' of a query can be scrutinised via the on-screen flags and date stamps, representing a dialogue between Investigator, CRA and CDM, and providing an in-built audit trail as stipulated by GCP/ICH guidelines. The e-CRF can be printed out once all checks are complete and returned to the site by the CRA at the final source data verification visit, where it is signed by the Investigator.

Some studies are inherently more suitable for RDE than others. It is important to assess the requirements of the study, for example the complexity of the data to be collected, the geographical location of the sites and the number of sites involved as well as training requirements. In general, RDE will prove to be most viable for simple studies with a large number of patients recruited at a small number of sites, particularly if the site is likely to be used by the sponsor company on a regular basis. Training and support of the site is also then more easily coordinated. Phase I studies lend themselves particularly well to the RDE process, since all the necessary elements are likely to be situated in a confined, easily regulated area.

Electronic Diaries

Data can also be captured remotely from electronic diaries supplied to patients utilising hand-held 'notepad' computer technology. Traditional paper-based patient diaries are notoriously inaccurate due to problems of patient compliance. Electronic diaries can be programmed to prompt patients to comply with the treatment regimen, and allow review of compliance since entry of data can be 'date-stamped'. Provided that diary data are downloaded at the end of each visit, assessment of compliance can be notified to the Investigator quickly enough that remedial action can be taken before the end of the study. This is of course dependent on the patients remembering to bring the electronic diary with them to the visit. Swift access to diary data also gives the sponsor earlier notification of adverse experiences. Training is an important precursor to effective use of electronic diaries. The Investigator must receive training from the CRA both in the operation of the equipment to capture the data and in the data transfer process which uploads the data from the diary. The Investigator must then be responsible for training the patient in the use of the equipment and in understanding the instructions. It is helpful if there is an in-built tutorial so that the patient can be tested in his or her understanding of the instructions prior to the start of the trial.

FACTORS INFLUENCING CHOICE OF DATA CAPTURE METHOD

The following factors might be considered when assessing the relative merits of the different data capture strategies.

1. *Initial costs.* Including outlay for new hardware and software, bespoke programming, training of Investigators, CRAs, CDM staff, process revision and documentation (new SOPs), validation of all new interfaces, security, organisational disruption.
2. *Ongoing costs.* Including training, support, e.g., provision of helpdesk, servicing, maintenance, communications, backups, ongoing validation.
3. *Accuracy.* Data quality, i.e., similarity of data to source data, ease of error identification.
4. *Speed.* Reduced time to database lock, lag times, set-up times, rapidity of entry onto database, accessibility of sponsor to data, potential for integrated validation.
5. *Security.* Patient anonymity and confidentiality, encryption, intellectual property/innovative ideas of sponsor, competitor interest.
6. *Flexibility.* Simplicity, adaptability to changing requirements/ environments (globalisation), compatibility with existing systems, reliability.
7. *Regulatory.* GCP/ICH requirements to be maintained, SOPs, audit trails.

The relative importance of each of these factors will of course depend on the individual company's goals, users, budget and study design. The traditional single option of manual input from a paper CRF onto a database has now been joined by technologies which have brought the ideal of 'point of generation' data capture to reality. These new technologies have wide-ranging potential advantages, specifically improved data quality, reduced in-house resourcing/ processing time and speedier access to data, but may prove prohibitively expensive in terms of hardware and software requirements, training and support costs, unless a true assessment of need has been determined.

FUTURE PROSPECTS

Remote Data Entry via the Internet

The potential of the Internet for use in CDM cannot be over-estimated. Set-up and access costs are cheap in comparison with the RDE methods mentioned above, and are becoming cheaper all the time. Many GPs and hospitals are already in possession of a suitable PC and telephone line and in theory it should be possible to give them access to the Internet at relatively little expense. The requirements would include a telephone line, modem and an Internet browser, which is the software used to read World Wide Web (WWW) pages. Of course in practice, the logistics are likely to be less simple. Security issues would need to be overcome by supplying encryption software, both to protect patient confidentiality and to preserve the sponsor's claim to original ideas and data. Testing of data entry and transfer mechanisms would also be mandatory for assurance of security. In addition, support and maintenance of the whole system would be difficult to administer if the PC belonged to the site and the rest of the hardware was loaned from the sponsor. It would be prudent of the sponsor to organise site audits of hardware and electronic transmission capability during the planning stages of a study, that is prior to the first patient being recruited and the associated need for immediate data capture. Suitability for the intended study could then be assessed after completion of a planned validation procedure, and preventive measures put in place to avoid potential corruption of data. An inventory of hardware would also be advisable, to document which components were the property of the sponsor. Resource would also be required for retrieval of equipment at the end of the study, unless a site maintains a regular association with the sponsor.

The Investigator and/or designated site staff would require password-protected accounts on the Sponsor's server, and would be able to access a specific website related to the clinical trial in which they were participating. The website might contain information about the trial, such as the protocol, recent amendments and advice, and the electronic CRF pages.

Clinical data could then be entered into the electronic CRF and pass directly to the sponsor's server. Simple checks on the data could be run in real-time, alerting the enterer to obvious range errors or inconsistencies, but more sophisticated edit checks may be less practical. A solution to this would be that more complicated cross-table checks could be run overnight, perhaps even utilising the processing power of the remote-based PC if edit check programs were downloaded from the sponsor's central server. Queries arising from the overnight validation process could be automatically electronically mailed to the site, alerting them to the fact that data entered the previous day required review. The conventional time delays of data entry and query turnaround would be drastically reduced, with the additional benefit that the Investigator would be addressing queries whilst the data were still fresh in his mind.

The great advantage of the Internet is thus the speed of communication possible. There would be a two-way benefit, for example the trial site could more quickly alert the sponsor of SAEs, whilst the sponsor could inform all sites, whatever their location, of new developments and instructions relating to the trial, thereby increasing the likelihood that any revised practices were implemented simultaneously. Compared with other methods of RDE, it is very quick and cheap to set up Internet-based systems, with the added value that interaction with standard software is both feasible and easy to validate.

There is less of a training issue with use of the Internet because the technology is simple and user friendly ('point and click') and therefore fast for novices to learn. This might be an important factor to consider if in the future an Investigator was involved in several trials for different sponsors, all utilising slightly different variations of RDE technology. The situation would be much more straightforward if all studies were managed on the Internet.

Direct Access to Medical Records

In the future, clinical research staff including those involved in CDM may be able to gain access to certain areas of GP or hospital databases, thus potentially negating the need for even electronic CRFs in certain circumstances. This would necessitate storage of medical records in a standard format for maximum effectiveness, and require encryption to totally anonymise each record. The issue of guaranteeing a patient's absolute right to anonymity is currently a highly debated topic and is likely to take some time to reach a resolution satisfactory to all concerned parties. There would be cost savings to the sponsor in that hardware would no longer be required at remote sites, there would be no ongoing need for support and maintenance and no training requirements for site staff.

Smart Cards

Another possible way of speeding up the capture of an individual patient's medical data would be to store these details on a 'smart card'. A patient's medical history, family medical history, details of past medications and previous participation in clinical trials could then be transferred automatically, and the card could be updated regularly with laboratory results, vital signs and changes to medication regimen. This idea again has implications with regard to patient anonymity and confidentiality, if the data were insufficiently protected.

Working from Home

The general trend towards working from home, whereby employees work at least part of their hours at home, has significant cost savings for the employer organisation and is made a step closer for CDM staff by the new technologies such as imaging, RDE and the Internet. We are likely to see increasing numbers of CDM staff able to complete their data management tasks from a home PC with modem link.

CONCLUSION

The scope of data capture requirements will vary widely between different companies engaging in CDM. For smaller concerns, traditional data entry from paper CRFs by data entry operators at a central location may still prove to be the most effective system when all factors are taken into account. However, larger companies which have pursued globalisation strategies and so benefited by the reduction in duration of their clinical trials, have established that data capture methods must be more efficient. As such, techniques such as remote data entry are becoming increasingly more widespread. The associated changes in the CDM process and ensuing restructuring of some elements of the organisation mean that the roles of those employed in CDM may become increasingly blurred with those of their colleagues in Clinical Monitoring and Application Development. The pace of development of technology is currently so rapid that there is the additional consideration for any company proposing to invest in new hardware and software of the hazard that it may become quickly out-of-date or redundant in a changing operational environment.

5 Planning and Implementation

CHRIS THOMAS

Covance Clinical and Periapproval Services Ltd, Maidenhead, Berks, UK

> I keep six honest serving men
> (They taught me all I knew);
> Their names are What and Why and When
> And How and Where and Who
> *Rudyard Kipling*

INTRODUCTION

A large proportion of the drug development process concerns the gathering and distribution of information during clinical trials and the data management function is pivotal in managing this information. Data management begins when the protocol is written and the data capture tool designed, and continues through to the study drug being licensed for the market place and beyond into post-marking surveillance. The earlier that the professional clinical data manager becomes involved in the process the more effectively the study will run. The key to a successful project is the quality of the project planning and the effective implementation of those plans.

The time spent at the beginning of a study putting together a comprehensive plan is one of the best investments of time in the life cycle of the study. It takes a good deal of self-discipline to resist the pressures to get on with the job in hand and to take time out for the planning stage. The most successful studies are those where the data management staff have been involved, along with other disciplines, at the earliest possible stages.

A good plan is a living document that is continually reviewed and has inbuilt checks and balances. The project plan covers the Why, What, When, How, Where and Who of a project. Once a good plan is in place, implementing the plan becomes a matter of following the steps and timings laid out in the plan, reviewing and monitoring its progress, ensuring that appropriate measures are in place for this purpose and taking corrective action when necessary to maintain control, which may involve making modifications to the plan.

Clinical Data Management. Second Edition. Edited by R.K. Rondel, S.A. Varley and C.F. Webb.
© 2000 John Wiley & Sons, Ltd

Whilst the focus of this chapter is the data management planning for a study, this cannot be dealt with in isolation and consideration must always be given to all other disciplines involved throughout the study. This chapter describes how the data management component of a typical clinical trial should be planned and implemented. The planning stage consists of a careful analysis of the business needs, which leads on to definition of the project objectives, timelines, top level budget and the assumptions and constraints affecting these. Once the objectives are clear, the project strategy, including a detailed plan covering the tasks to be performed, the milestone timings and the detailed budget (if appropriate), can be formulated. Resource planning can then take place and the project organisation can be set up.

Implementation consists of putting these plans into operation and using effective monitoring, review and control processes to ensure that the project runs to time, to budget and to the required quality (Figure 5.1).

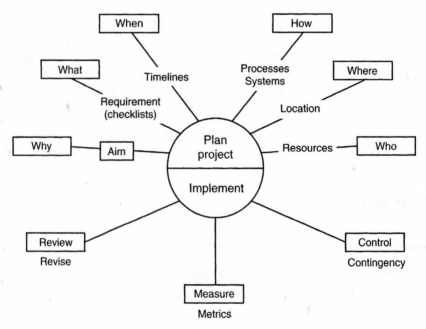

Figure 5.1 Planning/implementation satellite

PLANNING

Effective planning can determine the feasibility of a project and can help to evaluate different options and processes. It enables the project manager to estimate and organise resources and suitable support, to establish appropriate lines of communication, to decide on and use the best processes and systems, to identify the necessary tools to be able to control and monitor progress, to understand the budget and to identify risks and develop contingency plans.

'Why'—Understanding the Aim

Why is the study being conducted?

Every clinical data management programme, be it a single clinical trial or an integrated drug development programme spanning several phases of drug development, is conducted to meet a specific set of needs, which are owned by the 'sponsor'. The sponsor may be another department within the same pharmaceutical company or, in the case of a CRO (Clinical Research Organisation), another company. Usually the needs will be related to regulatory submissions or to marketing department requirements and effective planning of such projects relies on a clear and agreed understanding of these needs.

For single clinical trials much of this need will be stated in the study protocol. The protocol is an important source of information for the project plan; it will state the aim of the clinical trial, provide information of study timings and whether interim analyses are required. For other projects it may be necessary to explore and define these needs with a regulatory, marketing or other appropriate body.

The term clinical trial may be used to cover one study or a series of studies. Each can be considered to be a project in its own right and, as such, can benefit from the application of project management techniques.

'What', 'When' and 'How'

Once the need for the project has been understood and agreed it is then possible to define what the project will deliver. These deliverables need to be described in as much detail as is possible at this stage.

Specification of deliverables should include a clear indication of what is to be done, when, how and by whom. Developing timelines in clinical data management projects, where deadlines for regulatory submissions or marketing activities can be highly significant to the commercial success of a product, is a skilled project management activity. Similarly, specifying the required quality of the deliverable and the budget required to complete the project will always be a compromise, although most clinical data management projects will have to comply with ICH/GCP guidelines.

Data Management interactions may be wholly within a company or, in the case of a Contract Research Organisation (CRO), may be internal and external. Before beginning to gather information for the project plan, it is important that the data manager realises the time constraints on their internal and external customers so that these can be considered in the planning process.

At this stage it is also necessary to set out any other assumptions and constraints that might apply to the planning of the project, other than those related to time, quality or cost. For instance, it may be necessary to assume the availability of investigators in certain countries during holiday periods or the availability of fax machines at all sites for faxing queries. A constraint might be that clinical data may arrive as a bolus towards the end of the study or that lab data might arrive in paper format from some countries and in electronic format from others. There are many more examples of assumptions and constraints (which are not noted here) but which might need to be taken into account when planning a project.

A further issue in setting out what is to be done, and something that should be carefully specified, is how progress on the project will be reported back to the sponsor. Such reporting is important, not only to provide reassurance about progress, but also to check that assumptions, constraints and indeed project needs have not significantly altered.

Once detailed specifications have been drawn up these should be agreed with whoever will be the recipient of the deliverable. When these have been agreed, the detailed tasks that must be performed to produce the deliverable can be planned. There are many project management techniques for this, including bar charts and Gantt charts, but the essential planning activity is to produce a plan of the various tasks that can be used effectively to monitor progress and detect, in a timely manner, when this is not in accordance with the plan.

Regular review of the specifications throughout the life of the project will ensure that both the sponsors changing requirements and changes consequential on the progress of the study can be taken into account wherever necessary.

Key features of the scheduling plan will be milestones that identify significant steps towards completion of the deliverable.

What—the Requirements

When the aim of the study has been established it is time to gather information on the requirements for the deliverables. Where is the best place to start gathering this information and what do we need to consider? For example if the work has come from an external customer then there will be a contract which will give details of the customer's requirements and the scope of the project.

When starting to define the requirements for a study there are certain areas that are general to all studies and can form the basis of the plan. One of the most basic questions we can ask is, what is the end product? The end product may be a Clinical Study Report, a Statistical Report or a Clean Database.

Once the overall scope of the project has been agreed, a budget can be established. The project can be broken down into broad tasks and the ownership of these tasks can be agreed together with the interdependency of these tasks. Risks can be assessed and contingency can be built into the plan.

What are the other considerations which will need to be part of the plan? Standards need to be established so that progress can be monitored and there is a reference point at the implementation stage. The scope of the study and the endpoint will dictate many of the requirements for the processing of the study and the timelines within which this processing must be performed.

In order to be sure that all the relevant information has been gathered and that the same information is collected for each study, standard checklists can be recommended, an example is shown in Figure 5.2.

PROJECT OVERVIEW

Drug name
Therapeutic area

Indication
Project type   ☐ Phase I   ☐ Phase II   ☐ Phase III   ☐ Phase IV   ☐ PMS

Total patients (n)   Drop out %
No. of countries   No. of centres

PROTOCOL/CRF

Is protocol available?   ☐ Yes
                               ☐ Draft   Dated:
                               ☐ Final   Dated:
                         ☐ No

Is protocol input/review required?   ☐ Yes   When by?
                               ☐ No

How will amendments be issued?
Is input required into design of the CRF?   ☐ Yes
                               ☐ Standard modules
                               ☐ Available electronically?
                               ☐ Other, specify
                         ☐ No

Does the database need to be compatible with other databases?
                  ☐ Yes   ☐ No   ☐ N/A

Is CRF available?   ☐ Yes   ☐ Draft   Dated:
                                     ☐ Final   Dated:

Figure 5.2 Example: checklist for establishing requirements

(continued over)

SCOPE AND TIMELINES

Project endpoints: ☐ Data tape   ☐ SAS format, version   ☐ Other
                    ☐ Statistical report ☐ Clinical trial report (CTR)
                    ☐ Interim(s)   When:

Target dates FPI   FPO
              First data to Data Centre   LPO
              Last data to Data Centre   Final query reply to Data Centre
              Final file   Final report

DATA MANAGEMENT DETAILS

Data source   ☐ CRF   No. of pages:
                               ☐ Data tape format:
                               ☐ Other
Laboratory data   ☐ Yes
   ☐ Central labs   ☐ Electronic transmission   ☐ Local labs   ☐ Reference

                                                                Ranges:
   ☐ Other

Microbiology   ☐ Yes   ☐ No

Other data   ☐ Diary cards   ☐ ECG/EEG
                ☐ Quality of life (QOL)   ☐ Other, specify

Translations required?   ☐ Yes   ☐ No

Data availability   ☐ Ongoing   ☐ Other, specify
Database structure
Is specification available? ☐ Yes   ☐ No

Dictionaries   ☐ Autoencoding   ☐ Manual   ☐ N/A

                          ☐ COSTART   ☐ WHOART
                             Version: Version:
                                ☐ AEs   ☐ AEs
                                ☐ Diseases   ☐ Diseases

                          ☐ ICD-9   ☐ WHO DRUG
                             Version: Version:
                                ☐ AEs   ☐ Drugs
                                ☐ Diseases

Figure 5.2 (*continued*)

PROJECT COMPLETION

QA/QC required   ☐ Database audit   ☐ Error rate < 0.5%
☐ Other, specify   ☐ N/A

☐ CRF review   ☐ 2–3% of CRFs
☐ Other, specify   ☐ N/A

☐ Key fields   ☐ Deaths   ☐ AEs
☐ Withdrawals   ☐ Demography
☐ Laboratory data   ☐ Other, specify

☐ N/A

Archiving   ☐

GENERAL

General process flow diagram: ☐ Standard
Are regular meetings, e.g. conference calls required?   ☐ Yes   ☐ No
Are there any specific technical requirements?   ☐ Yes   ☐ No
Who will review draft tables/listings/figures?   Specify:

Is technical or therapeutic training required?   ☐ Yes   ☐ No

---

SOPs

Which SOPs will be followed?

DOCUMENTATION/INFORMATION TO BE OBTAINED

List of contacts and areas of responsibilities   ☐ Yes   ☐ No
Names of project team

Annotated CRF/database structure   ☐ Yes   ☐ No   ☐ N/A
Validation check specifications   ☐ Yes   ☐ No   ☐ N/A
Query flow, i.e. who, when and query turnaround time

TIMELINES

Have the timelines allowed for a SAP review?   ☐ Yes   ☐ No   ☐ N/A

Figure 5.2 *(continued)*

STATUS REPORTS

What information is required for the status report?

What report format is required?

How often are the reports required?   ☐ Monthly   ☐ Other, specify

Are regular listings, e.g. AE listings, required and
if so what format should they be in?   ☐ Yes   ☐ No
                                             Specify:
Who should the status reports be circulated to?

CRF

How many copies of No Carbon Required (NCR) will the CRF be?
                                ☐ 3 part NCR   ☐ Other, specify

Which copy will Data Centre receive?   ☐ 2nd NCR copy   ☐ Other, specify

Can Data Centre staff write on the copy received?   ☐ Yes   ☐ No

When will the CRF be finalised?   Date:

RANDOMISATION

When will the study be unblinded?   ☐ Final file
                                    ☐ For interim analysis
                                        details must be discussed with project statistician
                                    ☐ N/A

In what format will randomisation schedule be received?
                ☐ Electronic   ☐ Paper   ☐ Other, specify

Is it acceptable to get an independent programmer
to validate the schedule prior to final file?   ☐ Yes   ☐ No   ☐ N/A

SERIOUS ADVERSE EVENTS (SAE)

Who will hold the SAE database?   ☐ Specify

Who will reconcile discrepancies between the CRF/SAE database?
Is the CRF the definitive version of the SAE report?   ☐ Yes   ☐ No

Figure 5.2   (*continued*)

DICTIONARY CODING

Should the codes be written on the CRF? ☐ Yes ☐ No ☐ N/A
Who will deal with the 'no hits'? Specify:

Will the coded terms be reviewed on an ongoing basis or before final file?

☐ Ongoing How often?
☐ Prior to final file
☐ N/A

LABORATORY DATA

If laboratories are used, how many laboratories will there be?

☐ N/A

If central laboratories are used, will the electronic data come directly to Data Centre?

☐ Yes ☐ No ☐ N/A

If central laboratories are used, is the electronic copy the definitive version?

☐ Yes ☐ No ☐ N/A

If central laboratories are used, what is the format of the data?

What is the route for querying laboratory data?

☐ N/A

Figure 5.2 (*continued*)

When—the Timelines

The scope and the deliverables for a project will define the final timeline and, in order to meet this, the plan must include milestones with accompanying timelines. These timelines are no good in isolation and the plan must also allocate responsibility for delivery according to time. When timelines are established it is then possible to determine which tasks fall on the critical path.

Timelines which need to be established are:

- Time when final protocol and case record form (CRF) are available. This defines when project plans can be finalised
- First patient into the study. This indicates when the initial data will be available
- First patient completes study. This enables the following timelines to be defined
- Time for receipt of first data
- Time from patient visit to receipt of data

- Time from receipt of data to data on database
- Time from receipt of data to issue of queries
- Time for query turnaround
- Time for receipt of lab transfers or data from other sources
- Last patient completes trial
- Time from last patient visit to receipt of last CRF
- Time for locked database

There will also be other milestones which will need to be fitted into the overall timelines. Establishing realistic timelines and building in contingency at this stage can be vital to the success of the study.

How—the Process

The process will form a large part of the project plan and can only be decided once the scope of the project is known. Once a process flow has been proposed the systems that will be used can be decided and the tools necessary to monitor the progress and performance of the project can be put into place.

Although every company has standard processes it is always necessary to tailor these for the specific requirements of a study. The first thing to establish is the type of data and in what format the data are to be received. In a fairly straightforward study it may be that the CRFs are to be received by courier directly from site and the only other data to be received at the data centre are laboratory data.

Here are some of the possible sources of data to be considered:

- CRFs by fax
- CRFs by courier
- CRFs by post
- Central laboratory data received via e-mail link
- Central laboratory data received on diskette via courier or mail
- Scans received by courier
- ECG data received by courier
- Holter data received electronically
- Assessments received from a reader panel
- Diary cards received by courier or mail
- SAE database for reconciliation received electronically or in paper format

Once it has been established what data are to be received, from where and in what format, the beginnings of a data flow diagram (see Figure 5.3) will emerge and this will enable appropriate tracking systems to be suggested. The tracking process will encompass notification of the arrival of data and its acknowledgement and its progress through the process.

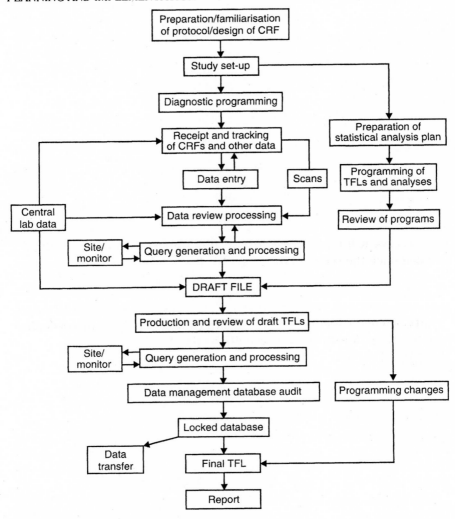

Figure 5.3 Example of simple dataflow diagram

The receipt of data is just the beginning of the flow through the system and the data manager next needs to establish the processes to be used in order to plan the next step in the chain.

If data have been received in the traditional form of paper CRFs, the next process to consider is the method of entry on to the database. This may be by traditional data entry methods, using double data entry or entry and verification procedures or it may be via a scanning and Optical Character Recognition (OCR) process, where the pages are scanned and data entry is performed from an image on only those parts of the CRF that are unsuitable for OCR methodology. The flow may differ depending on the process used.

The next major cycle which impacts on people outside the data management forum and needs to form part of the upfront plan, is the flow of queries. Who will queries be sent to and how will they be sent? Will they be sent directly to site or will they go via a monitor? This may not be the same for the whole study but may vary from country to country. Queries and query replies may be sent by courier, by post, be faxed or sent electronically. This flow needs to be decided upon and the associated process, including the tracking of queries and responses, defined.

The requirement for interim analyses needs to be taken into account as this can impact on the structure of the project team and the processes required. Should an interim be required where it is necessary to unblind the data this would impact on process and resource, as it would be necessary to have a separate team to work on the unblinded interim so that the core team can maintain their blinded status for the continual processing of the data beyond the interim analysis.

Other considerations are to establish which data will need to be coded using dictionaries and which dictionaries will be used. It must be established at the planning phase of the study how the 'no hits', or terms that do not code to a dictionary term at the coding process, will be dealt with as this is a task that is critical to the timelines for a locked database and may be critical on an ongoing basis if regular safety updates are required. Procedures must also be in place for handling updates to the dictionaries in use during the lifetime of the study.

If the data management function is to perform the SAE/AE reconciliation then this must also be built into the project plan. Sometimes this task is performed by a safety group, in which case it is necessary to know when they require listings from the CRF database.

Once the overall process for the project has been agreed it is necessary to document which SOPs will be used and whether there are any known deviations from these at the outset of the study.

An essential part of the process flow is the type and timing of Quality Control (QC) steps and the timing of any Quality Assurance (QA) audits. These need to be built into the project plan.

How—the Systems

The nature of the end product will indicate where the lines of communication need to be established. It is important that the data manager liaises closely from the beginning of the project with the project representatives from the other disciplines involved in the study. Well-planned communication links within the project team are essential for the smooth running of a study as the team may be spread across sites and countries. Electronic mail provides 24-hour and 7-days-a-week coverage and links will need to be established upfront.

How else can modern technology help with the exchange of information during a study? Systems can either be developed in-house or can be bought and modified for use within a company. An example is an interactive voice response system, using the telephone system, to obtain information which is stored in a database and can be used to provide information to both clinical and data management during a study. This information can be used in the review cycle of the implementation process.

Systems are available which can pull together study information from various sources which can then be accessed by study personnel to give details of the status of the study. If this method is to be used then the information that will be required throughout the study needs to be carefully considered at the planning stage to ensure it is being collected and is in an appropriate format.

The data manager will need to liaise closely with the programming and statistical groups to decide the structure of the database. How this is structured may depend on the final format in which the data are required. This information will have been collected at the early meetings, which may be with internal or external customers.

If the data management for a study is being conducted by a CRO, the CRO will need to consider whether the format that is required by the client should govern the initial structure of the database, or whether it would be more efficient to use internal standards and convert the data to the required structure after processing, for delivery to the client. With this in mind a test data transfer should be built into the overall project plan.

After deciding on the structure of the database the method of entering the data into the database must be decided. This will depend on how the data have initially been captured. If data have been captured remotely, that is at the investigator site, then part of the plan will be to decide how and when this will be loaded into the database. This may well also be true for laboratory data from central laboratories which is to be received electronically and for any other data received in this way.

If the data capture has been using traditional paper CRFs there are still options to be considered. Traditional data entry and verification or double data entry is generally the first thought, but it may be possible to scan the data directly into the database or to use a combination of scanning and conventional data entry from the scanned image. These options need to be considered at the very early planning stages of the study and it will only be possible to use the more modern technology if data management has been involved at the protocol and CRF design stage.

Once the media and the systems for database design and data entry have been decided, the next considerations are the systems that will be used for cleaning the data. How much of the clean-up process will be manual and how much will be able to be done electronically? Decisions on the type and number of computerised checks (known as validation checks, edit checks or diagnostic checks) will depend on the size and complexity of the study.

There are systems on the market which can provide tools for planning the study and updating the plan on an ongoing basis. Microsoft Project is an example of such a tool. Tasks, milestones and dependencies can be plugged into this package and a graphical representation of the project plan can be produced.

Other systems which need to be thought about at the planning stage are those which will help to track the budget and the resource requirement. These systems are essential for the effective implementation of the study.

The ideal system is one that links tasks and timelines with resource and budget, as this will enable the project to be tracked in the most efficient way.

Where—the Location

Location may be one of the early considerations and could depend on a few factors. If your company is a multinational company and the study being planned is a global study, there are questions that need to be asked and decisions that need to be made at the planning stage. This also applies if you are a CRO and are working with one or more external clients.

Points requiring consideration are:

- Where is the source of most of the data?
- Where are the rest of the project team?
- Where is the best data management resource available?
- Where is the database located?
- Where is the client located?

Who—the Resource Plan (Figure 5.4)

Although this comes at the end of the planning section, it is probably the most important section, for without the people in the project team none of the steps in the project plan would be able to be executed. Having the right number of appropriately qualified people available at the right time is an art as well as a science.

When planning the data management project team the data manager may have the responsibility for estimating the data entry, administrative support and data coordination requirements.

When looking at resource requirements some things to consider are:

- Experience of the therapeutic area
- Experience in data management

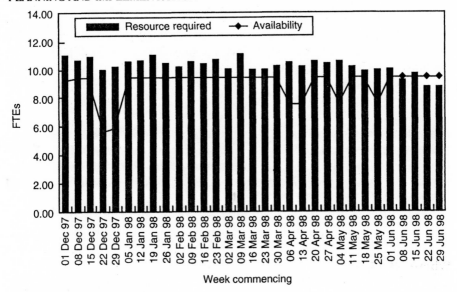

Figure 5.4 Resource graph

- Specialist skills
- Availability
- Expected flow of data
- Number of pages to be processed (this will give hours required for tasks and hence numbers of people needed)

The points above list some of the business requirements for estimating resource but there are also other considerations, for instance, cost may be an issue when a more senior person than was originally planned undertakes a series of tasks. The staff in our various data entry and data management departments are crucial to our projects as they are the ones performing the tasks that enable our projects to come in on time, on budget and to the required quality standard, therefore it is essential that their needs are also considered when putting together the project team.

A contented and well-trained team will always give of their best to a project so part of the planning process should be to plan for staff development as well as for the effective and timely execution of the project. A new study can be viewed as an opportunity to broaden the skills and experience base of the staff as well as to consolidate knowledge already gained.

What are some of the opportunities provided to staff when a new project is being planned?

- New therapeutic area
- New technology being used

- New process being used
- Increased functional responsibility
- Develop communication skills through liaison with other departments
- Supervisory responsibility
- Learn new tasks
- Enhance organisational skills

A good project plan will have taken these factors into consideration when planning the resource for the study, thus identifying the best people for the job both from the project perspective and from the staff development angle. The aim of the plan should be to retain a well-motivated team throughout the lifetime of the project.

As with the rest of the project plan, the resource plan will need to be adaptable to the needs of the project. Resource requirements will need revising on a regular basis as they are affected by such things as data flow, numbers of queries and query resolution rate. A change from the expected in any one of these factors can mean over- or under-utilisation of the project team. For example, less resource may be needed at the early stages of a study because of erratic data flow but, in order to cope with a large bolus towards the end, a large number of people need to be available; these people need to be familiar with the study, as at times of heavy workload there is seldom time to train.

Having now established the Why, What, When, How, Where and Who in the form of a project plan, we are in a position to move on to the next stage, the implementation phase.

IMPLEMENTATION OF THE PLANS

Now the time has been invested in putting together a comprehensive plan for the project, success depends on the thoughtful implementation of the plan. What are the key factors in the implementation process? Implementation of the plan will be discussed under the following headings:

- Review
- Measure
- Control

Review

The plan that has been constructed is a living document and constant review of all the steps in the plan allows adjustments to be made. What should be reviewed?

- Progress against timelines and budget
- Process efficiency
- Quality of product
- Resource—numbers and type
          team motivation

These are just some suggestions of key areas which, upon review, will provide a good indication of the progress of the project and will indicate other checks and balances that may need to be put into place.

When should review take place? During the implementation phase review of the plan will be continual, but there will be some parameters which should be reviewed and measured at specified timepoints in order for actions to be taken.

Constant assessment of the process and the product will provide information on the progress of the project. There are various methods that can be employed as part of this process and key to all of these is a good communication network and the ability to listen to the messages coming through this network, and to assess the impact on the project.

Feedback can come from many sources and the opportunity to gain this feedback should be built into the original plan. This is gained through team meetings, when the progress of the study against the plan can be discussed, and through audits which can highlight issues with the process.

Measure

In order to be able to measure the progress of a study realistic standards will have been established as part of the original plan. These will relate to the review process. Standards can be set up at the beginning of a study for some of the factors noted below and systems must then be in place to capture information which can be reviewed against the original standards.

Good metrics can provide information on performance, quality, resource issues, and so on and will highlight areas where corrective action can be taken. Useful metrics for the data manager which can be set up are:

- CRF retrieval rate
- Queries by country, patient, investigator and type
- Query turnaround time
- Time to DE
- Time for review

Some of these measures allow the data manager to identify early any shortfalls in the receipt of CRFs and the consequent impact on resource and timelines. Metrics on queries provide information on CRF design, training issues and the quality of the data and enable the data manager to provide feedback to the appropriate source.

Metrics on processing times enable the data manager to review processes and assess the impact on timelines and budget and also give the opportunity to assess bottlenecks early and adapt processes where necessary.

Control

Once a review cycle is in place and meaningful metrics are set up the data manager is in a position to control the study by taking appropriate corrective action where necessary.

What actions can be taken?

1. *Renegotiate.* If the metrics show that CRFs are not being retrieved and are not arriving at the data centre in an agreed period of time in order to meet timelines, then it may be possible to renegotiate final timelines, or, if timelines cannot move then maybe the deliverables at the timeline can be negotiated, e.g., only priority tables to be ready initially with the rest to follow at an agreed date.
2. *Move resource.* Information on data flow and work volume and the consequent updating of the resource plan may indicate a necessity for redistribution of resource. It may be possible to move resource from another project or it may be necessary to recruit more professional staff.
3. *Provide incentives.* Team meetings may indicate low morale due to a prolonged period of tedious tasks or review of CRF flow metrics may indicate a large amount of work to be done in a short time. These sorts of pressures on the team require imaginative solutions to keep the study plans on course; a flexible approach and recognition of differing needs within the team are essential. Incentives to increase motivation may be many and varied, monetary reward may be important to one team member, whilst extra time off may mean more to another, and promise of a social event at the end of the study may drive others on.

   Maintaining motivation throughout a long and difficult study is a challenge in itself and throughout the implementation of the plan the good data manager will constantly be assessing the opportunities for personal development that are offered to the study team.

4. *Change the process.* An overall view of the project may indicate a potential budget or time overrun and this could make a process change a consideration. A review of the metrics associated with data entry and review time would show where most gains could be made from a revised process. If the revised process involves removing some

of the traditional steps then the effect on quality must be carefully thought through.

These are just some of the actions that can be taken when an issue is highlighted through the review of the project plan.

SUMMARY

The planning and implementation of a project from a data management perspective involves many considerations. Asking the Why, When, What, Where, Who and How questions in a structured way will provide the information necessary to formulate the plan, and reviewing and measuring against the standards created by the plan and early actioning of any discrepancies is one of the keys to successful implementation. The main key to success is the realisation that the best laid plans are only as good as the interaction and communication between the people who are responsible for their implementation.

ACKNOWLEDGEMENT

The quotation from the *Just So Stories* by Rudyard Kipling at the start of this chapter is reproduced by permission of A. P. Watt Ltd, on behalf of the National Trust.

6 Data Validation

PANKAJ 'PANNI' PATEL

SmithKline Beecham Pharmaceuticals, Harlow, Essex, UK

INTRODUCTION

The primary objective of Clinical Data Management (CDM) is to ensure timely delivery of high-quality data which are necessary to satisfy both good clinical practice (GCP) requirements and the statistical analysis and reporting requirements. CDM data validation activities play a critical role within the drug development programme involving many people, multiple systems and several data transfers. The quality of the data validation process has a direct impact on the quality of data presented as part of an NDA submission.

There is a general misconception that data validation activities commence when clinical trial data are presented to the sponsor's data management department. The author will attempt to dispel this somewhat narrow view and discuss various stages of data validation activities which actually start when the investigator records the data on the case report form (CRF) and when the final medical report is issued as part of the overall clinical trial data handing and reporting process.

CDM REQUIREMENT IN GCP

CDM requirements within the ICH and EU CPMP GCP guidelines are not defined in any great detail, resulting in lack of clarity, or indeed misrepresentation. The FDA Code of Federal Regulations contains no mention of CDM! This should be considered as a major concern, given that CDM plays a vital role in protecting data integrity, and is charged with producing high-quality databases that meet clinical and regulatory requirements. However, the GCP guidelines do devote a chapter to the 'data handling' aspects, including the requirement of quality control/quality assurance mechanisms to ensure reliable data capture and subsequent processing.

Clinical Data Management. Second Edition. Edited by R.K. Rondel, S.A. Varley and C.F. Webb.
© 2000 John Wiley & Sons, Ltd

DATA VALIDATION PROCESS DURING THE CONDUCT OF A CLINICAL TRIAL

It is the sponsor's responsibility to implement and maintain quality assurance and quality control mechanisms at each stage of the data validation process to ensure data are generated and processed in compliance with the study protocol and GCP requirements.

What is the definition of data validation? It is a defined number of steps needed to turn the original or 'raw' item or items into the finished item, that is to turn CRF data into a clean database. These steps should ensure that the database is accurate, consistent and a true representation of the patient's profile.

Where does the data validation step start? Is it at the investigator site, when the data are first recorded on the CRF or does it begin when the CRF is presented to the sponsor company's CDM department? It starts at the investigator site and stops when the final medical report for the study has been issued by the sponsor company.

Data Validation Steps Performed by the Investigator

The GCP guidelines are quite clear on when the data validation step starts; the ICH guidelines state: 'The investigator should ensure the accuracy, completeness, legibility, and timeliness for the data reported to the sponsor in the CRFs and in all required reports.' The investigator should ensure that any data reported on the CRF are consistent with the patient's medical records and, where applicable, discrepancies should be explained. The CRF should be signed and dated by the investigator and/or the investigator's designate. In addition, all corrections on a CRF should be dated, initialled, and must be made in a way which does not obscure the original value.

Patient diary card data can be an important source of information about drug compliance, drug efficacy and daily activities. However, diary data can be very unreliable and it is imperative that the investigator reviews the diary's completion with the patient for completeness and accuracy of data recorded.

The sponsor should ensure investigator training and education on the need to accurately record data on CRFs and the impact this has on the overall quality of the clinical trial. A perfect data management system can do little to improve sloppy data produced at the investigator site.

Data Validation Steps Performed by the Monitor

GCP states that the 'monitor should check the CRF entries with the source documents and inform the investigator of any errors/omissions' and 'assure that all data are correctly and completely recorded and reported'.

This requirement is achieved through Source Data Verification (SDV), the process by which the information reported on the CRF by the investigator is compared with the original medical records to ensure it is complete and accurate. SDV is a fundamental step in the data validation process to ensure data integrity and maintain quality of data captured at source. Through the SDV process, the monitor should confirm accurate transcription of data from source files to the CRF and that the CRF contains all the relevant information about the patient's participation in the clinical trial.

There are two methods of SDV: Direct Access—the monitor is given direct access to the actual source document, and conducts an independent comparison versus the CRF; Indirect Access—the monitor is not allowed access either to the actual or to the photocopied source document. Key variables are chosen for which the investigator or member of staff reads the source document entry while the sponsor compares it with the CRF entry. This method is the most time-consuming but ensures the highest level of patient confidentiality.

Direct access to source documents must be the preferred choice in order to maintain data integrity and improve quality of data at source (i.e. at the investigator site). Sponsors should exclude investigators who do not allow direct access by sponsor and regulatory personnel to source documents. The USA FDA have recognised the importance of reviewing source documents and as such demand direct access to these documents. The responsibilities of both the sponsor and the investigator in SDV must be finalised at the outset of the clinical trial with a view to ensuring there are no misunderstandings of the requirements of SDV.

SDV is an integral part of data validation procedures, as required by GCP, and one could argue that if it is not possible to verify data in CRF as part of SDV due to unavailability of source documents, serious consideration should be given to excluding the data from the final study report.

Once the CRFs have gone through the SDV process, they are sent to the sponsor's CDM site for subsequent processing.

Data Validation Steps Performed by CDM

CDM data validation activities are an integral part of GCP and fundamental to the delivery of high-quality data for statistical analyses and reporting. Attention should be focused on ensuring that the data are a reasonable representation of what actually happened at the investigator site. The aim is to transform data recorded on CRFs into information that can be used in the final clinical report from which the right conclusions about the new drug can be made. Figure 6.1 represents a generic model for processing CRFs through CDM's data validation activities. Data clarification queries are issued to the investigator at various stages in the process, in particular, as a result of pre-entry review, data entry, and the running of edit checks.

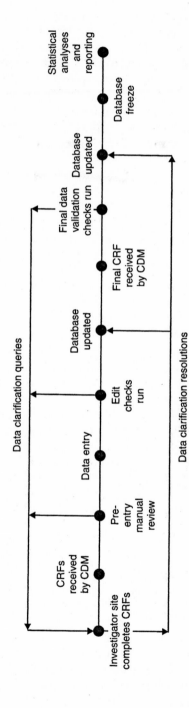

Figure 6.1 CDM data validation activities

CDM data validation guidelines should be developed to ensure data are processed in such a way as to maximise data integrity and to deliver high-quality data for analyses and reporting.

Process for defining and implementing edit checks

Edit checks consisting of manual and computer checks need to be performed on the data to ensure the database is accurate and consistent. The definition stage consists of producing an Edit Check Specifications (ECS) document and the implementation stage involves the programming and testing of the checks.

Figure 6.2 represents a generic model for defining and implementing ECS checks for which the data management is to be conducted by the sponsor company's own CDM group. The finalisation of the ECS document is the responsibility of the ECS Team, consisting of all functional groups who have a vested interest in the data generated from the clinical trial. In particular, the clinical and statistical groups are key players of the ECS Team, whose input in the development of the ECS document is critical to ensuring adequate checks are defined and implemented in the cleaning effort to deliver as high-quality database.

The first step in the process is for the clinical data manager to prepare and circulate a draft ECS document to the ECS Team, subsequent to which a document review meeting is held to finalise the document. It is essential all members of the ECS Team attend the meeting so the implications of the checks can be clearly understood. However, there may be a need for a further meeting if approval by all team members is not obtained. At this meeting all outstanding issues are resolved and the document signed-off.

Once the ECS document has been signed-off, the next phase is to complete the Edit Check programs. Sufficient time should also be allocated for the testing of the programs through the use of robust data prior to running the programs on live data. Test data should be created for all ECS checks specified, comprising both good and bad data to ensure only bad data are located in the output.

Figure 6.3 represents a generic model for defining and implementing Edit Checks for studies which are outsourced to Contract Research Organisations (CROs). The main differences to the in-house model are:

- The clinical data manager at the CRO is responsible for preparing and circulating the ECS document to the ECS Team
- The CRO is responsible for the programming and testing of the ECS checks

It should be noted that the need to ensure an ECS Team is set up applies equally to outsourced studies as for in-house studies. In addition, the timelines are the same as for in-house studies.

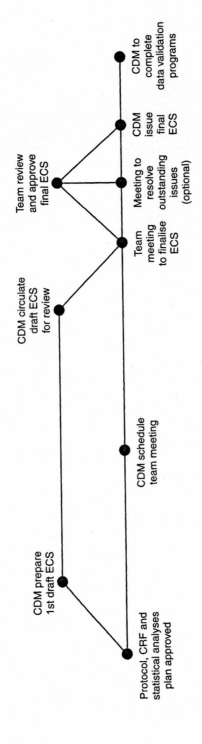

Figure 6.2 ECS finalisation process for in-house studies

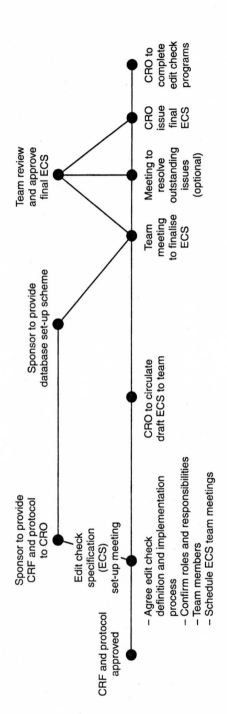

Figure 6.3 ECS finalisation process for studies contracted to CRSs

Any changes to the ECS document post finalisation need to be reviewed and approved by the ECS Team prior to implementation, irrespective of whether a study is in-house or contracted to a CRO. The clinical data manager should complete a 'request for amendment to ECS' form (see Figure 6.4), outlining the impact of the proposed change. It is essential that

---

REQUEST FOR AMENDMENT TO EDIT CHECK SPECIFICATION (ECS)

Sponsor study number:

CRF page numbers plus section:

Change: ☐ New specification – specific new edit check number

☐ Change/amendment to existing edit check specification (specify edit check number)

Reason/Impact

Approved: Yes/No   If 'Yes':

Planned date of implementation:................   Actual date of implementation:...............

Approved by representative member of:

Sponsor study team   ....

CRO data manager   ....

Figure 6.4 Request for amendment to ECS form

the impact on the statistical analyses plan and database be assessed, together with whatever back validation may be required as a result of the change in ECS.

The ECS document should itemise all manual and computer checks which will be performed on the data at either pre-entry review or post-entry. General assumptions as to how to handle dates, timefields, text strings, partial dates, units, continental decimals/commas and so on all need to be specified. Any derived data points should also be included in the document, that would wherever possible impact on computer checks. An example of an ECS format and content is represented in Figure 6.5.

EDIT CHECK SPECIFICATION DOCUMENT

DEMOGRAPHY: EDIT CHECKS

CRF module: DEMOG
Page: 1

1(a)   List if date of birth is missing

(b)   If DOB is missing then output:

(c)   'Please provide the patient's date of birth'

2(a)   List if study date – date of birth is ≤18 and ≥65.
       If age is not within range then query. If query confirms that the date of birth is correct then record this as a protocol violator in the data handling file

(b)   If DAT – DOB is ≤18 or ≥65 then output:

(c)   'Please confirm patient's date of birth'

(a) English terminology, (b) Technical terminology, (c) Investigator query text

Page 1 of XXX

Figure 6.5 Example of demography ECS page

Timelines for defining and implementing edit checks

The ECS finalisation process should commence after the protocol CRF have been finalised. The objective is to ensure that all checks are defined and implemented upfront, within a matter of weeks, and prior to the first CRF in-house. This helps to promote in-stream validation of CRF data and timely issue of any data clarification queries to the investigator sites.

Factors affecting quality of data

There are a number of factors which have an underlying impact on the overall quality of the data collected. These considerations warrant further discussion.

1. *CRF design.* CRFs need to be carefully prepared to collect data completely and accurately. Both the protocol and the CRF need to be designed in parallel to ensure consistency between the two. The CRF should allow collection of the data as requested in the protocol and the format should follow the protocol's treatment procedure. Adequate quality control procedures need to be implemented to ensure timings of visits and examinations match and that duplicated data are not being captured in different places. If the CRF does not allow data capture as requested by the protocol then errors are built into the study instead of quality, which would inevitably result in a high number of queries being generated as the CRF is processed.
2. *Field monitoring guidelines.* The quality of field monitoring guidelines has a direct correlation to the quality of data presented to the sponsor's CDM department and, subsequently, the volume of queries that need to be generated. Field monitoring guidelines should be developed in parallel with the CDM's data validation guidelines to ensure consistency of data monitoring and cleaning between the monitor and CDM. Field monitoring guidelines should be developed to ensure data integrity, and to check that the transcription of data from source documents to CRF is correct, complete and reliable.
3. *Source Data Verification (SDV).* As previously discussed, SDV is a critical phase of the data validation process, without which the integrity and quality of data would suffer. SDV is an effective way to ensure that the data reported by the investigator to the sponsor are accurate and valid.
4. *Missing data/CRF pages.* GCP guidelines clearly state that 'appropriate measures should be taken by the monitor to avoid overlooking missing data . . .'. However, large boluses of queries often get generated by CDM to retrieve missing data.

5. *Date conventions.* For multicentre clinical trials, differing date conventions being used by various investigators can present problems when it comes to entering the data on the database. It is vital that this issue is recognised at the outset of the clinical trial during the CRF development phase.

6. *Electronic laboratory data.* The main considerations are reconciling electronic laboratory data to the database:

   - How do you match a patient's screening lab sample when the patient's unique identifier is yet to be generated?
   - What course of action should be taken if the patient's demography details on the electronic lab data do not match the demography details recorded on the patient's CRF?
   - What units are going to be used? will these be familiar to the investigator?

There are further considerations for multicentre clinical trials:

- How do you deal with variations of tests used by different labs?
- Should conversion factors be used to make multiple ranges compatible or for a central laboratory's appropriateness of reference ranges for a patient population spanning across different countries?

QUALITY CONTROL AND QUALITY ASSURANCE OF CDM PROCESSES

Both the ICH GCP and EU GCP guidelines state 'Quality control must be applied to each stage of data handling'. The CDM process is quite complicated and can involve many people and multiple systems. It is important, therefore, to have an effective, quality-controlled system so that the process runs smoothly and efficiently. One possible way of ensuring that the CDM process is operating effectively and conducted to GCP requirements is through audits. It is important to have written policy that describes the auditing process and has been agreed by senior managers in data management. The policy should describe the range of audits to be performed and whether they are study-specific or system audits. It may specify that audits be performed by sampling across all clinical projects and all phases of a clinical trial program. Depending on the type of audit, sampling could also focus on other criteria, such as the critical data collected during the clinical trial. It is important to note that data management audits should be no different from audits conducted in any other area working to GCP standards.

In the mid to late 1980s, the FDA in the US, followed by France and Germany, began asking sponsor companies to have written SOPs as part of the GCP. The impetus for this came from several drug withdrawals, such as benoxaprofen, from the market and the media publicity about side effects of recently introduced products such as non-steroidal anti-inflammatory drugs.

In the early 1990s, several countries belonging to the EU followed suit with similar requirements. Those involved include the UK, Japan, the Nordic countries; Canada, EU member states, Spain and also the World Health Organisation. The FDA Code of Federal Regulations (CFR) and CPMP GCP guidelines stipulate the establishment of operational SOPs for conducting and monitoring clinical trials. CDM plays a vital role in protecting data integrity and the need to ensure that standard operating procedures (SOPs) are defined that encompass all aspects of the clinical trials' CDM process, which helps assure adherence to the FDA CFR and CPMP GCP guidelines and regulatory requirements.

These SOPs should not state all the details of these guidelines but should highlight the key points and present systematic ways of performing CDM activities to ensure compliance to the guidelines. SOPs are a tool which ensures the generation of quality data to support drug development. Drug development that does not conform the internationally accepted standard of GCP cannot be justified on ethical, moral, or economic grounds.

SOPs concerning the preparation of documents such as protocols, study reports, safety summaries and Investigational New Drug applications must encompass all GCP and regulatory requirements. Some typical CDM SOPs which ensure compliance to the above mentioned regulations include:

- Generation and Maintenance of Study File documentation
- CDM QC/Audit procedures
- Database design
- Query generation and resolution
- Data entry
- Dictionary coding
- Document Management including archiving
- Data Validation activities
- CRO selection and monitoring
- Database Freeze
- Systems validation and maintenance

CDM DATA VALIDATION IN THE FUTURE

In the quest to reduce development times of new drugs, new technologies and working practices are being tried and tested within CDM; for example, pen-based systems, optical imaging, voice recognition and, last but not least, remote data entry (RDE). These new systems have a direct impact on the data validation process. If we were to look at RDE, the investigator would enter data directly into the RDE system via electronic CRFs. The core of the edit checks could be implemented within the RDE software. Thus, the majority of the validation checks would be performed in 'real-time' at the investigator site. RDE would streamline processes and make data capture more efficient by displacing activities which are a bottleneck or by removing those which do not provide significant added value.

In the future, the success of new systems such as those mentioned above will be measured in terms of:

- Time savings (data flow from investigator site to sponsor, processing time)
- Reduction in resource requirements (with sponsor's clinical and CDM groups)
- Improvement in Data Quality
- Endorsement by regulatory authorities

SUMMARY

CDMs are charged with producing high-quality databases that meet clinical and regulatory requirements. The quality of a clinical trial determines the acceptability of the results and care must be taken to ensure that high standards of quality are present both in the clinical trial design and in the integrity and interpretation of data. To this end, all participants in the clinical trial have a role to play in safeguarding data integrity. As discussed, data validation activities start at the investigator site and end with a statement in clinical or expert reports to indicate that the clinical trial was conducted in accordance with GCP and that the report provides a complete and accurate account of the data collected during the trial.

7 Quality Assurance and Clinical Data Management

HEATHER CAMPBELL and JOHN SWEATMAN

Covance Clinical Development, Horsham, West Sussex, UK

INTRODUCTION

Ever since the finalisation of the International Conference of Harmonisation (ICH) GCP guideline in 1996, the implications have been very clear. No longer would the Regulatory Authorities be content to accept that the investigator site was the only target for high-quality standards in a clinical trial. The new proposal for a European Parliament and Council Directive on the implementation of Good Clinical Practice (97/0197 (COD))[1] describes the need for and importance of a clear paper trail for any clinical trial. In the same section on 'Verification of Compliance' the Directive describes the importance of the 'audit' of the study. In the many complex clinical trials being conducted today, the handling of clinical data outside the investigator site is of equal importance. In fact, some agencies, especially the Food and Drug Administration (FDA) have always taken an interest in the manner that clinical data were collected and analysed. The FDA *Compliance Program Guidance Manuals:* 'Clinical Investigators' (7348.810)[2] and 'Sponsors, Contract Research Organisations and Monitors' (7348.811)[3] require the Food and Drug Administration (FDA) Inspector to establish how the clinical data are going to be entered into the computer system and then analysed.

In any submission process, the clinical study report forms a vital part of the mechanism to get a new product onto the market. The development of the report commences not when the first medical writer prepares the title page but when the first entry takes place in the Case Report Form (CRF). Some may argue correctly that the process starts earlier when the protocol is developed, or when the CRF is designed and the staff at the investigator site are trained. All these processes require rigorous execution if the initial risks, however small, taken by the subject in a trial are to be justified. The role of the Quality Assurance (QA) group in this process is ensuring that the clinical data presented and interpreted in the clinical

Clinical Data Management. Second Edition. Edited by R.K. Rondel, S.A. Varley and C.F. Webb.
© 2000 John Wiley & Sons, Ltd

study report reflect a true picture of what took place in the trial. One of the main roles of the QA group is as an independent auditing group.

It is true that in the non-drug industry, the organisation that has a QA group may benefit by being more efficient, producing quality products or service. Frequently, the presence of a QA group is perceived as of marginal importance, certainly in the view of senior management. However, there is no doubt that the inclusion of quality in the culture of a company or organisation is a requirement of any operation conducting clinical trials. The last principle of ICH GCP requires that there are 'systems with procedures that assure the quality of every aspect of the trial'.

In order to form a clear picture of where QA fits into the clinical data management part of a clinical trial some definitions and comments are required for Quality Control (QC), QA, audit and the responsibilities of the QA group.

QUALITY CONTROL

The definition in the ICH GCP Guideline for QC is:

> The operational techniques and activities undertaken within the quality assurance system to verify the requirements for quality of the trial-related activities have been fulfilled[4].

This means that clinical data management must have documented evidence of what activities have been carried out throughout the trial to ensure the quality of the clinical data. QC tasks are the responsibility of the personnel handling the clinical data. In some cases, it is the actual group designated within clinical data management to conduct these tasks.

It must be remembered that QA auditing is not QC and the responsibility for fully checking transcription, calculations, interpretation and reporting must remain with operational clinical monitors and clinical data management personnel—'the experts'.

The QA group is responsible for taking 'snapshots' of the study at critical times and places. The information obtained will allow data management to extrapolate findings forming a picture of the quality and integrity of the data on which to base decisions.

QUALITY ASSURANCE

The definition given in the ICH GCP guideline for QA is:

> All those planned and systematic actions that are established to ensure that the trial is performed and the 'clinical' data are generated, documented

(recorded), and reported in compliance with GCP and the applicable regulatory requirement(s)[4].

This means in practical terms that clinical data management must have written procedures in place which will allow an independent group to audit against the actual processes taking place in the handling of clinical data. The documentation detailing what has happened during that trial should be present. The same group may have already reviewed the CRF, the protocol, and in some cases have trained the Investigator and his/her staff. The auditors may have visited the sites to audit the actual process of collecting clinical data by the Investigator and his/her staff.

Independent QA should be built into the clinical data management system and carried out concurrently with other clinical data management activities.

AUDIT

The definition in the ICH GCP guideline for an audit is:

A systematic and independent examination of trial related activities and documents to determine whether the evaluated trial related activities were conducted, and the 'clinical' data were recorded, analysed and accurately reported according to the protocol, sponsor's standard operating procedures (SOPs), GCP, and the applicable regulatory requirement(s)[4].

All key aspects of an audit are covered by this definition. All audits should be defined by an audit plan and the main scope should be recorded in the resulting audit report. Normally, key questions will have been listed before the audit has commenced and the auditor should be encouraged to restrict his/her attention to the audit's scope. However, too much rigidness can create the 'tick list' mentality which allows the CRF to match the clinical database listings but does not note that its storage is under a leaking roof; that is a lack of flexibility in the auditing process can mean that serious deficiencies are missed or fail to be addressed. The European Network of GCP Auditors and other GCP Experts have published an *Optional Guideline for GCP Compliance and Quality Systems Auditing*[5] which provides a basis to conduct any audit.

THE QUALITY ASSURANCE GROUP

QA auditing is the responsibility of an independent group which reviews clinical data at defined times to assure that procedures have been followed in accordance with approved quality procedures and that the quality of the clinical data is acceptable. The benefits of such a group auditing early in the process are that ambiguities or inconsistencies can be identified, documented and, more importantly, acted upon before impacting too heavily on the final product. This often results in making the documentation more user friendly and saves time or confusion during the study as well as assuring GCP is being complied with.

Historically the QA group spent its limited resources auditing at investigator sites with occasional audits 'in-house' to review the final report. In some cases, QA were undertaking a QC role and may have been seen and used as a safety net, involved only at the end of the process when it was too late to make a constructive difference to a project. In the past it was common for the QA group to audit prior to clinical database lock to provide a 'final seal of approval'. If problems were found at this stage, timelines would have to be extended, especially if there were queries which needed to be resolved at the investigator site.

The QA group should not hold up the clinical data flow; they should be auditing at intervals throughout the trial. At such audits they should be able to assure that procedures are adequate and are being followed. The task of the QC checks falls on the clinical data management personnel, since they are the operational personnel and know how the clinical data should be handled.

As already mentioned, it is beneficial for the QA group to be involved throughout the clinical trial process. The QA personnel should be consulted at the protocol and CRF design stage. This independent audit is essential to ensure that all possible pitfalls are avoided and GCP complied with. Auditors can then commence formal audits at the investigator sites when the clinical trial recruitment commences. The group can continue the auditing process on the clinical database in-house, completing a full review of the clinical data management process by auditing the handling of CRF data.

The QA group can use their broad experience to provide advice about the planned data management procedures. They can give an independent viewpoint, uninfluenced by other project concerns or pressures. In order for the group to be used to its fullest potential, regular audit reports should be issued to management. Such reports should highlight timeliness, completeness, reliability and consistency of the clinical data collected.

Regular audits of clinical data management systems (see section on Process Audits) may reduce accidental or deliberate corruption of the clinical data. It is important that audit findings are clear and precise so that they can be correctly followed up. This also ensures that future studies can benefit from changes incorporated into the process.

Another important factor in ensuring an error-free clinical trial is communication. Problems highlighted by audits of the clinical data management and clinical monitoring groups, early in the process, can be communicated to them. This reduces the impact on the final product.

TRAINING OF THE QA PERSONNEL

Before we discuss in some detail what processes should be present, some consideration should be given to the auditing personnel and how they are trained.

The selection of QA personnel is difficult. Auditors should be meticulous, analytical, good communicators and good trainers. Communication can involve 'one to one' situations, but often the auditor needs to be able to address a group. In addition, they are required to be disciplined enough to audit with thoroughness clinical data listings and tables against CRFs, and the clinical study report against source documentation. All personnel must have a full knowledge of the many facets of the clinical trial process and GCP. Frequently, in large institutions, the personnel conducting in-house data management audits are personnel involved in the data management and so the audit is really a QC activity. In order for such an audit to be regarded as a QA activity it must be performed by an independent auditor.

The selected individual should never be made responsible for the conduct of an audit until they have been fully trained and have reached a level of confidence acceptable both to themselves and to their management. The training should be based on a series of training sessions, often attending the same sessions as site monitors and data management personnel, until they are fully familiar with the theory behind the clinical trial process. In addition, many specialised external courses, such as those organised by the Drug Information Association (DIA) and the British Association for Research Quality Assurance (BARQA), provide additional training in a wider field of QA.

However, the most important part of the training is that carried out with other experienced auditors either in mock audits or as an attendee at a real audit. New personnel should be trained using real listings, tables and clinical study reports, which have already been audited by an experienced auditor. This allows for a comparison to be made between the trainee auditor's findings and the experienced auditor's findings. For cost-conscious management, time taken to complete tasks will be longer with new personnel and should be budgeted for.

INVESTIGATOR SITE AUDITS

A full description of the events that take place at an investigator site audit is not within the scope of this chapter but does need to be considered briefly. Considerable time is spent at the site establishing that correct documentation exists for regulatory and Independent Ethics Committee/Institutional Review Board (IEC/IRB) approval for the site, that the consent has been obtained correctly from each patient and that the study drug has been supplied to the patients correctly. All these items are important for GCP compliance and for any successful submission and will also feature in the clinical study report. However, from the point of view of clinical data management, the following aspects are critical if the clinical data are to be suitable for successful analysis.

The CRF

The CRF should be carefully designed to answer the questions posed by the protocol and to allow the appropriate safety data to be collected and recorded. There should be a clear definition of all data variables (e.g. diseases, adverse events, efficacy endpoints). Clinical data management can help in this quest by reviewing the draft protocol and CRF in conjunction with QA. This is particularly important if new CRF modules are being used which are different from those previously used or there have been problems with the previous template. Auditors constantly note that some of the questions asked are not completed by the Investigator, either because this part of the test or examination was never done or because the Investigator feels that it is an inappropriate question. The designer, even if medically qualified, sitting at his/her desk away from the intensive care ward or general practitioner's surgery should determine before the study commences what is essential and also what would be 'nice' to have but is not essential. The designer should also remember that the clinical data will need to be read before being entered into a clinical database. It should be in a format that allows easy completion by both the Investigator and his/her staff and easy understanding by the data entry individuals. The statisticians may also wish to comment if the data are collected electronically by remote data entry and will require manipulation before analysis. A good reference point for the design of CRFs is Gill Lawrence's review on CRF design[6].

The Protocol

The protocol should be easily understood in order for it to be followed by the Investigator and his/her staff. In spite of ICH GCP (Section 6), many protocols still appear to have been put together by several committees, often appear to have been written for different indications and for a different country, and therefore are very difficult to understand. Frequently amendments are required because of poor preparation of the protocol rather than due to issues which arise during the conduct of the clinical research. It may be a sensible approach to retrieve parts that have been well written and are relevant to the new study from a previous protocol but very careful editing is required. QA should always be part of the reviewing team. An experienced auditor will be familiar with the many pitfalls that will occur at the investigator site when a poorly designed protocol is used. When the protocol is badly written the resulting effect is the collection of poor-quality clinical data.

The Training of the Site Personnel

Training of site personnel is of paramount importance and should be done before a study commences. The Investigators' meeting, the pre-study visit and the initiation visit by the monitor will help prevent misunderstandings and ensure that the clinical data recorded in the CRF will provide the scientific information needed for regulatory submissions. Some pharmaceutical companies provide training in GCP to investigators and their staff in addition to any training that they may undergo for a specific protocol. Many investigators and their staff are prepared to give up their time for this type of training. QA should have a role in the training of site staff including the investigators. They should be present at the Investigators' meeting, and their audit findings from past and present studies should influence how clinical data management and clinical staff train the Investigator.

Source Data Verification

ICH GCP states that the definition for documentation is 'all records, in any form (including, but not limited to, written, electronic, magnetic, and optical records, and scans, x-rays and electrocardiograms) that describe or record the methods, conduct, and/or results of a trial, the factors affecting a trial, and the actions taken'. The monitor needs to ensure that there are source documents available and that the clinical data in the CRF match the source documents. At the beginning of the study, there should be clear guidance as to what source data will be required to be provided by the Investigator and this should be documented in the protocol. If the clinical data are not accurate and correct, there is little point in collecting the data. QA and, perhaps more importantly, inspectors from the regulatory authorities, will check that this process has taken place when site audits/inspections are conducted.

Monitors

These key staff should be well trained and given enough time and resource to ensure that the clinical data coming from the site are accurate and that the CRF has been completed correctly. They will be ultimately responsible for ensuring that the investigator and the site staff are trained properly. CRFs arriving in-house which require queries to be generated and sent back to the site cause delays, expense and frustration on the part of clinical data management and often the investigational staff. The site personnel believe that they have answered all the questions until they find additional ones in the post, perhaps several months after the particular visit that has generated the query. In addition, there is always the temptation to answer the query in-house in spite of the need for the endorsement by the investigator (ICH GCP 4.9.3).

CLINICAL DATA MANAGEMENT AUDITS

Before a study starts the following items should be addressed:

- Review of relevant quality procedures
- Preparation of protocol
- Design and preparation of CRF
- Allocation of staff and responsibilities
- Establishment of data security requirements
- Adequate office space
- Validated computer systems
- Archives (both current and long term)

It is beneficial to address the above in a clinical data management plan which ensures the documenting of processes to be followed during the data management process. It also guarantees, if followed, that an audit trail will exist and thus the study can be recreated if required.

Audits of the clinical data management area often consist of five distinct types: study documentation, complete CRFs, key variables, tables, figures and listings, and clinical study report audits. Such audits are normally conducted in-house.

STUDY DOCUMENTATION AUDITS

Clinical trial data require documentation that supports the Sponsor's claims to the regulatory agency when it is submitted for drug licensing. In many organisations there exists one project file containing both clinical data management and clinical monitoring documents. Document review is carried out throughout clinical trial using the ICH GCP essential document checklist. The auditor's philosophy will always be 'if it is not documented, it did not happen'. Therefore documentation has to be accurate and give a true picture of what happened during the clinical trial. In order for this to be the case the clinical data management team has to implement certain recorded checks throughout the life of the study. The clinical data management documentation will include the current protocol and its amendments, the receipt of the CRFs from the site, QC checklist for the data files, the preparation of the database, change control documents, unfreezing-refreezing file request forms, and the CVs, training records and job descriptions. Study documentation should be reviewed continuously throughout the clinical data management process. This is to ensure that there is a clear and concise record of the activities of the clinical data management group. The auditors are assuring that ICH GCP has been followed in parallel to ensuring that quality procedures are in place and being followed. This type of audit should not be seen as a filing exercise. It is important that at any time during the clinical trial there is documentation in place describing what has happened.

Such documentation is the primary record of all activities carried out by the clinical data management personnel in the execution of a study. Study documentation should be organised in such a way that it is accessible and easy to follow. If audits are started early in the process it can be ascertained quickly whether adequate documentation is being kept to give a true picture of what is happening in the process.

DATA AUDITS

The early audits by the QA group are conducted by reviewing study documentation so that if there are any missing areas the situation can either be resolved or the deviation documented. Above all, problems can be prevented from happening again.

CRFs should be reviewed by auditors early in the clinical data management process. Although driven by the clinical database, all documentation around the clinical data should be reviewed. The auditor is looking at the processes involved in getting the clinical data from the Investigator to the database. By doing this type of audit early in the process, the auditor can highlight any gaps in the QC activities and any GCP non-compliance, early enough for deficiencies to be corrected to reduce any impact on the final clinical database. This will also help towards producing a high-quality product and ensuring timelines are met.

The CRFs to be audited should be selected from different sites and countries so that the process of handling clinical data can be examined across the data sources. CRFs should be selected to cover all areas of the clinical data management process, that is, 'just data-entered', computer data validation checks completed, queries sent out, queries returned. This will give a true picture of how the data are being handled and whether there is adequate documentation in place and adequate quality control procedures. The percentage of CRFs to be audited depends on the size and complexity of the study. A simple small study such as an asthma study with 50 patients and five sites would probably only need five CRFs to be audited in order to get a picture of how the clinical data are being handled. Whereas a larger, more complex study with 3000 patients and 100 sites may required 50+ CRFs to be audited.

The auditor should be provided with all the study-specific documentation such as the final signed protocol, and the final version of the clinical data handling conventions, including data entry guidelines. This will ensure that they do not raise unnecessary queries and also gives them the assurance that such documentation exists and is being followed. All audit findings should be written clearly and precisely so that the auditee understands completely what has been found. If at any time the auditor feels that they are finding too many ambiguities or mistakes then the audit should be curtailed and a senior member of the clinical data management team informed. A decision then needs to be made on whether there is a systematic breakdown of the process or whether no particular breakdown can be identified. It could result in all the clinical data needing to be re-reviewed. If this audit has been done early in the process then there should be plenty of time before database lock to correct process problems.

An audit of the key variables is an important exercise prior to database lock. Key variables are dictated by the protocol and the project statistician, not the auditor. They normally consist of safety and primary efficacy clinical data as a minimum. It is essential that those variables specified are also those identified by clinical data management. The audit should then take place on a similar size population as the CRF audit. The 100% checks should be completed as part of the quality control process and the audit should be assuring that this process has taken place. Often it is beneficial to pick some patients previously audited at the CRF stage to assure that the key variables have been consistently handled and that any problems identified have now been resolved. When auditing the key variables the procedure is similar to the CRF audit with the main emphasis being on a review of the process and the documentation.

Another aspect of clinical data review is coding and the world of coding is a complicated place. Rules need to be laid out early on and specifications clearly given to the coders. The dictionaries used frequently at the first level are in-house, the codes are then often broken down into COS-TART and WHO-ART preferred terms. These dictionaries can be extremely constricting as often the verbatim term used by the Investigator does not match any of the terms found in them. It is hoped that in the future there will be a dictionary that is recognised worldwide, but this at present is still in a draft format.

When dealing with coding there should be a great deal of emphasis on quality control and those involved should understand the variables that they are coding and why they are coding at all. More and more companies are now adopting a policy of having a dedicated group of professionals who concentrate solely on coding. These personnel are usually medically trained and have a thorough understanding of the coding dictionaries. An important factor of having one central team performing the coding means that the coding is standardised and the clinical database is held in a central and uniform manner. The QA audit consists of a check to ensure that guidelines and quality control procedures are being followed.

It is now frequently the situation that coding is computer assisted and this has made coding easier on a practical level[7]. One of the main benefits is that looking up codes and later reference is easier. It also helps towards coding consistency as frequently referenced codes can easily be accessed.

Coding is used to provide a more effective way of analysing certain data collected. Codes can be used to present clinical data in a uniform and therefore easier way, but any misinterpretation of data meaning must be avoided. The existence of controlled guidelines and quality procedures and trained personnel prevents such misinterpretation. The QA audit can give the further assurance that the data can be regarded as a true representation of what the investigator collected on site. If many errors occur in the coding of clinical data, then this will affect the final clinical study report.

TABLES, FIGURES AND LISTINGS AUDITS

The process for the production of tables, listings and figures should also be audited early. This ensures that there are adequate documented quality control procedures in place and that they are being followed. As with the database audits, if problems can be found early on then changes can be implemented before there is an impact on the final product.

Final tables, figures and listings are audited by the QA group for programming, accuracy and also to ensure that the statistical analysis, as described in the protocol, has been followed. Often this results in a number 'crunching' exercise by the auditors. Documentation behind the production of the tables, figures and listings is also reviewed to ensure that validation has taken place and has been documented clearly. The main aims of such an audit are to provide assurance that the listings are a true reflection of the CRF, the tables are a true representation of the data found in the listings, and the figures are a true representation of the data found either in the tables or listings. The auditor is also looking to ensure that the programmers and statisticians are following documented procedures that adhere to ICH GCP, the final, signed protocol and statistical analysis plan.

A handover meeting should be held between the programmer, statistician and auditor to ensure there is no confusion regarding what tables, listings and figures are to be audited. A complete list should be provided to the auditor and if possible a cross-reference given between tables and listings, listings and figures, figures and tables. Often the same program is used to produce more than one table and it is helpful to the auditor if this information can also be made available to them. The auditor should have reviewed the protocol and statistical analysis plan prior to the audit in order to gain sufficient knowledge about the study. These documents are then reviewed throughout the audit to ensure that the final product exactly meets the requirements and to ensure the relevant quality procedures have been followed.

If a randomisation list is applicable, this is checked against the appropriate listing, also the procedures followed to break the randomisation code are reviewed. A complete CRF is checked against the listings to ensure that the programming is correct and that they truly represent what has been recorded by the investigator. All titles between tables, figures and listings are checked for consistency and accuracy with the statistical analysis plan.

All fields are checked for misspellings and any 'odd looking' values within a listing are investigated. This particularly applies to laboratory clinical data. All footnotes are reviewed for sense and suitability, and any flagged items are checked to ensure there is an explanatory footnote. Numbers are checked within the tables for accuracy. Checking should also be completed between tables and listings for such clinical data as adverse events and withdrawal details. As with clinical database audits the audit findings must be written clearly and precisely so that any resolutions required can be implemented.

CLINICAL STUDY REPORT AUDITS

The final clinical study report is audited to assure its integrity and accurate reflection of the clinical trial. All factual statements are checked against the medical writer's source and all documentation supplied is checked for its authenticity. The audit is also ensuring that the report is a true reflection of the study design outlined in the protocol. All numbers referred to from the tables and listings are checked for accuracy against the appropriate tables and listings. The process for auditing the report is similar to the tables, listings and figures audit in that the final, signed protocol and statistical analysis plan and quality procedures followed, are reviewed throughout the audit. After the report has been reviewed page by page for accuracy against source documentation, it is read thoroughly for general sense. The audit findings are again written clearly and precisely so that the audience can understand them and take the appropriate action in a timely fashion.

ERROR METRICS

The *Concise Oxford English Dictionary*[8] definition of an effort is a 'mistake or the condition of being wrong in conduct or judgement'.

Many auditing groups create elaborate error metrics in order to give a statistical meaning to the problems they have found in clinical data. The usefulness of errors can only be established if there is some structure behind their meaning. It is possible to have a very high error rate but on investigation it can be seen that the errors only concern non-critical data and so to spend time on resolving them would be wasteful. If the definition for an error is not clearly established then it can lead to misunderstandings between auditors and clinical data management. The actual calculation of the errors also needs to be statistically acceptable. This is when a statistician's skills are very necessary and valuable.

It is more beneficial often to review errors for systematic problems. A pattern of clinical data entry errors or a high error rate can highlight certain process problems. If these are highlighted early in the clinical data collection then resolutions can be implemented before too much data is adversely affected. It cannot be repeated often enough that error rates are only useful if they mean the same to all personnel looking at them and if the error criteria are also clear.

AUDIT CERTIFICATES

ICH GCP states that an audit certificate is 'a declaration of confirmation by the auditor that an audit has taken place'. The auditor can never state that everything contained in the clinical database, tables, figures and listings or clinical study report is 100% accurate and that there are no errors existing. They can state that they have carried out audits and that as far as they can reasonably determine the clinical database, tables, listings and figures or clinical study report are a true reflection of what happened in that trial.

CLINICAL DATA MANAGEMENT TRAINING

The QA group can help an organisation to improve customer satisfaction and reduce costs by implementing a quality system. This puts more emphasis on the group's role in helping to provide the means to achieve continuous improvements in performance. QA and QC, as already stated, are integral parts of the clinical trial process. It is essential that a proactive mechanism be implemented to promote high-quality clinical data acquisition and reporting. It is important that personnel working in clinical data management provide feedback on QC issues and are able to contribute to process improvement. This can only happen if these personnel are trained and kept up to date with procedures.

The QA group should be involved in training and should assure that adequate training takes place by performing regular documented audits. Through the auditing of training documentation and the processes the QA group can highlight any training needs to management to ensure that training requirements are met.

Auditors can be involved in quality procedure training, holding workshops to explain the importance of such procedures. They should also be involved in training in the principles of GCP. Often they are able to give examples of actual incidents which graphically describe the importance of GCP.

REGULATORY AUTHORITY INSPECTIONS

Frequently, the QA group are the hosts for the Inspections of the regulatory agencies. The request from the regulatory authority to inspect a specific project will usually be sent to the sponsor. In the case of international trials, this could be the local country office of the sponsor and the request requires to be relayed to the office where the data management has been carried out. The QA group will usually ensure that all the appropriate staff are prepared, that there is a room, ideally somewhat remote from the everyday business of the institute, and a photocopier, translator, and document collector available. Clear instructions should be given to the staff involved in the Inspection. Questions from the inspectors should be answered with honesty, with as much clarity as possible and without unrequested additional information.

If the support and training of QA has been effective, no surprises should come from the Inspectors' comments at the end of the Inspection. Previous audits by QA should have revealed most of the deficiencies. The frequently quoted deficiencies include the lack of original documents, protocol non-adherence and inability to identify staff involved in the Project. If problems are found, FDA inspectors will look in depth at the systems involved, including whether the computer system has been validated.

QUALITY SYSTEM

In the introduction we commented on the requirement of ICH GCP to have systems in place which 'assure the quality of every aspect of the trial' (ICH

GCP 2.13). Without some kind of quality management system it is difficult to envisage compliance with this GCP requirement.

TOTAL QUALITY MANAGEMENT (TQM)

TQM is an approach that can be used by the management of an organisation which is centred on quality. It ensures the involvement of all staff and aims at achieving long-term success by customer satisfaction, benefiting all members of the organisation, and society, and providing a mechanism for continuous improvement.

In all 'apparently' progressive organisations, various efforts are made to create a culture of 'quality' using some form of TQM. There is nothing new to the concept of implementation of the often considered mystic term of 'quality'. In 1951, Feigenbaum wrote a book on *Total Quality Control*[9]. In Japan, in the 1960s, the so-called 'quality circles' were developed to ensure the personal involvement of factory workers in quality management and problem solving. At the same time, in the US, the 'zero defect concept' was being applied to Pershing missiles, producing them without defects in the stipulated time.

The implication of TQM in clinical research is that QC will be carried out by all staff. If successful, QC should extend from the initial design to the final 'product', that is the clinical study report. QC should also extend to all aspects of the study, including the training of the individuals involved, the payment of staff and investigators, the quality of the paper used in the manufacturing of the CRF and all the essential but 'peripheral' tasks. However, until the rigour of ISO 9000 was established, TQM remained a vague concept to most ordinary members of staff.

ISO 9000

ISO 9000 is a series of quality management and quality assurance standards and guidelines. The series is written from the perspective of a service or product supplier. The standards have been designed for application to all industries but the relevant standard for GCP is that of ISO 9001 *Quality systems—Model for quality assurance in design, development, production, installation, and servicing*[10]. It provides the framework for a quality system which can assure that clinical data are handled in an error-free manner[11]. Such a system involves the training of study personnel, and comprehensive documentation of the operations and procedures that all personnel are following. Some describe the system as a bureaucratic nightmare, but this is only true when intelligence has not been applied to the standard. For example, ISO 9001 can encourage the design of concise CRFs since it will prescribe both the appropriate checklist, and the need for the right people to review and approve the form. It will also prevent the CRF from being designed before a near-final draft of the protocol has been prepared.

The system should assign responsibility for different aspects of quality monitoring, and ensure periodic audits of the clinical database and procedures against source documents. It should also regularly report on details of clinical data quality that identify sources of errors and delays that limit accuracy and timelines of the production of a complete clinical database. There should also be provision for corrective actions to be implemented and the system should be revised or redesigned if deemed necessary.

PROCESS AUDITS

One of the features of any quality management system is that audit of processes should be performed, as well as those audits related to specific protocols. One could argue that to conduct any audit even specific to a protocol will involve auditing the process as well. This is often true but frequently the protocol-specific audit will not highlight a general deficiency. The process of clinical data entry may, in a protocol-specific audit, show that data have been successfully entered into the database. It will not necessarily show that the staff have no documented training and, worse still, that the computer system, of which the clinical data entry is part, has not been correctly validated. Process audits should be conducted on all clinical data management processes at least once a year and more often if changes are taking place or deficiencies have been highlighted.

REMOTE CLINICAL DATA ELECTRONIC CAPTURE

The role of QA in clinical data management has been described essentially for a paper system. Increasingly, various hard and software packages will allow clinical data to be transferred into the clinical database with limited involvement of human input. Personnel in QA will need to establish that the data, perhaps entered by the investigator or read by a scanner, cannot be changed by unauthorised personnel or without authorised documentation. An audit trail will need to be available as would be required for a paper-based system. The manner in which the data arrive at the database where the analysis will take place is open to numerous pitfalls. For example, the problems of laboratory data being merged into a second database illustrate the need to be vigilant. The validation of the computer system to be used for data collection will need to be addressed.

COMPUTER VALIDATION

Computer validation is a process which documents that a computer system reproducibly performs the functions it was designed to do[12]. To achieve sufficient comfort in any system to meet this criterion and to satisfy the regulatory authorities, it will not be sufficient to establish that the software has been properly written and tested. The FDA have suggested in their new draft *Guidance for Industry* document that a computer system is one that includes 'computer hardware, software, and associated documents that generate, collect, maintain, or transmit in digit form information related to the conduct of a clinical trial[13]. Validation must include the original requirements, any modifications made after the system was designed, the security of the system, and the training of computer staff. The records of the testing of the design are part of the validation documentation. Written procedures for the operation and maintenance of the system will need to be present and the auditor will need to be assured that a full change-control process is followed. Any vendor software must be checked to establish that it, too, has been validated. Visits by client auditors to the vendor supplier will become commonplace. In the past, in QA, it was rare to find a specialist in computer validation auditing but this cannot be the case in the future. Increasingly, the general auditor will not only be skilled in data management auditing but also will have experience of computer validation auditing. For larger QA groups, a specialist computer auditor will be part of the team.

THE FUTURE

Three aspects will dominate the future for the QA of clinical data management.

First, the impact of various remote clinical data entry systems, the use of scanners to read the written word, and paperless and computerised clinical data management, will serve to reduce some of the more tedious aspects of QC. It should also eliminate some of the human elements of transferring clinical data from paper to paper and from paper to computer. Electronic Signatures consisting of a computer data compilation of a series of symbols will act as a legally binding equivalent of the individual's handwritten signature. A new role for the QA group will develop since some QA activities will be reduced, but this will be countered by increased auditing requirements for computer validation processes, extending to the vendors of the software and hardware. Electronic packages will often be the final product being submitted to the regulatory authorities for submissions, and the resulting listings and tables will be subjected to vigorous interrogation by those authorities. Again, QA will need to be present, reviewing clinical data, that will be more and more frequently on-line with the clinical data management staff and those preparing clinical study reports. The Assurance of Quality becomes even more important with the advent of harmonisation globally for submissions, since the contents of any clinical study report may be used internationally in marketing applications.

Second, all the indications for the future imply a preoccupation with cost containment in the drug industry. Governments, insurers and in many cases the patients will require new drugs at the minimum cost. Management will constantly seek to reduce expenditure and any quality system which does not reduce or abolish 'rework' does not ensure time-lines are met, and is not in compliance with ICH GCP and other applicable guidelines/regulations will be far more exposed to scrutiny. Management may see its profit margins decline with the additional fear that the regulatory authorities will delay or stop the product reaching the market. Against this background, it can be predicted that QA will play an ever more important role in successful drug development.

Third, as a result of the above developments, the training of QA personnel will assume increasing importance and greater control of it will be instituted by both government and professional bodies. The authors envisage that for some of the QA processes only 'chartered' QA personnel will be eligible. These 'chartered' personnel will have undergone formal training in QA processes, acquired several years of experience and be subject to further examination by their peers before being 'chartered'.

CONCLUSION

QA is an essential part of the clinical data management process. The QA group has several tasks which include auditing, training and advising. It is essential that auditing is not restricted to the two areas of the investigator site audit and the final clinical study report but is conducted at other stages too. The auditor should not just be identifying non-compliance but should also be trying to influence decisions and processes before significant problems arise.

Training by the QA department of all members involved in the clinical trial process can benefit everyone, provided the selection and training of QA personnel is thorough and of a high standard.

Working together, clinical data management and QA groups can ensure that the final product is acceptable for submission.

REFERENCES

1. 'Proposal for a European Parliament and Council Directive on the approxima-tion of provisions laid down by law, regulation or administrative action relat-ing to the implementation of Good Clinical Practice in the conduct of clinical trials on medicinal products for human use'; 97/C 306/10; COM(97) 369 final; 97/0197 (COD), *Official J. Europ. Comm.* **C306**, 9.

2. Food and Drug Administration (1997) *Compliance Program Guidance Manual* (7348.B10), 'Clinical Investigators'.

3. Food and Drug Administration (1997) *Compliance Program Guidance Manual* (7348.811), 'Sponsors, Contract Research Organisations and Monitors'.

4. Note for Guidance on Good Clinical Practice (ICH Harmonised Tripartite Guideline) (CPMP/ICH/135/95), approved 17 July 1997.

5. European Network of GCP Auditors and other GCP Experts (1997) *Optional Guideline for Good Clinical Practice Compliance and Quality Systems Auditing.*

6. Lawrence, G. (1993) Case Record Form design. In *Clinical Data Management,* Eds R.K. Rondel, S.A. Yarley and C. Webb, Wiley, Chichester, pp. 133–152.

7. Fizames, C. (1997) How to improve the medical quality of the coding reports based on WHO-ART and COSTART use. *Drug Inform. J.,* **31**, 85–92.

8. *The Concise Oxford Dictionary of Current English* (1995) (Ed. Della), Thompson, Clarendon Press, 9th Edition, Oxford.

9. Feigenbaum, A.V. (1951) *Total Quality Control Engineering and Management,* McGraw-Hill, New York.

10. International Standard ISO 9001 (1994) *Quality systems—Model for quality as-surance in design, development, production, installation and servicing.* Interna-tional Standards Organisation, Geneva.

11. Sweeney, F. (1994) Merging GCP and ISO 9000 requirements—a source of synergy in quality management of clinical research. *Drug Inform. J.,* **28**, 1097–1104.

12. Double, M.E. and McKendry, M. (1989) *Computer Validation Compliance,* Inter-pharm, Buffalo Grove.

13. Food and Drug Administration (1997) *Guidance for Industry—Computerized Systems used in clinical trials.* Draft release for comment.

8 Performance Measures

JON WOOD

Phoenix International, Romford, Essex, UK

INTRODUCTION

There is a very well known business maxim: 'What gets measured gets done'.

'Time to market', 'Reduced cycle times', 'In-stream processing'—phrases we hear daily within a busy clinical data management department. Believe me, the race is on. The clinical development process is gaining momentum, the process flow is changing and the competition increases daily. *So what's the rush?*

Well, today's focus is on quality drug development and *speed*. Medicinal products are developed to save lives and to prolong and increase quality of life. And let's not forget the pharmaceutical companies' market share and profit margins. The individual process tasks for the development of an ethical pharmaceutical medicine number many thousand. Each task is a key component of the clinical development process, following a carefully planned regulatory route map, guiding the medical science and the planned clinical trials to achieve the ultimate milestone, marketing approval.

Data management forms a key task set within the clinical development process, providing quality databases for analysis, reporting and regulatory submission. The conduct of a clinical trial involves complex interplay between many teams with a multitude of processes taking their place on the critical path. The measurement of performance and productivity is key to the successful achievement of project goals, each minor milestone forging the path to the next on the road to registration.

A clear vision of all endpoints must be maintained constantly in order to achieve the primary objective. The aim of this chapter is to review the variety of possible indicators of performance measurement, reflecting many stages within the data management process flow and their use in optimising efficiency and in managing achievement of key milestones along the complex critical path.

Clinical Data Management. Second Edition. Edited by R.K. Rondel, S.A. Varley and C.F. Webb.
© 2000 John Wiley & Sons, Ltd

PERFORMANCE

Performance can be defined in many ways. It defines a measure of fitness for purpose and can be used as an overall measure of quality and productivity or work rate.

Within this chapter, three primary performance indicators will be reviewed: *productivity, quality* and *process cycle times.* In defining suitable performance measures for the data management process, a *standardised* set of process tasks must be clearly defined. The data management process flow is changing and developing quickly as new technology is introduced to the data collection process.

It is difficult to consistently define the process flow as there is often much variation across organisations, clinical phases and therapeutic areas. However, in order to define comprehensive performance standards, it is important to base our measurement tools on a common set of processes within data management which can be consistently interpreted across clinical phases, therapeutic areas and indeed organisations.

We aim to answer several key questions: 'Are we being productive?', 'Are we resourcing effectively?', 'Are we developing a quality product?' or 'Just how long do things really take?'.

DEFINING THE PROCESS FLOW

Figure 8.1 presents a flow chart defining the key elements of the data management process flow. A typical Phase I clinical pharmacology study and early Phase II studies are of short duration, data transfer and data processing often being performed on a completed patient basis. The numbers of subjects being recruited often do not exceed 24–48. More complex Phase III/ IV studies are generally of longer duration with up to a year or more for patient recruitment with a similar timeline for the treatment phase. Patient recruitment often ranges from 500 patients or more. It is the role of the project manager to clearly define the process flow with the project team. The project team will usually comprise a data management team leader, programmers, statisticians and clinical research monitors. In order to focus on performance measures, it is necessary to review the process tasks in more detail. A summary of key data management tasks is presented below and will be used as a focus for performance measurement:

1. *Data collection.* Clinical data from the investigator site may arrive in the data management department in the form of Case Report Forms (CRFs), either for completed patients or as individual or grouped visit batches. Data may also arrive in an electronic format, such as laboratory data from central laboratories, diary card data collected on

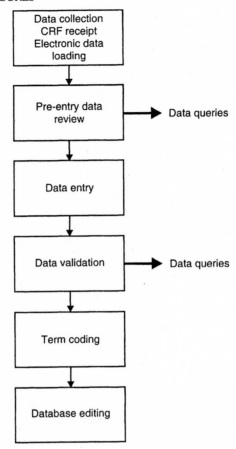

Figure 8.1

hand-held computers or via interactive voice response systems, or
more directly via remote data entry systems and remote data capture
solutions. However, in the majority of cases, clinical data still arrive in
paper format on CRFs.

2. *Pre-entry data review* (secondary monitoring). Often, a pre-entry manual review of all source CRF data is made to ensure completeness of
   data. Some data may be coded at this stage to support the data entry
   process. Data queries may also be raised at this stage.
3. *Data entry.* Following receipt of data from the investigator site, data
   are keyed or loaded onto the clinical database. Most data entry teams
   enter CRF data via an independent double data entry process with
   either a file extract and compare process or via an on-line verification
   process to ensure data quality at this key stage in the development of
   the database.

4. *Data validation.* Data are cleaned in a batch process using validation programmes which have been specified and developed before data entry commences. The majority of data queries are generated at this stage.
5. *Term coding.* Adverse event data, concurrent medications and medical conditions are often coded using standard dictionaries both using an autoencoder and via manual coding. Again, this is often a batch process.
6. *Database editing.* The developing database is edited following batch receipt of resolved data queries from the field.

Process tasks 1–6 are by no means comprehensive but typically summarise the in-process flow for data management. For a typical multivisit Phase III study, this process flow must be carefully orchestrated to maintain in-stream processing. This in-stream process is critical and can only be optimised by careful monitoring and review of all in-process tasks. Within the in-stream process flow, data are collected in a pre-defined batch format, reviewed, entered and validated in a defined cycle time. It is with the use of performance measures that we manage this in-stream process in detail. Managing the process flow also involves effective project management, communication, monitoring and rapid response to changes in data demands.

The role of the data management project manager is now becoming clearly defined. Effective project planning and monitoring is critical to the careful maintenance of the in-stream process. In today's timelines-driven environment, project management skills are becoming an important addition to the expanding data management tool set. Systems are also developing in line with ever-changing roles. Apart from the typical clinical relational database applications, integrated project management tools such as Clinical Trial Management Systems, Gantt and PERT charts and timesheet applications are becoming part of the standard suite of data management utilities. The focus is on planning and performance monitoring.

MEASURING PERFORMANCE

Metrics reporting is now a key function of the data management project manager or team leader. A defined set of quantitative measures can be presented to assist in management of the process flow. These measures can fall into three distinct categories:

- Status Reporting—measuring productivity against resources
- Measurement and reporting of quality
- Measurement and reporting of process cycle times

Status Reporting

The process tasks 1–6 can all be readily quantified and reported. The data management platform must also facilitate a tracking and reporting system in order to track process flow. The processing unit must be clearly defined. Examples of typical processing units are presented below:

(i)   Complete patient CRF.
(ii)   Pre-defined CRF visit batch.
(iii) Individual CRF visit.
(iv)   Individual CRF pages.

In addition, all data collected apart from the CRF, such as electronic lab data, diary cards, ECGs, pharmacokinetic data, patient questionnaires and so on, must also be tracked and reported. On-going processing measures such as the number of terms coded in the database and the numbers of individual data queries generated must similarly be tracked and reported.

The tracking and reporting system must facilitate logging of processing units at each key task in the process flow. Typically these are:

Process unit: for example CRF visit
● Received date of CRF visit in Data Management
● Double-entered date of CRF visit
● Verified date of CRF visit
● Validated date of CRF visit
● Date of 'clean' CRF visit

Process unit: Data Clarification Form (DCF)
● Query generation date
● Query resolution date

Logging of each CRF visit at the completion of each process task is often a manual process, but many data management groups now use bar code scanning to speed the process.

Figure 8.2 presents a typical format for the processing status report of a study within Data Management. The processing unit must be defined within the report. Status reports may be generated daily, weekly or monthly depending on the demands of the process flow and the importance of closely monitoring the work rate.

Regular weekly or monthly status reports simply present a 'snapshot' of the current processing status. It is more effective, however, to present the weekly or monthly processing status over time in the form of a histogram or bar chart. This provides the project manager with an effective visual measure of processing status and work flow over time. Productivity may be evaluated. An example of such a plot is presented in Figure 8.3. A

CRF VISIT SUMMARY STATUS REPORT

CLINICAL DATA MANAGEMENT

01-JAN-97

CRF VISIT STATUS	VISIT 1	VISIT 2	VISIT 3	VISIT 4	VISIT 5	VISIT 6	TOTAL
Received	97	86	57	42	14	4	**300**
Secondary reviewed	97	86	54	40	10	2	**289**
Double entered	97	86	54	36	10	2	**285**
Entry verified	97	86	52	36	10	2	**283**
Validated	97	79	50	30	6	2	**264**
Queries raised	83	68	36	23	2	2	**214**
Clean	56	36	22	12	0	0	**126**

Figure 8.2

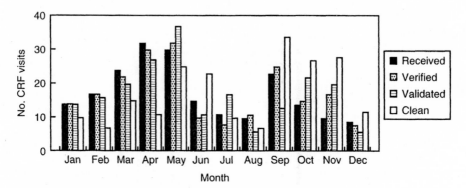

Figure 8.3

planned plot of processing status should reflect the status of patient recruitment in the field if an in-stream process is in place.

Effective communication with the clinical project manager is essential throughout the recruitment and data collection phase of any study. Many data management team leaders and project managers will also have access to a Clinical Trial Management System (CTMS). The CTMS is a parallel database providing up-to-the-minute information on all aspects of clinical trial activity. Key field-based information such as planned and actual patient recruitment dates, planned and actual patient study visit dates and clinical monitoring visits can be readily accessed by the data manager to provide a forward load for data retrieval and DCF resolution. This in-progress information is vital to the effective management of data flow and data processing resource. The CTMS may also provide immediate information on the status of serious adverse events and protocol violators before data are received and processed within the data management department.

Status reporting of data queries is also of great importance. Data collection from the field and data entry and management in-house constitute just one half of the data cycle. The other half involves the sometimes rather complex interchange of data queries in the form of DCFs generated through computerised data validation checks.

Data Quality

Data quality can also be an important measure of performance. Collecting 'clean' data begins during the protocol and data capture tool development stages. The data capture tool is more often than not a Case Report Form, and its design is fundamental to the collection of 'clean' data. Clear and concise CRF completion guidelines for the investigator as well as effective training through start-up visits and investigator meetings again facilitate the early capture of 'clean' data.

Increased performance of all data management processes is optimised by the receipt of high-quality data. Comprehensive primary monitoring on site by the clinical monitor also captures problems early, ensuring that the investigator can resolve patient data issues while they are still fresh in his mind. Monitoring guidelines may be developed by the data manager and clinical monitor in line with the comprehensive validation specification. These guidelines provide a focus for the clinical monitor, highlighting all important data issues to be reviewed on site. Status reports are often generated weekly, detailing all DCFs generated and those that are still outstanding. Data quality reports highlighting the numbers of data problems by type of data can also be very informative. Often, this information can highlight problems with the CRF design or indeed with investigator understanding.

This information must be captured and identified early on in the process flow to feedback and reduce the opportunities for data errors. Feedback may take the form of investigator newsletters or further overview meetings.

Data quality in the form of data queries can be presented as both primary and secondary monitoring queries. The number of primary monitoring queries, those identified by the clinical monitor and addressed at the investigator site during the monitoring visit, and the number of secondary monitoring queries, those raised during in-house validation review, can be presented in the form of a status report. A typical example is presented in Figure 8.4. It must be stressed, however, that this performance measure is often prone to misinterpretation. A high number of primary monitoring queries may reflect a poor CRF design, ineffective monitoring or indeed a

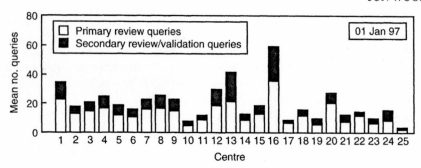

Figure 8.4

lack of investigator understanding. The focus, however, is clear, the objectives are to minimise and effect early capture of problems at source. The more data issues that are generated through the complex interchange of queries, the bigger the impact on process performance, leading to an associated increase in process cycle times.

Cycle Times

We have highlighted some key quantitative measures of processing status. Performance may be measured by review of processing status over time and by reductions in the number of data queries and improvement in data quality.

Performance may also be monitored by calculating and presenting cycle time measurements. The time taken to achieve key process tasks is critical and must be measured and monitored effectively to maintain the instream process flow. With mean total global cycle times in excess of three to four years from protocol approval to finalisation of report for many study designs, a high degree of performance within the data management phase is critical, reducing overall study cycle times.

The process tasks 1–6 all have assigned dates as recorded throughout the status logging process. In order to ensure in-stream processing, cycle time targets must be proposed and actively worked to. Of course, there are many contributing factors to the definition of cycle times:

- Study phase
    (i) Phase I studies typically comprise small numbers of subjects, typically 12–24 with a 15–30 page CRF. Data are normally collected in completed subjects and data can be entered and validated completely. In effect, during one complete processing cycle, all data queries for the subject may be generated for resolution.
    Typical cycle times:

⇒   CRF receipt to double data entry and verification: 48 hours
⇒   Verification to completion of validation: 48 hours
⇒   Query generation to resolution: 24 hours

These are merely examples of 'standard' cycle times and reflect the low volume of data and complete subject processing.

(ii)   Phase III/IV studies typically comprise much larger numbers of patients with a much larger page volume CRF. Data for a patient are also collected over a much longer time period, typically 6 months to a year and beyond. During the study set-up phase, it is often beneficial to pre-define the CRF visit batch structure for data collection to facilitate effective data processing. Data are collected in this batch format and entry, validation and database editing is performed on partially completed patients. Again, the focus is on in-stream processing and achieving process deliverables within these restraints forces the in-stream process flow. Typical cycle times:

⇒   CRF visit receipt to double data entry and verification: 5 days
⇒   Verification to completion of validation: 10 days
⇒   Query generation to resolution: 4 weeks

As already outlined in Figure 8.3, cycle time metrics may also be presented in a line plot illustrating cycle times over months for key process tasks. Figure 8.5 presents a plot such as this for three key metrics, time from receipt to verification, time from receipt to validation, and query resolution time. All cycle time metrics are calculated as a mean across all processing units. There are many issues affecting performance as reflected by increased cycle times. It may be appropriate to review both plots in Figures 8.3 and 8.5 together to investigate the process flow month on month. An increase in cycle time from data receipt to verification may be due to an increased volume of data collected in the field. Increased validation cycle times may be a reflection of data quality. Limited access to investigators due to holidays may also be reflected in increased query resolution cycle times.

Therapeutic area may have some impact on process cycle times. Studies in chemotherapy, transplantation and dementia typically comprise complex data capture tools and visit structures with multiple visits over one to two year's duration with a high volume of data points. Often, the data entry cycle times and validation cycle times are extended.

● Process design

We have already reviewed many of the key elements of the data management process flow. The design of the process flow is a critical

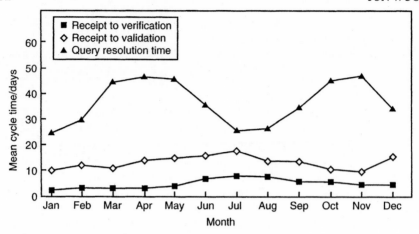

Figure 8.5

component of the study set-up task list. The collection, validation and database clean-up of any study involves effective interplay between Data Management, Clinical Research and the investigator and co-workers. It is important to define the process flow carefully and to obtain 'buy-in' and commitment from all measures of the project team. Cycle times must be defined at the study set-up phase, both for the data management process flow and for the query management within the clinical monitoring function. It is the effective generation and res-olution of data queries in an optimal cycle time that presents one of the greatest project management challenges. Monitoring performance throughout this important interchange of information is critical.

As an investigator's time becomes more limited, it is essential that each planned monitoring visit is as productive as possible. If the data management process flow is in-stream achieving defined cycle times, all data queries generated from the previous site data collection may be batched and addressed at the next monitoring visit. Data issues may be still fresh in the investigator's mind and resolution of often complex data queries is optimised.

Key tasks within the data management process flow may also be reviewed to increase performance and aid rapid query generation and resolution:

- Is double data entry really necessary?
- Limit the pre-entry secondary monitoring review
- Would validation review be faster by generating data listings than by reviewing often complex validation error reports?

Standardisation is often a key to optimal process design. Standardised data structures, database designs and validation codes will facilitate ease of processing and will ensure familiarity and minimise training requirements for all team members. Harmonised Standard Operating Procedures drive the standardisation process and ensure ease of understanding of all systems and processes. Parallel processing will also increase performance—entering, validating, coding and editing instream. A matrix structure for the data management team encourages flexibility and optimises communication and interactivity, again driving the in-stream process flow.

As already discussed, quality is also a key measure of performance and ongoing QC may also provide a key indication as to the effectiveness of data entry and validation.

SETTING THE BASELINE

We have reviewed a variety of quantitative measures and presentations of processing units within the data management process flow. In order to manage and respond to the process flow, it is important to clearly define and set the baseline for the measurement of performance. Example process cycle times have been proposed but just how do we measure these?

Many data management departments are now very familiar with the concept of timesheets and of collecting time per task data on a daily basis. During the study set-up phase, it is the role of the team leader or project manager within the data management team to define the budget and to allocate time to process tasks. Historical timesheet information can provide valuable data for the determination of process times. Typical study designs provide a framework for the assessment of key process times:

- How long to enter a CRF page or visit
- How long to validate and generate queries for a CRF visit
- How much data requires coding

Accurate assessments of process times may also be made by experienced data managers and data entry staff following review of the CRF. Once the assessments of process cycle times have been made, a project plan is developed to generate a budget for all data management tasks based on the process times per unit and the number of units anticipated. The budgeted number of hours must be planned out over the duration of the data management phase.

We have already summarised a typical group of data management tasks. These may be further refined to define a standard set of process tasks within data management. It is often appropriate to define a code list for the set of standard tasks. These may be set up within the timesheet application for the collection of data on a daily basis. A typical project plan with a standard task list is presented in Figure 8.6 with a budget number of hours

DATA MANAGEMENT TASK	TASK CODE	BUDGET HRS	TOTAL HRS TO DATE	ESTIMATED HRS TO COMPLETE	TOTAL + ESTIMATED HRS	JAN ACTUAL	JAN PLANNED	FEB ACTUAL	FEB PLANNED	MAR ACTUAL	MAR PLANNED
Database Development	DEVL	40	37	0	37	27	35	10	5		0
Validation Programming	PROG	40	23	0	23	15	35	8	5		0
Data Entry	DENT	70	15	40	55	0	0	15	30		40
Data Validation	VALD	20	11	35	46	0	0	11	15		35
Term Coding	CODE	15	3	10	13	0	0	3	5		10
Laboratory Data Loading	LABD	10	3	5	8	0	0	3	5		5
Database Editing	EDIT	20	2	15	17	0	0	2	5		15
Quality Control	QCON	10	2	5	7	0	0	2	5		5
Data Transfer	TRAN	5	0	5	5	0	0	0	0		5
TOTAL HRS		230	96	115	211	42	70	54	75		115

01-MAR-97

Figure 8.6

allocated to each process task over each month of the data management phase. This is our project plan and forms a key monitoring and decision-making tool, measuring performance by calculating actual versus budget hours for each task code.

Many timesheets systems today are available as network versions providing a standard graphical user interface. These may be available to all of the data management and data entry teams and can be set up with the standard data management task list. At the end of each day, each team member for a particular project will enter all hours 'logged' to each process task for that particular project. With a timesheet system such as this in place, the project manager or team leader can access and review all hours logged to each process task on a daily, weekly or monthly basis. These hours must be entered into the project management tool on a weekly or monthly basis and actual versus estimated hours per month must be reviewed. The project plan may be updated as often as necessary.

Estimated hours per task for remaining months must be reviewed as each month's actual hours are collected via the timesheet system. A status report such as the report format presented in Figure 8.2 may provide a measure of percent completion. As more timesheet data are collected it may become apparent that certain tasks are taking considerably longer than originally budgeted. This early information provides an opportunity to review the particular process task in detail and facilitates corrective action minimising process cycle times and driving in-stream processing. It may be possible to clearly define an actual process time per unit. Even though this time was a key assumption at the budget creation stage, often in reality more factors come into play. The project manager may have to look creatively for time savings with other process tasks to maintain the in-stream process flow. Increasing performance may be also effected by increasing resources. However, in many situations this is not possible and insufficient training or experience may lead to a reduction in data quality.

MILESTONES

Optimising process performance and maintaining in-stream processing drives the achievement of study goals and the meeting of critical milestones. If performance throughout the data processing phase is poor and in-stream cycle time targets are not being met, then end-of-study milestones will not be achieved.

There are several key milestones within the data management process flow:

LPLV   Last Patient Last Visit
LCI   Last CRF Data In-house

LQI   Last Query Issued
LQR   Last Query Received
DBR   Database Release
DBL   Database Lock

Once again, cycle times may be proposed, the critical phase being LPLV to DBL. The race is on. The study is finished, investigator sites are being closed out and the analysis and reporting phase is pivotal. Optimising performance and facilitating in-stream processing throughout the study phase means that this key cycle time to database lock is minimised.

ELECTRONIC DATA TRANSFER—ALL CHANGE

There is a great change ahead . . . at last. The new millennium will herald innovative advances in information capture and retrieval. The future of computerisation at the investigator site means that data capture will fundamentally change the way we manage clinical trial information. Performance will be demonstrated by process cycle times measured in hours and not in days or even weeks. Further development of guidelines defined by the harmonisation of GCP orchestrated by the International Conference on Harmonisation (ICH), will drive standardisation across the pharmaceutical industry. This is the key. The process flow *is* changing.

The volume of paper data comprising a regulatory submission and the requirement for coordinated review has accelerated the acceptance of electronic transfer of regulatory dossiers. Computer Assisted New Drug Applications (CANDAS) on PC CD ROM are becoming the norm. The way investigators operate and indeed the breed of investigators we are now working with is changing. Remote Data Entry (RDE) systems including Internet solutions will become commonplace. Instantaneous data access from anywhere in the world will be possible, carried by the power of the World Wide Web. The role of the Clinical Data Manager will evolve in this new environment where paper exchange will be limited. Rapid developments in new technology will be at the forefront of clinical research, maximising performance and reducing process cycle times. Many processes within the current data management flow are inefficient and time-consuming. In today's corporate empires, electronic information exchange is the lifeblood of growth and development. Clinical research will not be left behind.

SUMMARY

With the average number of clinical trials constituting a typical NDA submission often exceeding 50 comprising 3000–5000 patients, a complete global Phase I–IV programme may comprise 15 000–25 000 patients. Speed and quality are driven by increased performance throughout the data management process flow. The biometrics programme involving clinical data management and statistical reporting tasks often exceeds 30–40% of the overall cycle time from protocol development to finalisation of integrated clinical report. Any improvement in performance ultimately leads to reduced cycle times and accelerates the reporting phase.

Performance of many data management tasks can be actively and effectively measured, providing the project manager with all the necessary information to optimise the process flow and ensure in-stream processing and minimal cycle times.

Effective project management also requires key communication skills, closing the feedback loop and ensuring that all involved in the process flow actively participate in the reduction of process cycle times. As new technology and standardised processes drive the clinical research process further forward, a clearer understanding of project team management and procedures will maximise performance. Developing standardised performance measures is critical to the effective management of the data processing component of the development plan. The greatest impact on performance for the current data management process flow will be the introduction of network-based technology, distributing the data management model generating clinical databases on-line almost instantly. The next few years into the third millennium will see the greatest changes in clinical data management seen so far. These will be driven by technology and by the standards being set by the clinical data management businesses of today.

9 Data Presentation

M² Worldwide, Rockville, Maryland, USA

INTRODUCTION

After teams of scientists and researchers have designed an appropriate protocol for a clinical trial, conducted the study to collect the data and built the
database, the data must be reviewed for a variety of reasons. Data are reviewed by clinical researchers and data managers to ensure the integrity and
accuracy of the data, by quality assurance auditors to confirm the quality of
the data, by medical experts and biostatisticians to verify the efficacy and
safety of medicinal products, and eventually by regulatory authorities to
make decisions on which products are approved and which are not.

While a lot of thought is given to protocol design and conduct of the
study, not enough consideration is given to issues pertaining to data presentations. This chapter deals with the issues that must be addressed to
present or display the clinical research data in the best possible way.
Optimizing data presentation can only be achieved after careful consideration for the type of data display and the intent of the presentation.

It is the thorough review of clinical research data by regulatory authorities that results in new medicinal products being approved for widespread use. The consequences of this are improved health, reduced
diseases and often the difference between life and death for critically ill
patients. In addition millions of dollars in profits for pharmaceutical companies are at stake.

The recent boom in biotechnology and contract research companies
has made it possible for thousands of small companies to take innovative
new drugs from the laboratories to the patients in record time. The success of a clinical trial or clinical program often rests on presenting the
data appropriately. Hence sufficient thought must be given to the issues
pertaining to data presentation.

The remainder of the chapter is organized as follows:

- Clinical Research Issues for Data Presentations
- General Issues when Presenting Data

Clinical Data Management. Second Edition. Edited by R.K. Rondel, S.A. Varley and C.F. Webb.
© 2000 John Wiley & Sons, Ltd

- Two Schemata for Categorizing Data Presentations
- Types of Clinical Data
- Presentation of Raw Data
- Presentation of Summary Data
- Data Presentation for Validation
- Data Presentation for Analysis
- Conclusion
- Appendix—Sample Data Presentations

Throughout this chapter the terms data presentations and data displays are used interchangeably and apply to both the hardcopy or on-screen display. In addition the term new medicinal products applies to new drugs, biologics or devices.

CLINICAL RESEARCH ISSUES FOR DATA PRESENTATIONS

Before any new medicine can be made available to patients, it must go through a long and rigorous series of experiments on animals and humans called pre-clinical and clinical trials respectively. These trials are carefully designed by medical researchers and biostatisticians, and reviewed by regulatory authorities and ethics committees (Institutional Review Boards) before they are conducted.

Regulatory authorities such as the Food and Drug Administration (FDA—also referred to as the Agency) in the USA, the European Medicinal Evaluation Agency (EMEA) in Europe, and the Ministry of Health in Japan and in China authorize the conduct of clinical trials. These agencies ensure that clinical trials are conducted ethically and with the utmost regard to patients' safety while maintaining scientific integrity. Often these studies require some patients to be given a placebo (dummy medication, identical in all other respects to the investigational drug under consideration). All data gathered in these pre-clinical and clinical studies must be accurate and presented appropriately to address the hypothesis of interest.

Each clinical trial postulates a hypothesis and by gathering the data from a carefully designed clinical trial one can statistically analyze and present the data, allowing a reviewer to either reject the hypothesis or fail to do so. The hypothesis, also called null hypothesis, is what is widely accepted to be true or the standard of current belief, and the clinical trial is intended to result in data that either disprove it or fail to do so—the latter implying that the data did not provide sufficient evidence to disprove what is the standard belief (i.e. the drug is as effective as a placebo). Examples of null hypothesis are: (a) the mean reduction (from a pre-treatment baseline value) in Systolic Blood Pressure while taking Drug A (the Investigational Drug) is significantly greater than the mean reduction in Systolic Blood Pressure while on placebo; or (b) the percentage of patients who are cured after taking Drug A (the Investigational Drug) is the same as the percentage of patients cured after taking Drug B (a currently used approved drug).

Results from multiple pre-clinical and clinical trials are collated and presented to the appropriate regulatory authorities in order to obtain a license to market any new product. The application for new drugs presented to the FDA in the US is referred to as a New Drug Application (NDA). A license for getting a generic drug approved is called an Abbreviated NDA or (ANDA) while having an approval for a change in the labeling is achieved by filing a NDA or a Supplemental NDA (SNDA). In addition the approval of biologics requires a Product License Application or PLA. The FDA subsequently reviews the application and makes one of the following decisions: (a) approves the application, (b) asks for additional data before it can make a decision, or (c) rejects the application for marketing the new product.

To avoid any bias, clinical trials are often conducted in a blinded fashion. When this is done, neither the patients nor the individuals making assessments have any knowledge of the treatment the patient is receiving. The randomization codes or a list of what patient was given which treatment is only available to the drug packaging group and sometimes the Biostatisticians, who ensure its confidentiality. Often in clinical trials the Investigators are provided with 'code envelopes' or individual envelopes detailing for each patient the specific treatment that each one is being given. These code envelopes must be opened only in life-threatening situations. All code envelopes must be returned at the end of the study to the sponsor to confirm that the Investigators were blinded during the study. More recently code envelopes are being replaced by Interactive Voice Response (IVRS) systems.

Once the clinical trial is complete and the database has been validated the data manager locks the database and release it to the statisticians for analysis. After locking the database the packaging group/statisticians unblind the study by obtaining the randomization lists and determining which patient was assigned to which particular treatment group.

Just as the use of blinding avoids bias and is the standard for conducting sound statistical comparisons, the use of placebo or active controls allows for scientifically valid comparisons to be made with regard to the effectiveness and safety of the drug.

In addition, all statistical methods to be used and statistical tests to be performed must be specified in the protocol or in subsequent amendments prior to unblinding the study. This is to avoid 'looking' at the data and coming up with the 'best' analysis from the sponsor's perspective. This does not, however, preclude statisticians from further exploring unanticipated characteristics revealed by the data. These must, however, be clearly stated as such.

It is prudent to implement and test all analyses prior to unblinding the trial. This acts as a double check to ensure the quality and completeness of the database. It also allows the analysis to be programmed in parallel to conducting the study and cleaning the database rather than after locking the database.

To accurately determine the efficacy and safety of a medicine, not only must the data be gathered accurately, but once entered into a computer database, the data must undergo rigorous computerized completeness and consistency checks to ensure validity and analyzability. The primary objective of any clinical data management group is to create an accurate analyzable database that can be subjected to statistical analysis and subsequent determination of the effectiveness and safety of the new medicine.

It is also important to distinguish between database management systems and optimal database structure for data presentations. Databases are often constructed using relational database management systems such as Oracle®, SQL-Server®, Sybase®, Informix® or Ingres®. These focus on optimizing data storage, allowing transformations and minimizing data inconsistencies by normalizing the database to its third normal form. That is each column or field contains only one piece of information and each field depends on the primary key only and nothing but the primary key. However, for efficient data presentation, it is more helpful to have a denormalized database. Hence it is not unusual to build what are called 'analysis' SAS datasets (see Figure 9.1).

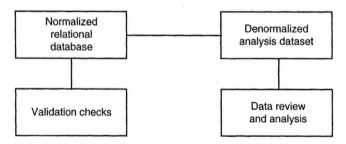

Figure 9.1   Use of a normalized vs. a denormalized database

GENERAL ISSUES

Presentation of clinical data is of paramount importance. It affects the health of all of us because it ultimately determines whether a pharmaceutical company can market its drug and recover its research and development investment. This presentation of data is often the culmination of years of research by teams of highly qualified scientists and the expenditure of hundreds of millions of dollars.

Data presentations can be formally generated for use by different reviewers or by ad hoc SQL (Structured Query Language) or SASASSIST® statements used by data managers. Although more careful thought must be given to data presentations implemented for different reviewers, it is good practice to make the ad hoc presentations coherent and self-contained without the use of clever abbreviations. This permits ease of understanding by others as well as by the individual generating the presentation at some later time.

Irrespective of the type of data presented or the intention of the presentation there are some essential things to remember.

First, make the presentation clear, concise and self-contained. Explicitly define whatever is necessary to allow the reviewer to understand the presentation. Do not leave out information essential to understanding the data. Place related information adjacent or close by, so the reviewer does not have to search all over the display or on multiple pages. Use appropriate descriptive titles indicating the content of the presentation and the population displayed. Use detailed column headers rather than internal abbreviated database variable names. Define units of measurement and translate (decode) coded values. Use footnotes to define approximations or any algorithms used. Avoid using clever coding schemes that can place more data on a page at the cost of making the review difficult.

The display in Figure 9.2 could easily be replaced by the one in Figure 9.3 with minimal additional effort.

Second, plan adequately and solicit input from people with appropriate expertise to ensure that the data presentation meets the needs of the reviewers. Develop shell displays and written specifications to allow the 'users/reviewers' of the data presentation to explicitly communicate with the 'creators/programmers' of the presentations. Often details that are

Listing 1 : Demographics data					
PTNO	TRT	SEX	AGE	RACE	HT/WT
1001	1	1	23	1	73/231
1002	2	2	29	2	67/198
1003	1	2	19	1	64/211
....	....	....	....	....	....

Figure 9.2 A poorly designed data presentation

Patient number	Treatment	Sex	Age (yrs)	Race[1]	Height (in)	Weight (lbs)
1001	Drug X	M	23	C	73	231
1002	Placebo	F	29	B	67	198
1003	Drug X	F	19	C	64	211
....	....	....	....	....	....	....
....	....	....	....	....	....	....

1 : C = Caucasian, B = Black, A = Asian, O = Other

Figure 9.3   A well-designed data presentation

unspecified may be made incorrectly by programmers or, worse still, set implicitly by defaults in the programs used to create the data displays.

Third, validate the program used to generate the presentations. Ad hoc queries to data could be simple SQL statements, but the moment one begins to write complex joins (merges) or data transformations, one must follow appropriate methodology pertaining to software development. These would include formal testing and validation before interpreting the data presented.

TWO SCHEMATA FOR CATEGORIZING DATA PRESENTATIONS

Data presentation can be broadly categorized in one of the following two schemata:

(A)   By type of data presented:
    (i)   raw data or individual patient data;
    (ii)   summary or aggregate data.
(B)   By intention of the presentation:
    (i)   for validating the data;
    (ii)   for reviewing or analyzing the data to determine the efficacy and safety of the drug.

These will be reviewed below with examples where appropriate.

TYPES OF CLINICAL DATA

Clinical data can be varied and for certain therapeutic areas or drugs often unique. However, historically there are certain data that are almost always captured in every protocol. These include:

(a)   Demographics data
(b)   Medical History
(c)   Coexistent diseases
(d)   Prior and concomitant Medications
(e)   Inclusion/Exclusion (entry) criteria
(f)   Drug accountability
(g)   Efficacy measurements
(h)   Adverse Experiences
(i)   Laboratory measurements (Hematology, Biochemistry, Urinalysis)
(j)   Vital Signs
(k)   Physical Exams

Examples of some of the above are in the Appendix at the end of this chapter.

Typically, medical history, coexistent diseases, medication use, entry criteria, adverse experience and physical exam data contain categorical data and involve displays of incidence rates of patients having an event or an abnormality. Most laboratory and vital signs data are continuous and involve displaying means, medians, standard errors and quartiles. Data in demographics, drug accountability and efficacy measurements and certain parameters in laboratory measurements would include both categorical and continuous data and would include both frequency displays and means, and so on.

Certain data such as Adverse Events (AEs), Medications and Labs are more difficult to handle and when presenting these due consideration should be given to the issues indicated below.

AEs and medications involve time-related events and it is important to know the start and stop times. In addition, based upon the design of the CRFs it may be necessary to collapse events that are captured as multiple events but are continuations of the same. It is also necessary to distinguish between a co-existent disease and an AE or between a prior medication and a concomitant medication. This is done by comparing the start and stop times of the event or medication with the time of randomization for each patient. FDA Guidelines provide for definitions of Treatment Emergent Signs and Symptoms (TESS). These are also sometimes referred to as New/Worsening AEs. In addition, usually AEs and medications are coded using an appropriate dictionary. Presentations of raw data should display both the raw/verbatim/reported terms and the coded terms. Incidence tables, however, must use the coded preferred terms.

Lab data can vary from one lab to another and unless a central lab is used it may be necessary to standardize the data, using an appropriate formula. In addition, presentations of lab data may involve both display of means and so on to see trends, and also incidence rates or shift tables to see how many abnormalities occurred in the different treatment groups at baseline and after randomization.

Since multiple subpopulations may be analyzed, usually all background data, demographics, medical history, coexistent diseases, prior medications and entry criteria are displayed for all subpopulations analyzed, while safety data, adverse experiences, laboratory data, vital signs and physical examination data are displayed for the safety subpopulation (all patients who received the study medication and have a safety assessment). Efficacy and drug compliance data are displayed for the intent-to-treat population (all patients who received study medication and have some efficacy assessments) and patients who completed the study per protocol.

If data are being presented in Integrated Summaries of Safety or Efficacy then often several subgroup analyses are implemented. These include demographic subgroups (Males, Females, All patients ≤65, All patients ≥65, etc.). In addition, subgroup analyses may also be presented for those who have a certain medical condition or disease to study drug–disease interactions, and for those taking a certain concomitant medication to see if there are any drug–drug interactions.

In addition, tabulations for AEs often are further subdivided by 'Severity of AE', 'Attribution to Study Drug', and so on, to better understand the safety profile of the medicinal product.

Programmers concerned with data presentation must understand the structure of the underlying database. Certain database designs allow for ease of presentation while others optimize storage and retrieval. Yet other designs minimize the possibility of creating inconsistencies.

Database designers are concerned with constructing efficient robust systems and often categorize the above into the following categories:

One record per patient: Demographics, medical history and entry criteria.
One record per patient per visit: Drug accountability, efficacy, laboratory data, vital signs and physical examinations.
Multiple records per patient per visit: Coexistent diseases, prior and concomitant medications and adverse events.

Medical history, entry criteria, laboratory and physical exam data may also be set up as multiple records per patient.

Once clinical data have been entered into an electronic database, they must be validated and then subsequently analyzed.

PRESENTATION OF RAW DATA

Raw data or individual patient data refers to a display of the actual data that were captured from the patient. Generally these are the actual measurements or the information provided from the patient. There are cases, however, when this may include derived fields (e.g., age-based upon the date patient entered the trial and their date of birth). Raw data may also be an aggregate of information captured that more accurately reflects the measurement (e.g., average of two or more blood pressure measurements). Raw data would include all the data collected and can be presented in one of two ways:

1. *'By Form' data listings*
These listings present similar data for all patients. Typically the data are sorted by: (i) treatment patient was assigned to; (ii) patient number; and (iii) visit when data were recorded. An example of a 'By Form' data listing for Demographics is given in Figure 9.3 above.

Listings similar to the one in Figure 9.3 could be done for other types of data.

Listings such as in Figure 9.3 are very useful in reviewing data of a certain type (from a particular CRF) for all patients. 'By Form' data listings may also be generated by selecting key data from different CRFs and presenting them in the above format to allow a review of the data across different patients. The objective of 'By Form' data listings is to review the selected data across all patients.

Current ICH guidelines specifically request data presentations for 'By Form' data listings of: (i) patients who died; (ii) had serious adverse events; (iii) discontinued the study; (iv) had a lab abnormality; and (v) were excluded from the efficacy analyses. In addition full 'By Form' patient listings are also submitted as an appendix in lieu of submitting all CRFs.

2. *Case Report Form Tabulations (CRT)/Patient Synopsis*
CRTs or Patient Synopses are very useful tools to get a summary of what happened to a particular patient. These displays select key data from all the data collected for a patient across all visits and present them concisely over one or more pages. A CRT allows a reviewer to quickly see all relevant information, since it is presented within a few pages. Ideally a Patient Synopsis should be one or at most two pages. These usually include demographics and key safety information for a given patient. In addition, it is possible to include data discrepancies for a given patient along with the synopsis.

An example of a Patient Synopsis is given in Figure 9.4.

PRESENTATION OF SUMMARY DATA

Presentation of summary or aggregate data allows one to draw conclusions from an ocean of data. Incidence rates of events and means allow a reviewer to see what happened across all patients who were given a particular treatment, and how this compares to patients who were given a placebo (or alternative treatment). This can be done at a specific time point or over time.

PATIENT SYNOPSIS

Pharma XYZ, Inc.   Pt. No.: 0102
November 11, 1997
Study: XYZ 97-01, Comparison of Drug X, Drug Y and Placebo

Age: 23 Yrs   Sex: Male   Race: Caucasian

Height (Baseline): 6 ft 2 in   Weight (Baseline): 210 lbs

Patient Status:
    Patient completed study with no protocol violations.

Key Study Dates:
        Date informed consent signed: 27 Jan 1997
        Date of first screening visit (−3):   01 Feb 1997
        Date of first dose: 03 Mar 1997
        Date of last dose: 22 Mar 1997
        Date of last study visit (4):   22 Mar 1997

Study Medication Information:
        Drug compliance: 98.9%
        Dates off medication:
            Patient was off study drug: 12 Mar 1997 and 15 Mar 1997

Medical History (Abnormal Findings at Baseline):
        ....
        ....

Physical Exam (Abnormal Findings at Baseline):
        ....
        ....

Prior Medications (Between 6 weeks prior to enrollment and randomization
visit):
        ....
        ....

Concomitant Medications (Between randomization and last study visit):
        ....
        ....

Abnormal Physical Exam findings after randomization:
        ....
        ....

Adverse Events:
        ....
        ....

All clinically significant Lab. values:
        ....
        ....

Comments:
        ....
        ....

Figure 9.4 A Patient Synopsis or summary

One way to QA (Quality Assurance) and better understand summary data at the cost of generating more data presentations is to complement each summary display with a listing of the raw data used to generate the summaries. This allows one to see the raw data used to compute means and so on or to see which patients were included in a group when displaying incidence rates. At least one major pharmaceutical company tries to do this for all summary presentations.

Presentation of summary data can be categorized as below:

1. *Tables of descriptive statistics*

Tables of descriptive statistics present incidence rates (frequency counts and percentages) and other simple descriptive statistics such as the mean, standard deviation, median and quartiles. These are usually generated during the statistical analysis but are often helpful during data validation to identify outliers or potential data discrepancies. The author is aware of at least one large pharmaceutical company whose data management department produces extensive descriptive statistics at the point of database lock. This is different than most companies where these listings are generated by the statisticians after database lock.

Descriptive statistics include mean ages of patients in each treatment group, the percentage of males and females in each treatment group, the number or percentage of patients experiencing adverse experiences in each treatment group, and so on.

Tables 9.1, 9.2 and 9.3 in the Appendix are all examples of descriptive statistics. Often skillful SAS programmers manage to combine the results from statistical hypothesis testing onto tables with descriptive statistics.

2. *Statistical analysis/modeling*

Statistical analysis/modeling deals with performing statistical inference or hypothesis testing. This is usually the forte of Biostatisticians, who in recent years have become a much sought after group. There are several good references in Biostatistics and readers interested in this should consult one of these.

3. *Figures, plots or graphs*

Like descriptive statistics, figures (also called plots or graphs) allow reviewers to visually review and easily understand what the data indicate. A simple plot of laboratory data over time for each treatment group can indicate whether the drug has any adverse effect on individuals. In addition, including lines to indicate normal ranges can also allow one to quickly grasp the extent of the effect of the drug (Figure 9.5).

Plots are useful for understanding continuous data, hence while plots of Adverse Events or other categorical data are usually not helpful, plots of lab data are often essential. Plotting lab data allows one to identify outliers and see trends as well as to see how many observations were above or below the Normal Ranges.

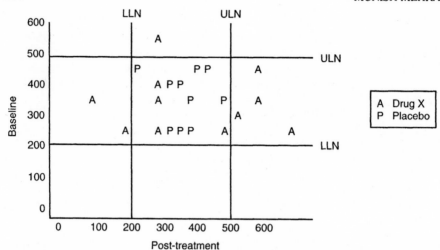

Figure 9.5 Plot of lab data. LLN: Lower limit of Normal; ULN: Upper limit of Normal

Plots may be generated for raw data (e.g., a patient's systolic blood pressure over time), for summary data (e.g., means across all patients for systolic blood pressure for each treatment group over time) or for statistical analyses (e.g., confidence intervals).

DATA PRESENTATION FOR VALIDATION

1. *Raw data or individual patient data*

Data presentations for validation should focus on identification of abnormal or potentially incorrect values. Hence either only the data outside a range or list of acceptable values should be displayed. If all data are printed then a flag (or symbol) should be printed next to the value to draw the reviewer's attention to the outliers.

Raw data may be presented either as 'By Form' listings, for example a print of all potentially discrepant demographic data. Alternatively raw data may be presented as a 'Patient Synopsis' or 'Case Report Form Tabulation'. These are summaries of all key data for a patient and would include the demographics data, concomitant medication information, adverse event data, comments and all other abnormalities. In addition, if potential discrepancies are flagged, a medical reviewer can quickly put a picture together of what happened to the patient and see if there are any inconsistencies in the information presented. These CRTs should be concise and should not try to print redundant information such as listing all inclusion/exclusion criteria, if the patient had met these criteria. See Figure 9.4 for a sample CRT.

2. *Summary or aggregate data to identify outliers*

When faced with a database of unknown quality, it is most helpful to quickly generate frequencies and a list of the outliers using PROC FREQ and PROC UNIVARIATE in SAS. This presents a 'quick and dirty' summary of the data. This idea may be extended to developing computer programs that provide descriptive summaries of the data, allowing a reviewer to quickly determine the quality of the database.

3. *Presentation for Quality Assurance*

Data presentations for QA must conform to the requirements per the QA plan written up by the auditors. When conducting a database audit this may be a print from the database of raw data listings for a percentage of patients.

It is usually easiest to write computer programs to generate these listings 'By Form'. However auditors prefer CRTs since CRFs are collated by patient and 'CRTs or synopsis' display data by patient. This amounts to more work for the programmers, but a lot less for the QA auditors.

Often a Patient Synopsis such as Figure 9.4 can allow QA auditors to compare key data in the database against those on the CRFs for selected patients very quickly.

DATA PRESENTATION FOR ANALYSIS

Once a database has been validated and deemed analyzable (i.e. all inconsistencies resolved and no erroneous values present), the statisticians generate statistical tables, figures, plots and summaries of statistical models fitted and tests performed. This allows formal determination of the efficacy and safety of the drug. Clinical trials must have enough patients and 'clean' data to make such a determination possible.

For further details of data presentations refer to the FDA Guideline for the format and content of the clinical and statistical sections of an NDA, July 1988 and the ICH draft guidelines on statistical principles for clinical trials, May 1997.

CONCLUSION

In conclusion, data presentation is an essential component of clinical data management and biostatistics. Clinical data managers must give sufficient thought to data presentation for easy review to ensure the accuracy of the data. Biostatisticians must realize that statistical modeling and hypothesis testing are of little use if the data are not presented in a manner that allows clinicians and other researchers to better understand the underlying phenomenon of interest—which is the efficacy and safety of the new medicinal product.

A well thought out data presentation can make both data validation and a review of the efficacy and safety of the data more accurate and efficient.

Appendix:
Sample Data Presentations

The following pages display some sample data presentations. Table 9.1 is an example of a table displaying continuous demographic data with the columns displaying the statistics, while the rows display the variables (parameters) and treatment groups. Tables 9.2 and 9.3 present categorical demographics and adverse events data respectively with the treatment groups and statistics as the columns and the variables and categories as the rows. Table 9.4 displays vital signs using a different format. Treatment groups are displayed as columns, but the variables and descriptive statistics are presented as rows.

In addition to displaying simple descriptive statistics it is also possible to include columns (or rows) displaying p-values from statistical hypothesis testing.

Table 9.1 Summary of demographics by treatment group (ITT Population)

Variable/Treatment group	N	Mean	SD	Minimum	Median	Maximum
Age (years)						
Approved Drug Y	396	33.0	11.21	12.0	30.0	72.0
New Drug X	396	31.6	10.50	12.0	29.0	57.0
Placebo	394	33.6	12.00	12.0	31.0	76.0
Total	1186	31.7	11.26	12.0	30.0	76.0
Height (in)						
Approved Drug Y	396	68.6	4.31	56.5	68.0	77.0
New Drug X	396	69.1	3.94	56.0	67.0	76.0
Placebo	394	67.5	3.92	59.0	66.0	76.0
Total	1186	68.1	4.08	56.0	67.0	77.0
Weight (lbs)						
Approved Drug Y	396	169.5	39.10	80.0	166.5	288.0
New Drug X	396	164.2	38.47	77.0	159.3	282.0
Placebo	394	165.0	38.05	100.0	157.0	290.0
Total	1186	164.5	38.59	77.0	160.0	290.0

Source: C:\PHARMAXYZ\XYZ-97-01\TABLE\TABLE.SAS(DEMOG.SD2)   OUTPUT: C:\PHARMAXYZ\XYZ-97-01\OUTPUT\DEMO1R.SD2 11NOV97 20:00

Table 9.2 Summary of demographics by treatment group (All randomized subjects)

| Variable/Category | Treatment group | | | | | | | |
| | Approved Drug Y | | New Drug X | | Placebo | | Total | |
	n	%	n	%	n	%	n	%
Gender								
Male	102	51.5	95	48.0	75	38.1	272	45.9
Female	96	48.5	103	52.0	122	61.9	321	54.1
Total	198		198		197		593	
Race								
Caucasian	144	72.7	147	74.2	139	70.6	430	72.5
Asian	7	3.5	6	3.0	8	4.1	21	3.5
Black	35	17.7	60	20.2	44	22.3	119	20.1
American Indian	0	0.0	1	0.5	0	0.0	1	0.2
Hispanic	10	5.1	3	1.5	3	1.5	16	2.7
Other	2	1.0	1	0.5	3	1.5	6	1.0
Total	198		198		197		593	

Source: C:\PHARMA\XYZ\XYZ-97-01\TABLE\TABLE2.SAS(DEMOG.SD2)   OUTPUT: C:\PHARMA\XYZ\XYZ_97-01\OUTPUT\DEMO2R.OUT   11NOV97   20:00

Table 9.3 Number and percent of subjects experiencing adverse events by treatment group, body system, and preferred term for all randomized subjects

| | Treatment group | | | | | | | | |
| | Approved Drug Y | | New Drug X | | Placebo | | Total | |
Body system/Preferred term	n	%	n	%	n	%	n	%
Total number of subjects	198		198		197		593	100
No. of Subj. with at least one AE	38	19.2	38	19.2	24	12.2	100	16.9
Body as a whole	26	13.1	12	6.1	15	7.6	53	8.9
HEADACHE	21	10.6	9	4.5	10	5.1	40	6.7
INFECTION	2	1.0	0	0.0	0	0.0	2	0.3
PAIN ABDOMEN	0	0.0	0	0.0	1	0.5	1	0.2
PAIN CHEST	0	0.0	1	0.5	0	0.0	1	0.2
Digestive	3	1.5	2	1.0	5	2.5	10	1.7
DIARRHEA	0	0.0	0	0.0	1	0.5	1	0.2
NAUSEA	2	1.0	2	1.0	4	2.0	8	1.3
NAUSEA VOMITING	1	0.5	0	0.0	2	1.0	3	0.5
Musculo-Skeletal	4	2.0	1	0.5	0	0.0	5	0.8
ARTHRALGIA	1	0.5	0	0.0	0	0.0	1	0.2
MYALGIA	1	0.5	0	0.0	0	0.0	1	0.2
Nervous	7	3.5	22	11.1	7	3.6	36	6.1
DIZZINESS	2	1.0	4	2.0	0	0.0	6	1.0
DRY MOUTH	1	0.5	1	0.5	0	0.0	2	0.3
NERVOUSNESS	2	1.0	1	0.5	1	0.5	4	0.7
PARESTHESIA	1	0.5	0	0.0	0	0.0	1	0.2
SOMNOLENCE	4	2.0	17	8.6	6	3.0	27	4.6

Pharma XYZ, Inc.
Study: XYZ 97-01
Comparison of New Drug X, Approved Drug Y, and Placebo
Population: (Evaluable subjects)

November 11, 1997
Final

Table 9.4 Summary of vital signs at baseline by treatment group

		Treatment group	
	Approved Drug Y	New Drug X	Placebo
Oral temperature (F)			
N,	243	251	235
Mean (SD)	95.5 (0.64)	98.4 (0.59)	97.6 (0.61)
Min, Max	94.3, 99.8	94.1, 100.2	95.1, 99.7
Heart rate (bpm)			
N	243	251	235
Mean (SD)	75.5 (8.44)	73.1 (9.88)	74.9 (8.11)
Min, Max	59, 104	62, 102	54, 106
Systolic BP (mmHg)			
N	243	251	235
Mean (SD)	113.5 (13.14)	114.3 (12.34)	112.8 (14.53)
Min, Max	86, 143	75, 139	79, 141
Diastolic BP (mmHg)			
N	243	251	235
Mean (SD)	73.2 (11.32)	72.1 (8.99)	73.2 (9.21)
Min, Max	59, 101	52, 105	49, 102

Source: C:\PHARMAXYZ\XYZ-97-01\TABLE\TABLE4.SAS(VS.SD2)   OUTPUT: C:\PHARMAXYZ\XYZ-97-01\OUTPUT\VS.OUT   11NOV97   20:00

10 Coding of Data—MedDRA and other Medical Terminologies

ELLIOT G. BROWN and LOUISE WOOD

EBC Ltd, High Barnet, Herts, and Medicines Control Agency, London, UK

INTRODUCTION

This chapter examines the way in which clinical data from various sources and phases in the regulatory life cycle of medicines are entered onto a computer database, analysed, presented and exchanged with other organisations. The process of capturing these data on a database is known by many as 'coding'. Until the early 1990s, it involved the selection of a word or phrase from a medical terminology and entry of the corresponding code (numeric, alphabetic or alphanumeric) onto a database. Coding was necessary because it required little space for storage on the database and made searching easier. However, the evolution of information technology over the last decade has meant that databases can easily accommodate text. This allows validation against a medical terminology at data entry, which enhances speed and accuracy. It obviates the need for searching through paper versions of the terminology to locate a code and prevents errors caused by incorrect keying in of numerical codes. The introduction of relational databases has allowed more sophisticated medical terminologies to be used. Despite these changes, the term 'coding' is still used to refer to data entry.

There is a plethora of medical terminologies available. Some were designed to encompass the whole of medical practice. For example, in the UK, Read Codes are the agreed standard for coding of medical terms in the National Health Service, whilst in the US, the Systemised Nomenclature of Medicine (SNOMED) is used widely. In addition there are many specialist medical terminologies and classifications, such as DSM-IV for psychiatric illnesses, classifications for tumours (ICD-oncology), laboratory and clinical observation coding (LOINC). However, the focus of this chapter is on medical terminologies which are used in the medicines regulatory environment. Brief outlines of the standard terminologies used are presented, but the emphasis is on the *Medical Dictionary for Regulatory Activities* (MedDRA), as this has been adopted by the International

Clinical Data Management. Second Edition. Edited by R.K. Rondel, S.A. Varley and C.F. Webb.
© 2000 John Wiley & Sons, Ltd

Conference on Harmonisation (ICH) as the standard medical terminology for regulatory communication.

WHY DO WE NEED TO CODE CLINICAL DATA?

For those involved in clinical research or pharmacovigilance in the pharmaceutical industry or regulatory authorities, the need is self-evident. However, for the reader who is new to these activities, it should be said that, in the course of our daily work, we deal with a variety of types of data from various sources. Often, there is a huge volume of data which has to be recorded and stored in a controlled manner, then retrieved, analysed and presented in a number of different formats in a reproducible fashion and for a variety of purposes.

For example, detailed information on adverse events for individual patients is collected in the course of clinical trials and post-marketing safety surveillance and may have to be communicated rapidly to regulatory authorities to meet legal obligations. Tabulations of data on safety and efficacy derived from clinical trials may need to be created to support applications for marketing authorisation of a new medicine; summary data may be needed to construct the standard product information comprising the Summary of Product Characteristics or product 'labelling'. In addition, we may need to review data compilations to search for signals of new adverse drug reactions (ADRs) and to present analyses of these in periodic safety update reports on marketed drugs. Similarly, these compilations may be required for responses to the internal and external enquiries on individual aspects of safety or efficacy which arise during the lifetime of a medicinal product. The types of data that are particularly relevant to this chapter include the patient's medical and social history, descriptions of adverse events and reactions together with concurrent illnesses and the therapeutic indications, contraindications, warnings and precautions associated with the use of a medicine.

It would be possible to store all this information as free text on a computer database, thus ensuring that the output from the database would match the input and hence comprise the multitude of ways that the data may have been recorded. Consider a patient with vertigo. A doctor noting the symptoms might have written 'has vertigo', 'feels vertiginous', 'feels as if spinning', 'spinning sensation', 'complains of room going round' and so forth. If we were subsequently required to identify all cases of vertigo, we would need to search for all the relevant different expressions captured in the free text. This would be time-consuming and it would be easy to miss some cases, for example those reported as room spinning. Furthermore, a colleague performing the same data analysis may obtain a different answer because he or she has used different search criteria.

Hence, although free text is often stored on a database, data entry is standardised by using a medical terminology. This links synonymous or similar terms and hence facilitates rapid, consistent and complete retrieval of information. The pyramidal structure of medical terminologies— a large number of terms at the bottom, tapering upwards via intermediate grouping levels to smaller numbers of classes or grouping categories at the top—enables large volumes of data to be summarised. Numbers of similar data points at any level can be counted and presented in a tabular form. Coded data can be readily searched, sorted and manipulated using a computer (see Table 10.1).

Table 10.1 Coding facilitates data management

Recording, storage of data
Data search and retrieval
Data manipulation and analysis
Counting and tabulation
Summarisation
Presentation in different formats
Reproducibility and standardisation

PROBLEMS IN CODING

Although the practice of coding is a ubiquitous and necessary activity in the pharmaceutical medical and regulatory environments, it is not without problems (see Table 10.2). Coding itself may be time-consuming. Terminologies may need to be updated frequently to respond to new requirements imposed by the data and effective maintenance can require considerable professional resource. At the MCA, for example, there is a weekly meeting of scientists and physicians to add new terms to the medical terminology used in its databases. For those organisations using static terminologies, the absence of an updating facility means that terms for which there is no appropriate match are coded inaccurately or risk matching in an inconsistent manner to existing terms.

Table 10.2 Coding may be problematic

Time-consuming, resource-intensive
Codes need updating, validating
Non-standardisation: communication problems
Lumping: lose specificity and original meaning
Splitting: difficult data retrieval and aggregation

Another difficulty arises because of the large number of terminologies in general use which deal with the same type of data. Thus, although there are standard terminologies for adverse reactions, such as COSTART or WHO-ART (see below), many pharmaceutical companies find that these are not extensive enough to cover their needs and they therefore customise these standard terminologies by adding their own terms. Needless to say, a customised standard terminology is not standard! Other organisations have preferred to create their own terminologies de novo.

Problems then arise when two organisations need to exchange data. Suppose that the terminology which I use lumps together all reports of all types of breathlessness and difficulties in breathing and calls them 'dyspnoea'—which is probably a reasonable thing to do in the context of a clinical trial, say. In some circles, I would be referred to as a 'lumper'. Your terminology—again perfectly reasonably—separates out dyspnoea, tachypnoea (rapid breathing) and orthopnoea (breathlessness on lying flat). This might be referred to as 'splitting' the terms. Unless you have access to my coding method, you will misunderstand me when I inform you that my database contains 25 cases of dyspnoea. Conversely, if you tell me that you have only 20 cases of dyspnoea on your database, I may not appreciate that there are additionally reports coded as orthopnoea or tachypnoea.

Many individual companies experience problems with compatibility of data because different medical terminologies are used in the clinical development and post-marketing departments or because different subsidiaries use different terminologies. Some companies use different coding dictionaries for adverse events in clinical trial and safety databases, hence the same event will be coded differently in each database.

Another aspect of this question of 'specificity' arises when we wish to retrieve data. Suppose we received 10 reports of blue vision occurring with a drug which is already known to cause blurred vision in some patients. If the specificity of our medical terminology was low, we might find that such cases were 'lumped' together with reports of blurred vision, scotoma, colour blindness, myopia, halo effect, tunnel vision—all of these being coded as 'vision disorder'. Indeed, our terminology may have no term which is more specific than vision disorder. We might then be unable to say how many reports of blue vision we really have, without looking at all the reports of vision disorder individually, which may be time-consuming and difficult. All that we know from reviewing coded data in our database is that we have 45 cases of vision disorder.

Looking at a printout from our database, staff who are unfamiliar with the dictionary structure might be falsely reassured into thinking that these 45 cases were all blurred vision, which they know the drug can cause, when in reality several of them constituted something new and unexpected. On the other hand, if we have large numbers of subdivisions of terms, that is a terminology of high granularity, we may experience problems when we try to retrieve data and to analyse and present them in tabular form. Because there are so many individual terms, which may be dispersed throughout a large terminology, we may forget to include some when trying to retrieve all related terms or conditions.

SOME STANDARD MEDICAL TERMINOLOGIES

Typically medical terminologies are organised into System Organ Classes which represent disorders of a body system and/or groups of organs which together perform a particular function. Preferred Terms are the basic units of the terminologies.

World Health Organisation Adverse Reaction Terminology (WHO-ART)

This terminology is widely used by regulatory authorities and, usually in modified, expanded format, by the pharmaceutical industry. It is available in English, French, Spanish, German and Portuguese and a Japanese adaptation (J-ART) is also available. The European translations are complete down to the Preferred Term level. The terminology is maintained and distributed by the WHO Uppsala Monitoring Centre.

WHO-ART is organised according to 32 System Organ Classes. Preferred Terms are included under one or more System Organ Classes and these are the basic unit for recording data for regulatory and pharmacovigilance purposes (see Table 10.3). Preferred Terms may be grouped together under High Level Terms, but many are not grouped in this way. At the lowest level in the terminology are the Included Terms, each of which is associated with a Preferred Term. Each System Organ Class is represented by a four-digit code. Additional four-digit codes are used to represent Preferred Terms. Each Included Term has a unique code, the first four digits of which are the Preferred Term code.

WHO-ART is available as paper or electronic versions. It is arranged in two listings. One of these is ordered by System Organ Class, showing first the High Level Terms in alphabetic order, with the linked Preferred Terms and Included Terms, then listing the unlinked Preferred Terms in alphabetical order with their associated Included Terms. The other list is shown in alphabetical order of Included Terms.

Advantages of WHO-ART include its simplicity, the logical numerical coding system and the fact that it is well known and has been widely used. Its relatively small size means that users can easily become familiar with its contents. Its specificity is poor, so that the medical meaning of the original report or case may be lost in coding. In addition, the poorly

Table 10.3 Extract from a WHO-ART SOC

SOC 1300 Urinary system disorders

HLT Renal function abnormal

PT	*0595 Albuminuria*	
IC		Proteinuria
		Bence Jones proteinuria
		Proteinuria aggravated
PT	*0598 Creatinine clearance decreased*	
PT	*0613 Polyuria*	
IC		Urine volume increased
		Diuresis excessive
PT	*0931 Kidney contracted*	
PT	*0618 Renal failure acute*	
IC		Renal failure acute ischaemic
		Renal shutdown acute
		Renal failure acute hypotensive
PT	*0619 Renal function abnormal*	
IC		Renal concentrating power decr
		Hyposthenuria
		Isosthenuria
		Kidney dysfunction
		Renal function tests NOS abnormal
		Urine specific gravity fixed
		Renal clearance low
		Renal failure aggravated
		Renal failure NOS
		Decreased fluid output
PT	*0620 Renal function abnormal glomer*	
PT	*0627 Urinary casts*	
IC		Cylinduria

SOC = System Organ Class
HLT = High Level Term
PT = Preferred Term
IC = Included Term

developed hierarchy means that in reality the only useful groupings for data retrieval and presentation are at the System Organ Class level.

Coding System for a Thesaurus of Adverse Reaction Terms (COSTART)

This terminology is maintained and distributed by the US Food and Drug Administration (FDA) and was used by them for drug safety surveillance prior to the advent of MedDRA. The so-called COSTART—'Glossary terms'—are represented by long alphabetic coding symbols. The expanded coding symbol is called the 'printed as' term—for example,

ADENOMA THYR for thyroid adenoma. Several Glossary terms are typically associated with one Coding Symbol—for example, PAIN ABDO is the Symbol associated with the Glossary terms abdominal cramp, abdominal discomfort, abdominal pain lower, abdominal pain upper, and so on (see Tables 10.4, 10.5). Glossary terms are used to identify the most appropriate COSTART Coding Symbol for entry onto a database. Since Glossary terms do not have unique codes, the precision of the original reported description is usually lost during coding.

Table 10.4 Illustration of a COSTART SOC

SOC MUSCULOSKELETAL

COSTART CODING SYMBOLS
Anomaly congen MS
Arthralgia
Arthritis
Arthritis pyogen
Arthritis rheumat
Arthrosis
Atrophy muscle
Bone dis
Bone fract spontan
Bone implant lysis
Bursitis
Chondrodyst
Cramps leg
Cramps legs
Epiphys clos delay
Epiphys clos premat
Fibro tendon
Fluorosis
Hem muscle
Joint dis
Myalgia
Myasthenia
(Etc.)

The COSTART terminology comprises 12 Body System Classes and is arranged according to several indices: a mid-level pathophysiological classification for retrieval purposes (see Table 10.6); lists of COSTART Coding Symbols and associated 'printed as' terms; and a number of search categories. These comprise clusters of terms for a variety of conditions such as application site reactions, collagen disorder, hypersensitivity, efficacy lack, neoplasia. In addition, there are maps showing equivalent WHO-ART Preferred Terms and COSTART Coding Symbols.

Table 10.5 Examples of COSTART Glossary terms with associated COSTART coding symbols

Glossary term	Coding symbol
Jaundice hemolytic	Anemia hemol
Jaundice hepatocellular	Hepatitis
Jaundice neonatal	Jaundice neonat
Jaw malformation	Anomaly congen MS
Jaw pain	Pain
Jitteriness	Nervousness
Joint ache	Arthralgia
Joint dislocation temperomandibular	Joint dis
Joint disorder	Joint dis
Joint effusion	Arthrosis
Joint inflammation	Arthritis
Joint malformation	Anomaly congen MS
Joint pain	Arthralgia
Joint stiffness	Joint dis
Joint swelling non-inflammatory	Arthrosis
	(Etc.)

International Classification of Diseases

This system is a hierarchical classification for statistical purposes, rather than a terminology per se, which was developed for the collection of morbidity and mortality data. There have been a number of revisions and versions over the years. Although it was not designed for regulatory use, there is currently extensive use of ICD-9, ICD-9-CM and ICD-10 in the pharmaceutical regulatory environment, primarily in the clinical trial context. The ICD classifications have a single variable axis whereby aetiology is the only grouping option, with the exception of a small proportion of terms covered by the 'dagger and asterisk' system which also allows for classification by manifestation.

In ICD-9, there are 17 chapters plus two supplementary classifications—External causes of injury and poisoning; Factors influencing health status and contact with health services. The chapter headings are similar to System Organ Classes, for example 'I. Infectious and Parasitic Diseases', 'VIII. Diseases of the Respiratory System', and so on. Each chapter is divided up into subgroups represented by discrete three digit codes, each code delimiting a more specific group of medical conditions. Thus, Infectious Diseases are covered by the codes 001–139, Mental Disorders by codes 290–319. Within the Infectious and Parasitic Diseases chapter, Cholera is 001, Typhoid and paratyphoid fevers 002, Other Salmonella infections 003, and so on.

Additional digits are used to represent more specific diseases, so that 001.1 is Cholera due to Vibrio cholerae. The four-digit codes ending .8

Table 10.6   Illustration of a COSTART mid-level system

Description	Mid-level code	Coding symbols
AIRWAYS DISEASE	PULMAIRWAY	Asthma Bronchiectasis Bronchosteno Cough dec Cough inc (Etc.)
INFECTION	PULMINFECT	Bronchiectasis Bronchiolitis Bronchitis Pneumonia Pneumonia aspir Pneumonia interstit (Etc.)
METABOLIC	PULMETABOLIC	Acidosis resp Alkalosis resp
NONSPECIFIC/GENERAL	PULMGEN	Apnea Cough dec Cough inc Dyspnea Edema lung (Etc.)
PLEURAL	PULMPLEURAL	Effus pleural Pleural dis Pneumothorax (Etc.)

refer to 'other' related conditions and .9 refer to conditions which are 'unspecified', such as unspecified mastoiditis (i.e. not stated whether acute, chronic, etc.).

In the 'dagger and asterisk' system, the asterisk (*) is placed in the chapter of the organ system to which the manifestation or complication relates. The dagger (†) is placed in the chapter relating to the diagnosis and underlying disease. For example, in Chapter X, Diseases of the Genitourinary System, we find '585 Chronic renal failure' and in association with it, 'Uraemic pericarditis † (420.0*)', and 'Uraemic neuropathy † (357.4*)'. Uraemic neuropathy is also included as the subsidiary term

'357.4* Polyneuropathy in other diseases classified elsewhere, Uraemic (585†)' in Chapter VI, Diseases of the Nervous System and Sense Organs, under the heading '357 Inflammatory and toxic neuropathy'. Similarly, in Chapter VII, Diseases of the Circulatory System, we find '420 Acute pericarditis', under which is the term '420.0* Pericarditis in diseases classified elsewhere. Uraemic (585†)'.

ICD-9-CM provides additional specificity by having five digit codes, so that Mastoiditis and related conditions are coded as 383, Acute mastoiditis is 383.0, Acute mastoiditis without complications is 383.00, whereas subperiosteal abscess of mastoid is 383.01 (see also Table 10.7).

Table 10.7 Illustration of the structure of ICD-9-CM

320–389 Diseases of the nervous system and sense organs
  330–337 Hereditary and degenerative diseases of the central nervous system
     335   Anterior horn cell disease
       335.2   Motor neuron disease
         335.2 0   Amyotrophic lateral sclerosis
         335.2 1   Progressive muscular atrophy
         335.2 2   Progressive bulbar palsy
                                          (etc.)

ICD-10, released in 1993, has an alphanumeric hierarchical coding scheme. As with ICD-9, there is a facility for multiaxiality highlighted with dagger and asterisk symbols—so that terms can be present in more than one chapter/System Organ Class—and the possibility of allocation of dual codes to individual terms. ICD-10 comprises three volumes. The first provides a tabular list including the classification at three- and four-character levels, a morphological classification of neoplasms, lists for mortality and morbidity, definitions and nomenclature regulations. A second volume includes an instruction manual and an alphabetical index is provided in the third volume.

Examples of the chapters are II. Neoplasms, V. Mental and Behavioural Disorders. The contents of the chapters are designated by a letter of the alphabet. For example, Chapter IV includes Endocrine, nutritional and metabolic diseases (E00–E90). These cover Disorders of thyroid gland (E00–E07), Diabetes mellitus (E10–E14), Other disorders of glucose regulations and pancreatic internal secretion, Disorders of other endocrine glands, Malnutrition, and so forth.

As an example of the structure, Disorders of thyroid gland E00–E07, are subdivided into seven categories, including: E00 Congenital iodine-deficiency syndrome, E01 Iodine-deficiency-related thyroid disorders and allied conditions, E02 Subclinical iodine-deficiency hypothyroidism, E03 Other hypothyroidism, E04 Other nontoxic goitre, and so on.

E06, Thyroiditis, excludes postpartum thyroiditis, which is present in the chapter covering pregnancy. It covers Acute thyroiditis E06.0, Subacute thyroiditis E06.1, Chronic thyroiditis with transient thyrotoxicosis E06.2, Autoimmune thyroiditis E06.3, and so on. Each of the four-letter/digit coded terms is associated with one or more lower level terms which do not have a code. For example, E06.3 Autoimmune thyroiditis has terms such as Hashimoto's thyroiditis, Hashitoxicosis, Lymphadenoid goitre, associated with it.

THE MEDICAL DICTIONARY FOR REGULATORY ACTIVITIES (MedDRA)

Background and Development

Perceived deficiencies in existing medical terminologies used for drug regulatory affairs include: a lack of specificity of data entry terms; limited data retrieval options because of poorly developed hierarchies; inadequate maintenance, such that the terminologies have not evolved in response to user needs. In addition, there is no medical or scientific rationale for using separate adverse drug reaction (ADR) and morbidity terminologies. It introduces unnecessary complexity to computer systems and to the tracking of events throughout a product's lifetime. Having recognised this, the UK Medicines Control Agency (MCA) developed its own unified medical terminology for regulatory affairs in the late 1980s and early 1990s. This is used in its ADROIT pharmacovigilance database and its product licence databases (PLUS). Several large pharmaceutical companies also developed their own medical terminologies as the increasing complexity of the pharmaceutical regulatory environment highlighted the shortcomings of existing terminologies. These were frequently based on existing systems such as ICD-9 and COSTART. With the advent of the European regulatory system and the EUDRA initiatives to facilitate electronic communication between regulatory authorities in European Union Member States, it was recognised that there was a need for a unified standard medical terminology across the European Union. The MEDDRA (*Medical Dictionary for Drug Regulatory Affairs*) project was set up by the MCA to further develop its medical terminology and to investigate whether such a terminology could support the exchange of regulatory data in Europe. A Working Party comprising representatives of the UK, French and Spanish regulatory authorities, together with participants from eight international pharmaceutical companies and the Pharmaceutical Research and Manufacturers of America (PhRMA), met for the first time in November 1993 to perform this task and were subsequently joined by observers from the

US FDA and the WHO Uppsala Monitoring Centre. The aims of the Working Party were to:

1. review the MCA's medical terminology and to modify it in order to produce a first draft of MEDDRA in electronic format for wider consultation;
2. work towards international acceptance for one terminology for use in drug regulation; to commence piloting the use of MEDDRA for a variety of regulatory purposes; and
3. propose options for the long-term maintenance of MEDDRA.

The project's objectives were endorsed by the EU Committee on Proprietary Medicinal Products in December 1993.

At a meeting in September 1994 held under the auspices of the Council for the International Organisation of Medical Sciences (CIOMS), representatives of regulatory authorities, WHO, international pharmaceutical companies and dictionary user groups agreed that MEDDRA version 1.0 should form the basis of a new international medical regulatory terminology and that the parties concerned should devote their efforts to this project. In addition, it was agreed that the ongoing project to define adverse reaction terms should continue separately under the aegis of CIOMS, but focus on MEDDRA rather than WHO-ART Preferred Terms.

The medical terminology project was progressed within the framework of ICH following the establishment of the medical terminology (M1) Expert Working Group (EWG) under the chairmanship of Dr Sue Wood. The M1 EWG comprised representatives of the FDA, the Japanese Ministry of Health and Welfare, the European Union and the pharmaceutical trade associations of the US, Japan and Europe, with the MCA acting as the Rapporteur for the EU. WHO were observers.

MEDDRA version 1.0 was released, free of charge, for testing in November 1994 to regulatory authorities worldwide and to pharmaceutical companies and associated organisations. Over 600 copies were distributed as part of this alpha test. Although only a short time was available for the test, there were 46 responses, reporting on a range of testing activities. In March 1995, the M1 EWG met for the first time and embarked upon a programme of activities leading to the EWG 'deliverables' of a terminology of agreed content and structure ('the implementable version') together with an agreed maintenance framework, with work continuing until July 1997.

It defined the scope of the terminology and its hierarchical levels, agreed its rules and conventions, developed the user manual, completed the incorporation of all data entry level terms from WHO-ART, COSTART, ICD-9, ICD-9-CM and the Japanese versions of WHO-ART (J-ART) and ICD-9 (MEDIS) and ensured that the multiaxial links in the terminology were appropriate and complete. In addition, it incorporated changes agreed as a result of the alpha test and the subsequent widespread consultation in the US and Japan. MEDDRA Version 1.5 was released in electronic format in February 1996 for further review and testing purposes. As a result of this, it was agreed that all levels in the hierarchy should be populated for all terms. The number of High Level Terms and High Level Group Terms was expanded to improve its utility for data retrieval and presentation purposes. The names of all the terms at the High Level Term and High Level Group Term levels were reviewed, and amended if necessary, to enhance transparency of the subsidiary terms.

There was also a major expansion and restructuring of the Neoplasms, Infections and infestations and Psychiatric disorders System Organ Classes, resulting in a considerable enlargement of the terminology at the lower levels. Restructuring of the Investigations System Organ Classes was also performed at this time to provide clinically relevant groupings for purposes of data retrieval.

The framework, organisational reporting structure and remit for the maintenance organisation were developed and the preparatory work for its recruitment via an open competitive tendering process was completed.

In July 1997, at the Fourth International Conference on Harmonisation, the ICH Steering Committee signed off the implementable version of the terminology (V2.0) and renamed it the *Medical Dictionary for Regulatory Activities* (MedDRA) terminology. It then fell to the ICH Steering Committee and its Tender Evaluation Panel to select the MedDRA Maintenance and Support Services Organisation, which in turn would distribute the terminology to future users and be responsible for its long-term maintenance.

At the time of writing, linguistic translations are complete down to and including Preferred Terms for French, Spanish and Japanese. Although the full terminology is written in British English, there are many American English alternatives among the Lowest Level Terms. German and Portuguese translations are planned. It is anticipated that the Maintenance and Support Services Organisation will provide additional translations if there is a business need to develop and support these.

MedDRA Scope and Utility

MedDRA was designed to be applicable to all phases (excluding animal toxicology) of development and post-authorisation activities of medicinal and biologically derived products, to post-authorisation activities, and to describe the health effects of medical devices. The terms in MedDRA cover medical diagnoses, symptoms and signs, ADRs, therapeutic indications, the names and qualitative results of laboratory, radiological and other investigations, surgical and medical procedures, and social circumstances.

MedDRA does not include a drug or device nomenclature or terms covering study design, pharmacokinetics or patient demographics. It does not include adjectives such as those describing disease severity or frequency, although qualifiers such as acute, chronic, recurrent are included in terms when clinically relevant. There are separate Preferred Terms for medical conditions and aggravation or exacerbation of the condition.

In the pre-registration phases of a product's life cycle, MedDRA may be used, for example, for recording adverse events and medical history in clinical trials, in the analysis and tabulations of data from these and in the expedited submission of adverse event data to government regulatory authorities. It may be used in constructing standard product information, such as Summaries of Product Characteristics or product labelling, and in registration files in support of applications for Marketing Authorisation/ New Drug Applications. After licensing, it is expected that MedDRA will be used in pharmacovigilance for the continuing evaluation of drug safety, for both expedited and periodic safety reporting. MedDRA is the preferred terminology for international electronic regulatory communication under the ICH M2 and E2B agreements.

The Structure of MedDRA

The structure of MedDRA is represented diagrammatically in Figure 10.1. As will be explained below, MedDRA is multiaxial as well as being hierarchical, so that Preferred Terms, with their associated Lowest Level Terms, may be represented under more than one System Organ Class. Table 10.8 shows the 26 MedDRA SOCs.

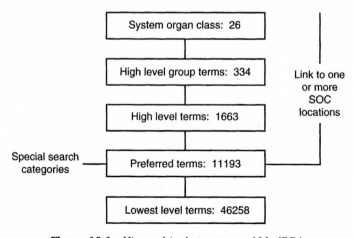

Figure 10.1   Hierarchical structure of MedDRA

Table 10.8 MedDRA System Organ Classes

Blood and lymphatic system disorders
Cardiac disorders
Congenital and familial/genetic disorders
Ear and labyrinth disorders
Endocrine disorders
Eye disorders
Gastrointestinal disorders
General disorders and administration site conditions
Hepato-biliary disorders
Immune system disorders
Infections and infestations
Injury and poisoning
Investigations
Metabolism and nutrition disorders
Musculoskeletal, connective tissue and bone disorders
Neoplasms benign and malignant (including cysts and polyps)
Nervous system disorders
Pregnancy, puerperium and perinatal disorders
Psychiatric disorders
Renal and urinary disorders
Reproductive system and breast disorders
Respiratory, thoracic and mediastinal disorders
Skin and subcutaneous tissue disorders
Social circumstances
Surgical and medical procedures
Vascular disorders

Each Preferred Term represents a separate, unique medical concept which is within the scope of MedDRA; it is the term preferred for use in the regulatory environment and is formatted according to MedDRA conventions. Preferred Terms are unambiguous, specific and self-descriptive. Eponymous terms are only used if recognised internationally. It should be noted that a Preferred Term may describe a single syndrome, even though a syndrome represents a collection of signs and symptoms. Each Preferred Term is duplicated as a Lowest Level Term and may be linked to one or more other Lowest Level Terms which are synonyms, lexical variants or alternative spellings of the Preferred Term. In addition, some Lowest Level Terms describe conditions which are more precise or specific than the Preferred Term to which they are linked; whilst not synonymous, they do not warrant Preferred Term status from a regulatory perspective. An example of a Preferred Term and some of the Lowest Level Terms which are linked to it is shown in Table 10.9. Pneumonitis allergic and Pneumonitis hypersensitivity are synonyms; Allergic pneumonitis and Pneumonitis allergic are lexical variants; Bagassosis and Baggasosis demonstrate differences in spelling; Malt worker's lung and Bird fancier's lung are different conditions which do not warrant a separate Preferred Term from a regulatory perspective. The Preferred Term Alveolitis allergic is duplicated at the lower level.

Table 10.9   MedDRA Alveolitis allergic PT, examples of Lowest Level Terms

Lowest Level Terms
Allergic pneumonitis
Alveolitis allergic
Alveolitis extrinsic
Bagassosis
Baggasosis
Bird fancier's lung
Extrinsic allergic alveolitis
Farmer's lung
Humidifier lung
Malt worker's lung
Maple bark-stripper's lung
Mushroom worker's lung
Other allergic pneumonitis
Other specified allergic alveolitis and pneumonitis
Paint stripper's asthma
Pneumonitis allergic
Pneumonitis hypersensitivity
Suberosis
Unspecified allergic alveolitis
Unspecified allergic alveolitis and pneumonitis
Ventilation pneumonitis
Woodworker's lung
(Etc.Etc.)

Each Preferred Term is represented only once under a particular System Organ Class, to which it is connected vertically via a single High Level Term (HLT), which in turn is fixed in location and represented only once in that System Organ Class under one High Level Group Term. However, the parallel vertical System Organ Class axes are not mutually exclusive; a Preferred Term may also be linked to secondary locations in one or more other System Organ Classes, in which it is again placed under a specified High Level Term and High Level Group Term, retaining its associated Lowest Level Terms. Having multiple locations for a Preferred Term within the terminology has the advantage that the way medical conditions are presented is not artificially constrained by their location. Terms may be sited according to aetiology, pathology, location, body function and so on. Thus, for example, 'cerebrovascular accident' may be represented in tabulations as a vascular or a neurological event, depending on context. Each

Preferred Term has a Primary System Organ Class to enable cumulative data to be presented without double counting of terms. Primary System Organ Classes are 'hard-wired' in MedDRA and allocated on the basis of defined conventions. The detailed MedDRA user guide explains the development of the terminology and defines hierarchical levels and the rationale and conventions for their use. It will be made available to users when MedDRA is distributed by the Maintenance and Support Services Organisation.

An important concept which may cause confusion is the fact that each Preferred Term has only one 'route' up the hierarchy within a given System Organ Class. Thus, for example, in the Investigations System Organ Class, the PT 'Prothrombin level decreased' appears under the High Level Term 'Coagulation and bleeding analyses'. Even though a decreased prothrombin level may also be a sign of severe hepatic dysfunction, this Preferred Term cannot also be represented under the High Level Term 'Liver function analyses' within the same System Organ Class.

A noteworthy convention applies to investigations. These are represented only in the Investigations System Organ Class; there are no secondary linkages. However, terms describing clinical conditions, for example hypoglycaemia, hyperkalaemia, are excluded from the Investigations System Organ Class: they are present only in other System Organ Classes such as Disorders of Metabolism and Nutrition. This has important implications for search strategies (see below). In the Investigations System Organ Class, there are commonly Preferred Terms to describe a high value, a normal value and a low value, as well as terms for the investigation parameter itself without qualification (e.g., serum sodium high, serum sodium low, serum sodium normal, serum sodium). The latter type of term may be useful in setting up database fields, in which numerical values may then be entered.

High Level Group Terms and High Level Terms are designed for data analysis, retrieval and presentation. They provide clinically relevant groupings of terms for drug regulatory purposes. However, attempts to make the 'contents' of a High Level Term or High Level Group Term transparent have resulted in some of the names of the High Level Terms or High Level Group Terms becoming rather cumbersome, for example the High Level Term 'Gastrointestinal necrosis and gangrene (excluding gangrenous hernia)' or the High Level Group Term 'Cognitive and attention disorders and disturbances (all forms)'. It may be that the maintenance organisation will consider standardising abbreviations for some of these group terms, if they do not sit comfortably as table sub-headings when used in the presentation of data in their present state.

MedDRA includes data entry terms from several sources. Version 2.0 includes all Preferred Terms and Included terms from the (WHO-ART, latest version) and its Japanese adaptation (J-ART, 1996), COSTART (5th

Edition) Printed As and Glossary Terms, HARTS (Release 2.2) terms, ICD-9 three and four-digit code terms and ICD-9-CM (4th revision) three, four and five digit code terms, as well as terms from the Japanese adaptation of ICD-9, MEDIS. These terms are included as Lowest Level Terms in Med-DRA: some are also Preferred Terms. Their source numerical codes or symbols are stored in attribute fields linked to the MedDRA terms. They have been included in order to facilitate the migration of legacy data at the time of transfer to using MedDRA. Vague, obsolete, mis-spelt or hybrid terms which have been 'inherited' from other terminologies are flagged as non-current. These are retained in MedDRA as Lowest Level Terms and can be used to preserve historical information, but will not be used for new data entry. It is planned that data entry terms from ICD-10 will be included in MedDRA at a later date. Each MedDRA term has an associated unique numerical code but there is no hierarchical sequence to these. It should be noted that the location of terms within MedDRA does not reflect their position in source hierarchies: it is not a metathesaurus.

Using MedDRA for Data Entry

Because of the large size of MedDRA, the selection of terms for data entry will generally require the use of an autoencoder and/or a computerised search programme. It is intended that data should be entered at the Med-DRA Lowest Level Term level in order to capture the specificity of the information on the source document. When a MedDRA Lowest Level Term or Preferred Term is selected for data entry, there is automatic up-posting within the hierarchy—that is assignment of Preferred Term, High Level Term, High Level Group Term, and location in primary System Organ Class together with secondary System Organ Class linkages. Hence, data entry staff are not selecting these on an ad hoc basis, which would result in inconsistencies.

Although the large number of Lowest Level Terms in MedDRA make the chances of an exact match with the recorded or verbatim term likely, there will still be a large proportion of instances where this is not the case. Under these circumstances, two approaches might be taken. Firstly, a search for words or parts of words in MedDRA which are similar to the verbatim term. If this does not produce an acceptable match, it is possible to search likely locations in the terminology based on suitable High Level Terms or High Level Group Terms for an appropriate Preferred Term and Lowest Level Term. For example, if we are looking for a term which is equivalent to the verbatim term 'acute GI distress', it would be logical to look in the MedDRA Gastrointestinal System Organ Class and on an intuitive basis, to see what Preferred Terms exist under the Gastrointestinal Symptoms and Signs High Level Term. The 'best fit' Lowest Level Term associated with the most suitable Preferred Term might be selected.

If a suitable Lowest Level Term does not exist, the Maintenance and Support Services Organisation may be requested to allocate a new term. However, prospective MedDRA users should be aware that strict guidance has been provided to the Maintenance and Support Services Organisation to prevent the uncontrolled proliferation at this lowest level. For example, new terms including anatomical location (e.g. facial wart, fracture 3rd middle phalanx) will not be permitted unless there are particular attributes relating to the body site which are important. Thus, oedema up to the knees might qualify for inclusion under the Preferred Term lower limb oedema, as it provides a specific implication for the severity of the condition, compared with, say ankle oedema.

Data Retrieval

We may wish to retrieve data from the database for one of a variety of purposes. For example, for tabulation of specific adverse events or instances of a particular condition in the patient medical history in a clinical trial. Alternatively, we might wish to identify the number of reports of similar or associated conditions which might constitute a signal of a new adverse reaction in the course of post-marketing surveillance, or perhaps in response to an enquiry from an outside party as to how many cases of a particular reaction have been reported.

Display of all the data in a pre-formatted table may produce the required answer for a single drug. Thus, a table might show all the data assembled according to System Organ Class, with display of all the populated High Level Group Terms, High Level Terms and their respective Preferred Terms. Counts can then be made of cases or reports at the different levels. Cases comprising related medical concepts may be retrieved by identifying relevant System Organ Classes, High Level Group Terms and then High Level Terms, selecting the appropriate Preferred Terms and then searching the database for the associated cases or reports. When doing this, it is essential to also retrieve any appropriate Preferred Terms from the Investigations System Organ Class.

There are some possible alternative approaches to data retrieval using MedDRA. What we need to do is to identify the Preferred Terms which we will then seek in the computer database. A decision must be made on whether to search only for terms located in a System Organ Class as their primary location, or to also include Preferred Terms linked to other primary System Organ Classes.

An example of a search using primary plus secondary locations might be in retrieving reports relevant to pulmonary oedema. Intuitively, a search might be based on the Respiratory disorders System Organ Class, which includes the High Level Group Term Lower respiratory tract disorders (excluding obstruction and infection)—see Table 10.10. Under this

High Level Group Term are the High Level Terms Lower respiratory tract inflammation and immunologic conditions, Lower respiratory tract radiation disorders, Occupational parenchymal lung disorders and Parenchymal lung disorders NEC (not elsewhere classified) as well as Pulmonary oedema (all forms)—see Table 10.11.

Table 10.10 MedDRA SOC Respiratory, thoracic and mediastinal disorders

HLGTs
Bronchial disorders exc.neoplasm
Congenital respiratory tract disorders
Disorders of thorax excl. lung and pleura
Lower respiratory tract disorders exc. obstruction & infection
Lower respiratory tract infections
Neonatal respiratory disorders
Neoplasms of respiratory tract
Pleural disorders
Pulmonary vascular disorders
Respiratory symptoms & signs
Upper respiratory tract disorders
Upper respiratory tract infections (all forms)

SOC   = System Organ Class
HLGT = High Level Group Term

Table 10.11 MedDRA HLGT Lower respiratory tract disorders excluding obstruction & infection

HLTs
Inflammatory and immunologic conditions
Lower respiratory tract radiation disorders
Occupational parenchymal lung disorders
Parenchymal lung disorders NEC
Pulmonary oedema (all forms)

HLGT = High Level Group Term
HLT = High Level Term

The latter High Level Term includes the Preferred Terms Adult respiratory distress syndrome, Capillary leak syndrome, Non-cardiogenic pulmonary oedema, Pulmonary congestion, Pulmonary oedema NOS (not otherwise specified) and Pulmonary oedema post-fume inhalation (Table 10.12). However, the Preferred Term Pulmonary oedema NOS is only situated in this High Level Term as a secondary site. Its primary location is in the Cardiac System Organ Class.

Table 10.12 MedDRA HLT: Pulmonary oedema (all forms)

PT	Primary SOC	Other SOCs	
Adult respiratory distress syndrome	Resp		
Capillary leak syndrome	Resp	Vasc	
Non-cardiogenic pulmonary oedema	Resp	Vasc	
Pulmonary congestion	Resp	Card	Vasc
Pulmonary oedema NOS	Card	Resp	
Pulmonary oedema post fume inhalation	Resp	Inj&P	

SOC = System Organ Class
HLT = High Level Term
PT = Preferred Term
NOS = Not Otherwise Specified
Resp = Respiratory disorders; Vasc = Vascular disorders; Card = Cardiac disorders
Inj&P = Injuries and Poisoning

Searching the Respiratory System Organ Class alone using Primary and Secondary locations would find the above terms. However, a search for cases of pulmonary oedema based on Primary System Organ Class locations would have to encompass both the Respiratory System Organ Class and the Cardiac System Organ Class in order to retrieve all the relevant terms. The Preferred Terms Left ventricular failure and Pulmonary oedema NOS are present in their primary location under the High Level Term Left ventricular failure (all forms), which is itself found under the High Level Group Term Heart failure (all forms) in the Cardiac disorders System Organ Class.

Tabulation of data according to body site using primary as well as secondary System Organ Class locations might duplicate cases associated with the Preferred Term Pulmonary oedema NOS, although this could be eliminated at the output stage.

Cases comprising related medical concepts may be retrieved by identifying relevant High Level Terms, and selecting the appropriate Preferred Terms. It is essential to also retrieve any appropriate Preferred Terms from the Investigations System Organ Class, for example to identify abnormalities on chest X-ray or in cardiac function tests.

If pulmonary oedema is likely to be a recurring issue, we might save a list of all the Preferred Terms we have identified, to facilitate future retrieval. Whilst this search would not be part of the agreed international terminology, MedDRA does include some pre-defined searches, known as Special Search Categories (SSCs). These comprise clusters of Preferred Terms which may cut across System Organ Classes. The Preferred Terms concerned are associated with broad clinical concepts which are not otherwise represented in one location in the terminology. Examples of SSCs are Haemorrhage and Anaphylaxis. An extract from the 103 Preferred Terms included in the Haemorrhage SSC is shown in Table 10.13.

Searching for terms included in Special Search Categories provides automatic identification of relevant cases. Fescharek described the use of MED-DRA version 1.0, especially SSCs, in searches to characterise the safety profile of biological products, based on spontaneous ADR reports.

Table 10.13   Extract from the 103 Preferred Terms in MedDRA's Haemorrhage Special Search Category

Adrenal haemorrhage
Anastomotic ulcer haemorrhage
Antepartum haemorrhage
Auricular haematoma
Bleeding tendency
Bleeding varicose vein
Blood in stool
Broad ligament haematoma
Breast haemorrhage
Cardiac tamponade
Cephalhaematoma
Cerebral haemorrhage neonatal
Choroidal haemorrhage
Colitis haemorrhagic
Colonic haematoma
Colonic haemorrhage
Conjunctival haemorrhage
Coronary artery atheroma haemorrhage
Cystitis haemorrhagic
Diarrhoea haemorrhagic
Duodenal haemorrhage
Duodenal ulcer haemorrhage
Duodenitis haemorrhagic
Dysfunctional uterine bleeding
Ear haemorrhage
Ecchymosis
Epistaxis
Exsanguination
Extradural haematoma
Eye haemorrhage

The Maintenance and Support Services Organisation (MSSO)

The MSSO has been selected and awarded a fixed-term renewable contract with the owners of MedDRA (the International Federation of Pharmaceutical Manufacturers Associations, in trust for the ICH Steering Committee). It will sublicense a Japanese Maintenance Organisation (JMO). Copies of MedDRA, in a variety of formats, and licences for its use will be available exclusively from the MSSO or JMO, for users in Japan. The maintenance framework, summarised in Figure 10.2, has been developed to ensure that

MedDRA will be available at a reasonable cost, that it will be updated at a frequency which is appropriate to the needs of users and that there is evolution in response to advances in medical and scientific knowledge and to changes in the regulatory environment. The cost of subscription to MedDRA will depend on a variety of factors, including the annual turnover of the subscriber and the level of services required (such as the number of new terms which may be added in a year, frequency of updates)

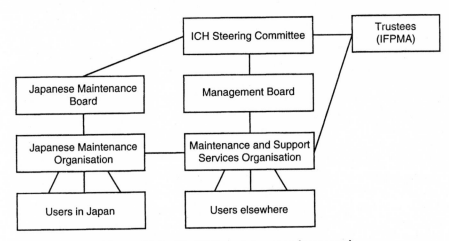

Figure 10.2   MedDRA maintenance framework

The MSSO will be accountable to users and will report to the Management Board. The latter will approve core service fees, the JMO sublicence fee and oversee the activities of the MSSO to ensure that it continues to meet user needs. There is provision for replacement of the MSSO if it proves unsatisfactory.

The MSSO will be responsible for the routine maintenance of the terminology and for ongoing development. Terms proposed for addition to MedDRA by individual users will only be added if they meet the pre-defined criteria for term additions and their hierarchical link will be subject to medical review by staff employed by the MSSO. Major changes to the terminology, for example the restructuring of a System Organ Class, will require consultation with users and the approval of the Management Board.

The MSSO will also provide training in the use of the terminology and technical support to users in migration of their legacy data from their existing medical terminology to MedDRA and in the implementation of MedDRA. Although the MSSO will be required contractually to provide these services, it will not have exclusive rights on these activities. Hence, the fees for these services will be market driven and not regulated by the Management Board.

At the time of writing, contractual arrangements with the selected MSSO have been finalised and it is anticipated that the MSSO and JMO will release MedDRA version 2.0 in the Spring of 1999.

Implementation

As noted above, MedDRA V2.0 was adopted as the standard medical terminology for regulatory communication in the ICH regions in July 1997. However, availability of the terminology has been restricted pending the appointment of the MSSO. In July 1997, Brown carried out a survey of how regulators in the EU, Japan and the US intended to use the terminology. Fifteen regulatory authorities responded. Most indicated that they were likely to use it for their own pharmacovigilance purposes within nine months of availability and would require companies to use it for expedited ADR reporting or in periodic safety updates within 21 months of availability. Plans to use MedDRA for purposes such as standard product information or marketing authorisation applications were less well advanced. There was no consensus as to what levels (Preferred Terms, Lowest Level Terms) should be used for the various regulatory purposes or whether these could replace original (verbatim) reported terms.

The European Agency for the Evaluation of Medicinal Products (EMEA) will use MedDRA version 2.0 for the EUDRAWATCH pharmacovigilance network, which is expected to be functional early in 1999. This will provide regulatory authorities in member states of the European Union with the facility to exchange ADR reports electronically with the EMEA. In Europe, pharmaceutical companies will be encouraged to submit expedited reports of adverse reactions electronically, using the ICH E2b and M2 standards for the data elements of the report and the mode of transmission, and MedDRA as the medical terminology. Since Brown's study was published, the EU regulatory authorities have decided that Lowest Level Terms should be used for electronic ADR reporting by pharmaceutical companies since transmission of data at the Lowest Level Term level provides the recipient with data of maximum specificity and the option of analysis at any level.

The FDA has implemented MedDRA V2.0 in its Adverse Event Reporting System (AERS) database and has indicated that it will mandate the use of MedDRA for electronic reporting from companies. It is likely that it will require Preferred Terms to be used for data submission. Concern has been voiced by companies about the divergent approach in Europe and the US and it is possible that further discussion on a harmonised agreement for the data exchange level may occur at ICH.

For countries outside the ICH framework, is seems likely that a conservative approach to the implementation of MedDRA will be adopted. At the 1998 annual meeting of Collaborating Centres participating in the WHO international drug safety monitoring programme, regulators from non-ICH countries proposed to review progress with MedDRA in the ICH countries and to carry out a programme of testing MedDRA compared with WHO-ART for purposes of retrieval and presentation of data from the WHO ADR database. However, it is to be hoped that all regulators will accept the use of MedDRA by companies in the analysis and presentation of data for pharmacovigilance and other regulatory activities.

As regards pharmaceutical companies and contract research organisations, the timing of implementation will presumably be determined by the demands of the regulatory authorities and internal factors, such as the establishment of new in-house clinical research and pharmacovigilance databases. Transferring legacy data to MedDRA should be straightforward where the data have been previously entered on a database using WHO-ART, COSTART, HARTS, ICD-9 or ICD-9-CM. In those cases, 1:1 matching between MedDRA LLTs and, for example, WHO-ART PTs or COSTART Printed As or Glossary Terms will be possible. Where legacy data have been entered on a database using an in-house terminology, it is still likely that there will be a large proportion of exact matches with MedDRA Lowest Level Terms, but there will need to be term-by-term reconciliation for non-matches. Companies intending to change to MedDRA will have to make important decisions on how best to make the transition and flexibility will need to be demonstrated by regulatory authorities in accepting the different approaches used.

Strengths and Weaknesses

Although published comparisons between MedDRA Version 2.0 and other terminologies are not available, there is an expectation that MedDRA will demonstrate several advantages over existing terminologies, based on the results of the testing of previous versions. In particular, medical validity and relevance to regulatory work are expected to be better than that provided by currently available standard terminologies and MedDRA's richness should prove an advantage over other terminologies in representing precise medical concepts.

Critically, MedDRA has been accepted internationally within the EU, US and Japan as the standard for regulatory communication. As familiarity with the terminology increases for both industry and regulators, there could be savings in time and resource in its use. Certainly, the Maintenance and Support Services Organisation should save time currently spent in maintaining in-house terminologies. However, of greater benefit would be regulatory acceptance of the reliability of company-encoded data without a need for re-coding prior to entry on a regulatory database.

MedDRA's size requires a computer for ease of handling, which could be a disadvantage for some potential users. Its size may be problematic for users in gaining familiarity with its content, and the lack of a logical code might pose a problem for some.

In terms of the daily work of those who will use MedDRA, once existing systems have been adapted and MedDRA installed, the impact is likely to be significant. Provided an auto encoder is used, data entry should be simpler and more accurate than with existing terminologies because the large number of Lowest Level Terms in MedDRA will facilitate exact matches with the original words used on the source documents. There should be less need for judgement in data entry, hence improving consistency at data input. Resource-intensive in-house dictionary updating exercises will no longer be required. On the other hand, data retrieval, analysis and presentation may be more complex with MedDRA, requiring a deeper understanding of medical terminology and of the medical concepts under investigation. There may well be a need for a more individual approach to analysing and presenting the data from each study or across studies in relation to each drug safety issue being analysed. The preparation of package inserts and summaries of product characteristics will probably be more complicated than formerly, especially in the US. Whereas, using the relatively small number of COSTART terms to code adverse events made inclusion of, say, all events occurring with an incidence of more than 1% a simple matter, this would probably be less straightforward using MedDRA. The large number of Preferred Terms in the latter means that, although more accurately represented than with COSTART, it may be less straightforward to provide cut-offs for inclusion in the package insert in an automated manner. The results from these endeavours, however, are likely to be considerably more meaningful and clinically relevant than those obtained with existing terminologies.

Although the hierarchical structure has been extensively used in the pharmacovigilance environment at the MCA, its utility in the aggregation and presentation of clinical trial data remains to be confirmed. Brown compared MEDDRA Version 1.5 with COSTART in coding adverse event terms from a Phase II dose-ranging clinical trial. No medically acceptable terms could be found for 10% of 378 different adverse event terms using COSTART Glossary terms. When using MedDRA Lowest Level Terms on the same data, only 2% of the adverse events could not be satisfactorily represented. Using the two terminologies to enter the same data resulted in apparent differences in the total numbers of different adverse events in the tabulations as well as in the frequency of individual events, according to whether COSTART or MedDRA was used.

White examined 204 verbatim adverse event reports for two marketed drugs and compared WHO-ART with MEDDRA Version 1.5 Preferred Terms in relation to the current labelling for the products. Hence, 'expectedness' of the adverse events for purposes of expedited regulatory reporting could be evaluated. Thirty-two terms (15.7%) were rated as medically significantly different between the terminologies, but without affecting the labelling. Ten terms (4.9%) were considered medically significantly different and affected expectedness in the labelling as did three other terms which were not medically significantly different. It was concluded that the increased specificity of MEDDRA at the Preferred Term level could result in increasing the number of adverse events which are unlabelled and hence require expedited reporting.

The nature and naming of the High Level Terms and High Level Group Terms in MedDRA poses a potential problem. These have been designed to ensure clinically appropriate groupings of subsidiary terms and have been named in such a manner as to make their contents transparent. However, the structure has not yet been validated in respect of functionality for data presentation and it may be that some adjustments will be found necessary. For example, all forms of vertigo can be retrieved under the High Level Term 'Cerebellar co-ordination and balance disturbance and vertigo', which included Preferred Terms, Epidemic vertigo, Vertigo CNS origin, Vertigo NEC (not elsewhere classified), Vertigo aggravated, Vertigo labyrinthine and Vertigo positional but there is no group term for data presentation which covers just all forms of vertigo. The High Level Term 'Cerebellar coordination and balance disturbance and vertigo' also includes Preferred Terms such as Ataxia NEC, Balance impaired NOS (not otherwise specified), Cerebellar ataxia, Cerebellar syndrome, Clumsiness, Clumsy child syndrome, and so on. It might prove useful to prepare a list of the most frequently occurring adverse events and items of medical history recorded in the tables from a variety of previously analysed clinical trials. This list could then be used to check that suitable group terms are available in MedDRA for use in analysing clinical trials in the future. If there are deficiencies, these should be presented to the Maintenance and Support Services Organisation for resolution.

The objective of the ICH M1 initiative was to develop a single medical terminology for regulatory activities which overcomes the limitations of current terminologies, is internationally acceptable, and is supported by appropriate arrangements for long-term maintenance. Only time will tell whether this has been achieved. Significant resources have been devoted to the development of MedDRA and the establishment of responsive maintenance arrangements which will allow any teething problems with the new tool to be addressed rapidly and ensure that MedDRA continues to meet changing user needs. Inevitably, implementation of any new medical terminology is a resource-intensive process. However, the ICH sponsors consider that the long-term benefits of improving the effectiveness and transparency of the regulatory process will outweigh the costs. It is anticipated that MedDRA will improve the quality of data available for analysis and decision making and facilitate the exchange of data by supporting electronic communication, hence speeding up the process of developing and licensing medicines and monitoring their safety.

ACKNOWLEDGEMENT

This chapter is dedicated to the memory of Dr Sue Wood, our late colleague and friend. Having recognised the deficiencies in existing terminologies and the need for a single medical terminology to support the analysis of data throughout the medicines regulatory process, Sue developed, with colleagues, the Medicines Control Agency's medical terminology. Subsequently she established the MEDDRA Working Party and chaired the M1 Expert Working Group of the International Conference on Harmonisation. Her leadership, vision, tenacity, drive and expertise were in large measure responsible for the development and adoption of the *Medical Dictionary for Regulatory Activities* and for many other major contributions to the safety of medicines internationally.

BIBLIOGRAPHY

Brown, E.G. (1996) Medical terminology: a view from Europe. In P.F.D. D'Arcy and D.W.G. Harron (eds), *Proceedings of the Third International Conference on Harmonisation*. Queens University Belfast Publications, pp. 500–503.

Brown, E.G. and Clark, E. (1996) Evaluation of MEDDRA in representing medicinal product data sheet information. *Pharmaceutical Medicine*, **10**, 1–8.

Brown, E.G. and David, M. (1998) The *Medical Dictionary for Regulatory Activities* (MedDRA): a survey of regulatory authority approaches to implementation. *Int. J. Pharm. Med.*, **12**, 23–27.

Brown, E.G., Wood, K.L. and Wood, S.M. (1999) *The Medical Dictionary for Regulatory Activities* (MedDRA). *Drug Safety*, **20**(2), 109–117.

Brown, D.R., Brown, E.G. and Moulvad, T.B. (1997) A comparison of two medical terminologies in coding and analysing clinical trial safety data. *Int. J. Pharm. Med.* **11**, 85–89.

Coding Symbols for a Thesaurus of Adverse Reaction Terms (1989) 3rd edn. US Food and Drug Administration, Rockville, MD, USA.

Fescharek, R., Dechert, G., Reichert. D. et al. (1996) Overall analysis of spontaneously reported adverse events: a worthwhile exercise or flogging a dead horse? *Pharmaceutical Medicine*, **10**, 71–86.

Huntley, K., Veverka, M.J. and Golden, M. (1995) The FDA's *Medical Dictionary for Drug Regulatory Affairs* Alpha Test. *Drug Information Journal*, **29**, 1133–1143.

International Classification of Diseases (1994) 9th revision. *Clinical Modification*. Medicode Publications, Utah, USA.

International Classification of Diseases (1977) 9th revision. World Health Organisation, Geneva.

International Statistical Classification of Diseases and Related Health Problems (1992) 10th revision. World Health Organisation, Geneva.

MEDDRA: setting a new standard in medical terminology (1997). [Editorial]. *Int. J. Pharm. Med.*, **11**, 248.

Mitchard, M. and Wood, L. (1996) *Regulatory Communications. European Pharmaceutical Law Notebooks*, **II**, 139–155.

ten Ham, M. (1996) WHO and international terminology. In P.F.D. D'Arcy and D.W.G. Harron (eds), *Proceedings of the Third International Conference on Harmonisation.* Queens University Belfast Publications, pp. 514–516.

Tsutani, K. (1996) View from Japan. In P.F.D. D'Arcy and D.W.G. Harron (eds), *Proceedings of the Third International Conference on Harmonisation.* Queens University Belfast Publications, pp. 503–512.

White, C. (1998) A preliminary assessment of the impact of MEDDRA on adverse event reports and product labelling. *DIA Journal*, **32**, 347–362.

WHO Adverse Reaction Terminology (1996) Collaborating Centre for International Drug Monitoring, Uppsala, Sweden.

Wood, K.L. (1994) The *Medical Dictionary for Drug Regulatory Affairs* (MEDDRA) Project. *Pharmacoepidemiology and Drug Safety*, **3**, 7–13.

Wood, K.L. (1996) Rapporteur's progress report. In P.F.D. D'Arcy and D.W.G. Harron (eds), *Proceedings of the Third International Conference on Harmonisation,* Queens University Belfast Publications, pp. 495–498.

Wood, K.L., Coulson, R.A. and Wood, S.M. (1995) MEDDRA: the basis for the new international medical terminology for regulatory purposes. *ESRA Rapporteur.* **2**, 12–15.

Wood, K.L. and Wood, S.M. (in press) The international medical terminology for regulatory activities: a tool to improve the utilisation of regulatory data and to support its communication within and between organisations. In M. Mitchard (ed.), *Electronic Communication Technologies: a Practical Guide for Healthcare Manufacturers.* Interpharm Press, Buffalo Grove, USA.

11 Database Design Issues for Central Laboratories

TOM TOLLENAERE

T2 Data Consult BVBA, Leuven, Belgium

INTRODUCTION

Database designers are taught to 'normalise' their data, to avoid inconsistencies in their databases. Although this is a good principle for many database applications, a clinical trials laboratory environment is somewhat different from, say, a classic production or sales environment. There are two reasons for these differences:

- Clinical trials must comply with specific standards and regulations for data handling
- The raw data that must be processed by clinical trials laboratories are often inconsistent

In this chapter we will try, mainly by means of simplified examples, to outline the issues related to database design for clinical laboratories, in a clinical trials context.

This chapter is organised as follows:

- In the first section we review the guidelines and regulations applicable to the use of computer systems for clinical trials laboratories
- In the second section we briefly introduce the principle of database normalisation, which is a standard approach towards the design of database systems
- In the third section we show by means of a simple example in a clinical trials context, why normalisation poses important problems, due to inconsistencies in the data
- In the fourth section, we try to summarise good datahandling principles for clinical trials laboratories. We do this based on the official guidelines

Clinical Data Management. Second Edition. Edited by R.K. Rondel, S.A. Varley and C.F. Webb.
© 2000 John Wiley & Sons, Ltd

and regulations, as well as on practical examples of inconsistencies frequently encountered by clinical trial laboratories

- In the fifth section, we cover another problem, unrelated to inconsistencies, that may influence database design for clinical trial laboratories
- Finally, in the sixth section, we show a number of database designs for audit trail systems, to allow recording of 'corrections' made to the data in order to resolve inconsistencies

APPLICABLE GUIDELINES AND REGULATIONS

Most clinical laboratories are familiar with the Good Laboratory Practices (GLP). With respect to the design and use of computer systems, in 1995, the OECD (Organisation for Economic Cooperation and Development) established a GLP Consensus document, entitled 'The Application of the Principles of GLP to Computerized Systems'[1]. However, the GLPs have been established primarily for animal research, and are hence not applicable to clinical trials work. In general, the applicable guidelines for clinical trials are the Good Clinical Practices (GCP). EC GCP was fairly vague about guidelines for the use of computer systems, but refers explicitly to the Good Manufacturing Principles (GMP) Annex 11 on 'Computerized Systems'. The new ICH GCP[2] merely states that systems should be validated, but does not define what 'validation' really implies, or which standards need to be followed. Finally, for the US there is FDA 21CFR11[3] on Electronic Records and Electronic Signatures, which defines standards for, for example, electronic audit trails.

Apart from GCP and GLP, there are other standards on the use of computerised systems, which some clinical trial laboratories may or may not consider to be applicable. For example, the US Environmental Protection Agency (EPA) has compiled the 'Good Automated Laboratory Practices' (GALPs)[4]. The ISO-9000 series has a guideline ISO 9000-3 specific for the development of software[5]. Strictly speaking, although each of these contains valuable guidelines, we consider GCP (and implicitly Annex 11) and 21CFR11 to be *the* guidelines for the development and use of computer systems for clinical trials laboratories.

As can be expected, there is a great deal of overlap between the various guidelines and regulations. For an overview of differences and similarities between all these regulations and guidelines we refer to Segalstad[6]. For this chapter, we will consider the ICH GCP, GMP Annex 11 and 21CFR11 as our main guidelines. However, the principles outlined in this chapter should fit, at least in spirit, into any quality system for computerised systems for clinical laboratories.

DATABASE NORMALISATION

The details of the principles of normalisation are beyond the scope of this chapter, but roughly speaking, in a normalised database, the data are split into a number of related tables, in order to minimise the duplication of information. The idea is that information which is not duplicated, is easier to maintain consistent. A classic example is the following: suppose we need to store information about articles in stock, knowing we are interested in the total (sales) value of the stock. An example of a non-normalised database containing this information would be as shown in Table 11.1.

Table 11.1

Table: Stock			
Article code	Price	Amount	Location
ABC	100	5	Shelf A
DEF	150	10	Shelf B
ABC	99	5	Shelf C

The problem with this database design is obvious: due to a (clerical?) error there is an inconsistency in the price for article ABC. Furthermore, if the price of an article were to change, one would have to update every 'record' in the stock table. The design shown in Table 11.2 does not suffer from this problem: this is a normalised design.

Table 11.2

Table: Articles		Table: Stock		
Article code	Price	Article code	Amount	Location
ABC	100	ABC	5	Shelf A
DEF	150	DEF	10	Shelf B
GHI	160	ABC	5	Shelf C

The advantages are clear:

- There is no duplicate information about the price of an article, hence there can be no inconsistencies
- Updating the price of an article only need to be done once, in the article table

The problem, however, is that from the Stock table, the value of the stock cannot directly be calculated. However, modern relational database systems, such as Oracle, Sybase, SQLServer or DB/2, have mechanisms to 'join' tables, as shown in the code below.

Query 1

```
select Stock.ArticleCode, Stock.Amount, Stock.Location,
 Articles.Price
  from Articles, Stock
    where Stock.ArticleCode = Articles.ArticleCode;
```

```
3 rows found :
ArticleCode  Amount  Location  Price
ABC               5  Shelf A     100
DEF              10  Shelf B     150
ABC               5  Shelf C     100
```

The example in Query 1 shows how the appropriate stock value information can be retrieved from the database. The 'language' used to query the database is known as SQL (Structured Query Language). When the 'select' statement is executed, the database system returns the information actually selected: in this example this data are printed between the dashed lines. In this example, the field 'ArticleCode' is used as a 'key' to 'link' or 'join' the two tables together.

DATABASE NORMALISATION AND INCONSISTENT DATA

In this section we will try to give some simple examples of cases in which 'traditional' database designs might lead to problems in a clinical trials laboratory environment. These examples will be used as a basis for the discussion in the remainder of the text.

Suppose our clinical trials database has been designed as follows: it consists of two tables, one containing patient identification (demographics), and one containing laboratory results for various visits of these patients. An example of this database is shown in Table 11.3.

Table 11.3

Table: Patients			Table: Results				
Patient number	Patient initials	Date of birth	Patient number	Visit	Visit date	Glucose	Total bilirubin
321	ABC	01/01/1960	321	V1	01/01/1997	12	5
456	DEF	02/02/1961	456	V2	02/02/1997	9	4
789	GHI	03/03/1962					

This database is normalised, to the extent that patients are uniquely defined, and they are identified by means of the patient number, or, in other words, the patient number is the 'primary key' in table Patients. If we query the database for the results of patient 'ABC' we obtain the correct data, for one visit, V1, as shown in Query 2.

Query 2

```
select results.Visit, results.VisitDate from results,
 patients
  where Patients.initials = 'ABC'
    and patients.PatientNumber = results. PatientNumber;
-----------------------------------------------------------------
1 row found :
Visit  VisitDate
V1     01/01/1997
-----------------------------------------------------------------
```

Suppose now the following happens: the sample for visit 2, patient ABC comes in, with a patient number '123', rather than '321'. Since the database is normalised, patient ABC can be in the database as either number '123' or '321', but not both. The data received by the central laboratory is inconsistent, and can hence not be entered into this database as such.

Problem: the data received cannot be entered into the database *Cause:* the design of the database cannot handle inconsistencies in the data

Suppose now that, fortunately, the investigator can be contacted, he confirms an error was made in the patient identification for visit 1, and the operators enter the sample for patient '123' and correct the mistake in the Patients table. The contents of the database resulting from these actions are shown in Table 11.4.

Table 11.4

Table: Patients			Table: Results				
Patient number	Patient initials	Date of birth	Patient number	Visit	Visit date	Glucose	Total bilirubin
123	ABC	01/01/1960	321	V1	01/01/1997	12	5
456	DEF	02/02/1961	456	V1	02/02/1997	9	4
789	GHI	03/03/1962	123	V2	03/03/1997	8	6

If the database is now queried for all results for patient 'ABC', the results for the first visit suddenly appear to be missing, as shown in Query 3.

Query 3

```
select results.Visit, results.VisitDate from results,
 patients
  where Patients.initials = 'ABC'
   and patients.PatientNumber = results.PatientNumber;
----------------------------------------------------------------
1 row found :
Visit   VisitDate
V2       03/03/1997
----------------------------------------------------------------
```

Problem:	data appear to be missing
Cause:	the design of the database is such that the operators cannot assess the consequences of the modifications they enter

As a matter of fact, the data are not really missing, but when the operators changed the patient number in the Patients table, they forgot to change the patient number for V1, 01/01/1997. The operators should have done this, as the patient number is the 'key' used to link the Results table with the Patients table. However, the use of keys is a database design issue, of which the operators are probably not aware—they shouldn't even be; this is probably beyond their expertise.

If the database were to be designed in a denormalised form, as shown in Table 11.5, the problem would have been different.

Table 11.5

Patient number	Patient initials	Date of birth	Visit	Visit date	Glucose	Total bilirubin
321	ABC	01/01/1960	V1	01/01/1997	12	5
456	DEF	02/02/1962	V2	02/02/1997	9	4
123	ABC	01/01/1960	V2	03/03/1997	8	6

This database design does not make it impossible to enter the data actually received by the central laboratory. If we query this database for patient 'ABC' we will find all results; if we query for patient '123' we will, as long as the error made at visit 1 is not corrected, only find results for visit 2. Both examples are shown in Query 4.

Query 4

```
select Visit, VisitDate from results
 where initials = 'ABC';
------------------------------------------------------------
2 rows found :
Visit   VisitDate
V1      01/01/1997
V2      03/03/1997
------------------------------------------------------------

select Visit, VisitDate from results
 where PatientNumber = 123;
------------------------------------------------------------
1 row found :
Visit   VisitDate
V2      03/03/1997
------------------------------------------------------------
```

DATA HANDLING PRINCIPLES FOR CLINICAL TRIALS LABORATORIES

As a basic rule, all data should be entered by the laboratory exactly as they are received, even if they are known or suspected to be erroneous or inconsistent. The laboratory is not 'owner' of the sample/patient identification data, and cannot assume any responsibility about these data: this is the investigator's responsibility. Upon detection of inconsistencies the lab should enter the data as is, contact the investigator (or have the monitor or sponsor contact the investigator), and await detailed written instructions about how to correct the inconsistency.

Mechanisms to handle and store corrections will be covered in the last section of this chapter. In the meantime, our clinical trials database systems should be able to store inconsistent data. From the examples above we already know that this involves the use of denormalised database designs, as normalised databases can by definition not store inconsistent data. The following subsections discuss some of the types of inconsistencies to be expected, and a number of classic database design techniques that should be avoided for clinical trials databases for clinical trials laboratories.

Making a list of what might be inconsistent is impossible: according to Murphy's Law, anything that can be inconsistent, will eventually be inconsistent. Still, some cases are typical.

Patient Initials

Patient initials are probably the major cause of inconsistencies. Consider the following list of initials for the same patient number at various visits:

- Visit 1: A–B
- Visit 2: AB
- Visit 3: B–A
- Visit 4: A☐B (in which ☐ denotes a space)

Although, certainly if other patient identifiers, such as sex and data of birth, are in all four cases the same, it may be very likely that these four cases concern the same patient, it is not for the laboratory to decide this.

Strictly speaking, these data should be entered as such, and should only be corrected after confirmation by the investigator. The point is that data entry operators should be trained not to make any assumptions on the data. As a matter of fact, these four initials might belong to four different patients, respectively, for example:

- Mrs Angstrom-Bergson
- Andy Bennet
- Mr Bennet-Anderson
- Anita Borg

Admittedly, it would be very unlikely for the same investigator to enrol these four patients, and mix up their sexes and dates of birth, but it is not impossible, and hence if the data entry operators make any assumptions about this, patient results might get mixed up.

Inconsistencies Between Different Patient Identifiers

Consider the following five forms, which are based on a case the author has come across. These are laboratory analysis request forms for three different visits of the same study, and two forms for an extension of that study.

In the example of these five forms we observe the following:

- Between visit 1 and visit 2, patient ABC/Male/01/01/1960's pre-randomisation number has changed. The data entry operators should not infer that form 1 and form 2 concern the same patient; form 2 might actually be for a patient with the pre-randomisation number 1234, which may be a different patient than ABC/Male/01/01/1960. The investigator has probably mixed up patient pre-randomisation numbers with patient demographics, but one cannot guess which of the two is

Form 1

Analysis request form
Study XYZ
Investigator: Dr. John Johnson

Visit 1
Week 1

Patient demographics		
Pre-randomisation number *1234*		
Patient initials *ABC*	Sex *Male*	Date of birth *01/01/1960*

Form 2

Analysis request form
Study XYZ
Investigator: Dr. John Johnson

Visit 2
Week 4

Patient demographics		
Pre-randomisation number *4321*	Randomisation number *9001*	
Patient initials *ABC*	Sex *Male*	Date of birth *01/01/1960*

Form 3

Analysis request form
Study XYZ
Investigator: Dr. John Johnson

Visit 3
Week 5

Patient demographics		
Pre-randomisation number *1234*	Randomisation number *9002*	
Patient initials *ABC*	Sex *Female*	Date of birth *01/01/1961*

Form 4

> **Analysis request form**
> **Study XYZ**
> Investigator: Dr. John Johnson   Visit 16
>   Week 21
>
> | Patient demographics | | |
> |---|---|---|
> | Pre-randomisation number | Randomisation number | Extension patient number |
> | *1234* | *9001* | *19001* |
> | Patient initials | Sex | Date of birth |
> | *ABC* | *Male* | *01/01/1960* |

Form 5

> **Analysis request form**
> **Study XYZ**
> Investigator: Dr. John Johnson   Visit 17
>   Week 22
>
> | Patient demographics | | |
> |---|---|---|
> | Pre-randomisation number | Randomisation number | Extension patient number |
> | *4321* | *9002* | *19002* |
> | Patient initials | Sex | Date of birth |
> | *ABC* | *Male* | *01/01/1960* |

correct. Actually, both may be correct: consider the case of identical twin brothers, with similar names, for example Albert and André Bergstrom-Carlsson

- Between visit 2 and visit 3 we observe the same initials, but different patient number and sex. Here we have even less reason to assume this concerns the same patient; as was indicated in the previous subsection, identical initials need not indicate the same patient
- Between form 4 and form 5 we have a complete mismatch: although initials, date of birth and sex are different, all three patient numbers are different. Again, no assumptions should be made, and the data should be entered as they appear on the request forms, awaiting confirmation about the patient's identification by the investigator

There is an additional problem with these forms, resulting from the design of the study: there are multiple patient numbers for various phases of the study: a pre-randomisation number, a randomisation number, and, for the extension, a third patient number.

A problem is that many (commercial) laboratory information systems (LIMs) can only handle one patient identification number. For these kinds of database systems, we are faced with two concerns:

1. As long as, for the appropriate visits, the 'links' between the different patient numbers are provided (on the request forms), and as long as these are filled out correctly by the investigator, the 'chain of identification' is complete. The problem is that for these visits only one identifier can be entered—whichever choice is made, operators need to do this consistently in the same way. Furthermore, quite often the sponsor demands that the results for the previous visit are printed on the laboratory reports. If only one patient number is kept in the database, then at some point patient numbers for previous visits will need to be changed in the database, otherwise, at the visit the patient number is changed, the system will not find any previous results for the new patient number. In the last section of this chapter we will discuss techniques for keeping track of changes to the data, but nonetheless, this poses a data management problem.
2. If, as is the case in our example, the 'link' between the different patient numbers is provided twice or more, the data at different visits may be (and will be eventually) inconsistent. In these cases, for systems that can handle only one patient number, the operators will be forced to make a choice, and hence will be forced to make assumptions they should not be making.

The bottom line is that database systems for clinical trials laboratories should be capable of capturing multiple patient numbers, and should be able to handle inconsistencies between these numbers.

Avoiding Enforced Uniqueness

In many database systems, tables can be set up such that certain fields, or combinations of fields, should be unique. The system will then prevent the entry of data that violate this uniqueness constraint. In general, it is not good practice for databases to hold clinical trials raw data. Some examples:

- Assumption: the whole of the patient's demographics (initials, sex and date of birth) should be unique (per investigator). We have earlier pointed out the case of identical twins with identical initials
- Assumption: visits are unique per patient. In practice this is not the case either, as investigators may decide to repeat a patient visit,

without using a repeat visit form. For many studies, request forms for
unscheduled visits are foreseen. For these visits, the assumption that
every patient can only have one unscheduled visit is invalid

The bottom line here is that any constraint on the uniqueness of data to be
entered into the system will result in inability to enter inconsistent data,
and hence should be avoided.

A related technique that should be avoided is limiting data values. In
some database systems the data to be entered into fields can be limited to
a list. An example is the coding of visits; as the sequence of visits is
defined in the protocol, the database designer might feel tempted to limit
the values for the visit coding to the ones listed in the protocol. For
example:

- Visit 1, Week -2
- Visit 2, Day 0
- Visit 3, Day 1
- Visit 4, Week 1
- Visit 5, Week 2

For this protocol, if the investigator decides, for whatever reason, to see a
patient on day 2, he might use a request form for any other visit, bar the
visit coding printed on the form, and 'invent' something like 'Visit 2a, Day
2'. If the laboratory database system has been designed to hold only visit
values out of the above list, the raw data actually received ('Visit 2a, Day
2') cannot be entered into the system.

UNEXPECTED RESULTS

The Problem

So far, we have covered problems with patient and sample identification.
For a clinical trials laboratory, these will be the major causes of concern
when designing databases for clinical trials laboratory results. There is,
however, one more issue that has become a practical problem for clinical
trials laboratories: when a study is set up, the study protocol lists the
laboratory analyses to be performed. Quite often, the clinical trials laboratory will set up a database to contain those results. In this results
database, 'placeholders' are foreseen for every expected result. For example, in Tables 11.4 and 11.5, for every visit, two results are expected,
one for glucose and one for total bilirubin.

However, quite often, when certain analyses yield exceptional values,
the lab. may decide to run additional, not-foreseen tests. An typical

example is a total bilirubin which is out of normal range, for which the laboratory's MD may decide to have a direct bilirubin run, even if this is not demanded by the protocol. The question is whether the laboratory database should be able to store this result.

There seems to be no international consensus on this problem. However, it should be clear that these additional results may have clinical significance, and hence should, in the patient safety interest, certainly be reported to the investigator. If the laboratory reports off the study database, and this database cannot store this result, some manual intervention may be needed. Therefore, it is the author's opinion that a good database design should allow unexpected results to be stored.

To what extent these additional results should be reported to the sponsor is also an unresolved issue: many sponsors demand the clinical trials laboratory to deliver the data in a pre-determined format, which may not foresee unexpected results. It is the author's opinion that these issues should be subject of pre-contract discussions between sponsor and laboratory.

How to Handle Unexpected Results

From a database system design point of view, there are basically two ways to approach this problem:

1. Write programs that detect the presence of unexpected results, and that dynamically and automatically add the appropriate fields to the database tables.
2. Design the database so that it can contain any number of results, expected or not.

The first solution does not really change the design of the database, but it changes the implementation of this design. Coding programs to do this demands some programmer ingenuity, and, depending on the development tools provided by the database system, may be quite expensive. In addition, this approach may lead to 'wasted' space in the database: when a field is added to a table, it is in principle added to all records of that table, whether this field is used for this records or not (actually, some modern relation database systems, like Oracle, have mechanisms to detect this, and are able to avoid this kind of waste of space).

The first solution leads to a radically different database design, which may be interesting to consider. In this design, every occurrence of a laboratory result is registered as a separate record, as shown in Table 11.6, which contains the same results as in Table 11.4, with an additional direct bilirubin.

Table 11.6

Table: Results				
Patient number	Visit	Visit date	Analysis	Value
321	V1	01/01/1997	Glucose	12
321	V1	01/01/1997	Bilirubin	5
321	V1	01/01/1997	DirectBilirubin	7
456	V2	02/02/1997	Glucose	9
456	V2	02/02/1997	Bilirubin	4

This kind of design, which is actually used by quite a few drug companies for their biostatistics databases, has the following features:

- Records only appear for analysis actually performed; if certain analyses are not to be done on certain visits, there will be no 'empty' fields in the records for these visits
- Additional, non-expected results can be captured without changing the actual table structure
- The design is more space-consuming than, e.g., the design shown in Table 11.4, as for every visit, multiple records are created, and in each of these records, the patient/visit identification is duplicated

Missing Values and Codes

As noted in the first 'feature' of the design in Table 11.6, a remark was made about 'missing values'. This subject is worth some further attention.

Suppose that in Table 11.5, for patient DEF, V2, the value for glucose is missing. In that case, it would be (for example, for an auditor) unclear what has happened. There are various possibilities:

- Perhaps this analysis has not been asked for by the protocol?
- Perhaps for some reason the laboratory has not performed this analysis, maybe the sample tube was broken by a laboratory technician and the sample got lost?
- Perhaps the analysis has been scheduled, but the result is not available yet? Maybe the laboratory ran out of reagent for this analysis, and will complete the analysis tomorrow?
- Perhaps two samples were required, one for the glucose analysis and one for the bilirubin analysis, and the bilirubin sample was never received by the laboratory (ignoring, for the sake of argument, the fact that bilirubin and glucose could be determined on the same sample)?
- Perhaps the analyser reported a bilirubin value below or above detection limits?

Basically, it is good practice never to have missing values in the results databases, and to code 'missing' results with the reason why the result is not there: each of the cases in the above list of potential reasons for missing results could be 'coded'.

There are various coding strategies; a number of these are discussed below.

Negative numbers

A classic coding strategy is the use of 'special' negative values, for example:

- −99: not demanded by protocol
- −98: no sample
- −97: pending
- etc. . . .

This approach has the advantage that negative numbers are numeric, and can easily be stored in numeric fields for results. The disadvantage is that the numbers chosen might, for certain (exotic?) analyses, be actually meaningful; this would make it impossible to distinguish between a 'missing' and an 'exotic' result.

Alphanumeric codes

An alternative would be to store all results as 'strings' of character. Codes for missing values can then be alphanumeric, for example:

- NotDone
- NoSample
- Pending
- etc. . . .

The disadvantage of this approach is that, when the data need to be formatted for delivery to the sponsor, the values will probably need to be converted back to numericals. However, some analysers report results as alphanumericals anyway, for example Urine colour might be reported as, 'Yellow', 'Straw', and so on. If a database design such as the one in Table 11.6 is used, in which the type or result is not a priori known (as a result the record may contain a result for no matter which analysis), one may have to provide for alphanumeric results anyway.

Others

Some database systems allow the coding of alphanumeric codes in numeric fields. For example, the SAS system can store the code '.A' (a '.'

followed by a single alphanumeric character) in any numeric field. If your laboratory's database system provides similar facilities, these can be used to store codes for missing results.

Reporting missing values to the sponsor

When the sponsor defines the format in which the laboratory should report the final data, quite often issues such as coding of missing values are overlooked. In many other cases, the coding demanded by the sponsor will be different from, or less extensive than, the coding used internally by the laboratory. In these cases (and also in the case discussed above, where alphanumeric fields are used to store numeric values) some transformations will be needed on the data. We will come back to this issue in the last subsection.

AUDIT TRAILS

In the previous sections we have established that (raw) data received by clinical trials laboratories are likely to be inconsistent, and that the database systems designed to capture these data should be capable of storing these inconsistencies. Evidently, these inconsistencies should be resolved, and accordingly the data should be corrected. This is the final subject for this chapter: how to handle corrections to (inconsistent) data?

GMP Annex 11.10 demands specifically that 'the system should record the identity of operators entering or confirming the data' and that 'Any alteration to an entry of critical data should . . . be recorded with the reason for the change. Consideration should be given to building into the system the creation of a complete record of all entries and amendments (an "audit trail")'.

Basically, there are two approaches towards designing database systems with audit trails. These will be discussed in the following subsections, but first we elaborate on the requirements of a good 'correction system' for storing audit trails.

Requirements for a Corrections System

A good system, which records all changes and corrections to the data, should fulfil the following requirements:

- The identity of the operator should be automatically recorded, and the operator should not be able to change this identification
- The time and date the correction is entered should be automatically recorded, and the operator should not be able to change this information

- The system should refuse the entry of a correction if no reason is entered
- The system should allow all fields in all records to be amended
- The system should allow deletion of records, for example to delete duplicate records
- It must be possible to 'undo' every correction, for example, it should be possible to 'undelete' an erroneously deleted record
- All changes and modifications should be recorded
- It should be possible to 'reconstruct' the status of the database as it was at any given point of time, and explain why this status is different from the status at any other point in time.

In the following two subsections we outline two design approaches for audit trail database systems.

Design 1

In this approach the system keeps for every table a 'table of previous records', containing a trail of all amended records, called the 'Audit Trail'. The system is summarised in Figure 11.1, and a simplified example is shown in Table 11.7.

In this example, it is possible to deduce what happened to the data in the Table Results:

- On 06/06/1997 operator Mary deleted the results for patient 456, visit 02/02/1997, on sponsor request. Although the data are no longer in Table Results, the deleted data can be found (and reinstated if necessary) in table ResultsTrail
- On 05/05/1997 operator John changed the patient number '321' for visit 01/01/1997 into '123', after confirmation by the investigator

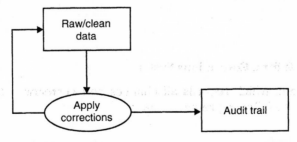

Figure 11.1 In this design the database is continuously updated. The original data in the database are the raw data, which, as more corrections are applied, become clean. For every correction that is applied, a 'trace' is written into the Audit Trail table. In this figure, database tables are shown as rectangles, and processes (operations to the data) are shown as ellipses

Table 11.7

Table Results

Patient number	Visit date	Glucose
123	01/01/1997	12
789	03/03/1997	8

Table ResultsTrail

Patient number	Visit date	Glucose	Correction date & time	Operator	Reason for change
456	02/02/1997	9	13:01 06/06/1997	Mary	Deleted record sponsor request fax ref. Study/06/06/97
321	01/01/1997	12	12:00 05/05/1997	John	Investigator confirmed incorrect patient number

Design 2

Although Design 1 fulfils all the requirements for a good correction system, a more elaborate design may be more appropriate. This design has the following features.

The correction system consists of three tables:

- The raw data, which are never modified
- A database of corrections
- A corrected database, which is a copy of the original raw data, to which the corrections are applied

The corrections table contains:

- An identification of the record(s) to be corrected
- The type of correction (modification, delete, undelete)
- Fields to be corrected
- New values of the corrected fields
- Time and date of the correction
- Identification of the operator making the corrections

In practice, this system works as follows: at regular times, for example every night, the corrected table is deleted, and a new corrected table is generated, taking into account the corrections entered during the day (evidently, if a new version of the corrected data is needed urgently, the regeneration process can be started at any time).

The process is summarised in Figure 11.2; a simplified example is presented in Table 11.8.

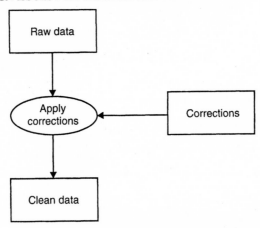

Figure 11.2 In this design the raw data are never touched. All corrections to be applied to the data are stored in a 'Corrections' table. At regular intervals, the corrections are applied to the raw data, and the result constitutes the 'Clean Data'

Actually, this approach is quite clean in its conception, as corrections are treated the same way as raw data: they are never changed; a correction to a correction is entered as a new correction. Two examples can be seen in Table 11.8:

- Mary erroneously deleted the record for patient 789. The fact that she did so, and afterwards placed the record back by means of the 'undelete' operation shown in the second record, can clearly be seen in the audit trail. The correction of the incorrect 'delete' is explicit in the trail, and is marked as 'undelete'
- John had to change the patient number 321 into 123, but made an error and changed it into 132. When he saw his own error, he corrected it by means of another correction, changing the 132 into 123. Again, this is clear and explicit in the audit trail

Comparing the Two Designs

The advantages of Design 2 over Design 1 are the following:

- The original raw data are never touched; this gives an extra degree of guarantee of the integrity of the raw data
- Furthermore, corrections are treated as raw data, in the sense that once entered, they are never changed, nor removed
- Restoring the state of the data at any given point in time is easier; this can be done by selecting the corrections up to a certain date, and the application of this selection of corrections then constitutes the data desired

Table 11.8

Table RawResults				Table CorrectedResults		
Patient number	Visit date	Date of birth		Patient number	Visit date	Glucose
321	01/01/1997	12		321	01/01/1997	12
456	02/02/1997	9		789	03/03/1997	8
789	03/03/1997	8				

Table Corrections

Record identification	Type	Field	New value	Correction date & time	Operator	Reason for change
PatientNumber = 789	delete	—	—	12:59 06/06/1997	Mary	Deleted record sponsor request fax ref. Study/06/06/97
PatientNumber = 789	undelete	—	—	13:00 06/06/97	Mary	Deleted wrong record
PatientNumber = 456	delete	—	—	13:01 06/06/1997	Mary	Deleted record sponsor request fax ref. Study/06/06/97
PatientNumber = 321	change	Patient Number	132	12:00 05/05/1997	John	Investigator confirmed incorrect patient number
PatientNumber = 132	change	Patient Number	123	12:01 05/05/1997	John	Made a wrong correction: changed patient 321 into 132 instead of 123

- The corrections themselves are explicit—unlike in Design 1, where the differences between original and corrected data must be deduced by comparing the trail and the latest version of the data
- This system makes it possible to correct multiple records by means of one 'correction'

Clean Databases

A final remark: we have shown earlier in this chapter that a normalised database design cannot capture the inconsistencies that are bound to occur in the raw data a clinical trials laboratory receives. However, the ultimate goal is to produce, by the end of the study, a clean database, to be delivered to the sponsor (or to a contract research organisation [CRO] responsible for the biostatistics part of the clinical trial). Evidently, if the final, clean data are consistent, they can be represented and delivered in the form of a normalised database, as is quite often demanded by some sponsors.

As was mentioned before, when data need to be prepared for delivery to the sponsor or a contract research organisation, the laboratory will need to perform additional transformations. Hence, we can extend Figure 11.2 as shown in Figure 11.3.

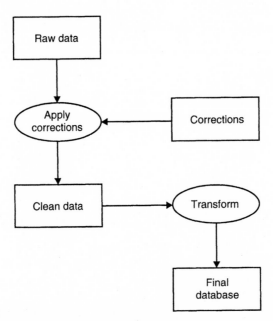

Figure 11.3   This figure shows all the manipulations that happen to the data. The figure is identical to Figure 11.2 but an additional process is added: that of transforming the 'clean' data into a (perhaps) normalised version, and the translation of codes to the format wanted by the sponsor or CRO

CONCLUSIONS

In this chapter we have shown that the design of database systems for clinical trials laboratories poses some specific problems, not (frequently) found for classic database applications in other industries. Most of the issues raised here stem from inconsistencies in the raw data received by the laboratory. We have shown that a normalised database system cannot capture inconsistent raw data as they are received by the laboratory.

Furthermore, we have touched upon some other issues that may influence the database design for clinical trials laboratories: unexpected and missing results.

Finally, we have presented two outlines of designs for database systems to store audit trails. These are important in a clinical trials context as, according to regulations, all corrections to (inconsistent) data need to be fully traceable.

It should be clear that a thorough understanding of the peculiarities of a clinical trials laboratory environment, as well as an understanding of the applicable guidelines and regulations, are prerequisite to good data management for clinical trials. It is the author's hope that this chapter may contribute to a better understanding of these important issues.

REFERENCES

1. OECD (1995) GLP Consensus Document: The Application of the Principles of GLP to Computerized Systems, OECD Series on Principles of Good Laboratory Practice and Compliance Monitoring Number 10, Paris.
2. ICH (1996) Harmonised Tripartite Guideline for Good Clinical Practice, International Conference on Harmonisation of Technical Requirements For Registration of Pharmaceuticals for Human Use.
3. FDA 21CFR Part 11 (1997) Electronic Records; Electronic Signatures; Final Rule. *Federal Register*, **62**, 54, 13429, 20 March.
4. EPA (1990) Good Automated Laboratory Practices, Office for Information Resource Management, US Environmental Protection Agency, Research Triangle Part, NC, Draft.
5. ISO (1991) ISO 9000-3, Quality Management and Quality Assurance Standards, Part 3, Guidelines for the application of ISO 9001 to the development, supply and maintenance of Software, International Standards Organisation, Geneva.
6. Segalstad, Siri H. (1995) Quality Assurance of Computer Systems: What is needed to Comply with ISO 9000, GMP, GLP and GCP? *Laboratory Automation & Information Management*, **31**, 11–24.

12 Computer Systems

LOUISE PALMA

Berlex Laboratories Inc., Montville, NJ, USA

INTRODUCTION

Clinical Data Management has been undergoing considerable changes over the past few years. Consolidations and acquisitions are occurring throughout the industry, resulting in companies with various data management departments functioning around the world. Also, the industry is calling for greater efficiency, quality improvement, lower costs and decreased timelines in the conduct of clinical trials. In response to these demands, Data Management (DM) is broadening our expertise in new processes and systems and as a result becoming more computer literate. Technology can contribute significantly to meeting our goals and the increasing demands in the management of clinical data. The FDA and European regulatory agencies have also become increasingly interested in the utilization of new technologies for their review. This trend will undoubtedly increase as we continue to become more competitive and gain more knowledge of the new technologies and processes surrounding them, together with the increasing pace of computer development.

All companies conducting clinical research, including pharmaceutical, biotech, medical device and contract research organizations, have been undergoing major changes in their clinical data management systems to accommodate the growing needs and demands of the industry. There are various new systems that have been developed recently which are trying to ease the processing of what is considered to be some of the most difficult and complex data. The industry trend seems to be going in the direction of relational database management systems and client server platforms. However, most companies are using commercial software packages because in-house development is costly overall. There are still a number of companies which continue to develop and build systems. The business need is a major factor when determining whether or not to go with new technology.

DM is aware of the benefits of new processes and technologies and should expect to see some of them either short term or long term. Some benefits include:

Clinical Data Management. Second Edition. Edited by R.K. Rondel, S.A. Varley and C.F. Webb.
© 2000 John Wiley & Sons, Ltd

- Reduction in cycle time from protocol development to report
- Improved Regulatory Compliance (complete audit trails, CANDAs)
- Improved data integrity and quality, tracking techniques
- Improved efficiency and utilization of resources
- Facilitated clinical research monitoring capabilities
- Improved project management and planning capabilities
- Reduction or maintenance of project costs

Once a decision has been made to reevaluate the systems in Clinical Data Management (CDM), a present state analysis should be conducted. This should include the present strengths and weaknesses of the current systems, so a gap analysis against the systems under consideration can be done. This will help establish where you are versus where you want to be.

One of the first steps following this decision is to define ways of establishing how to select and evaluate the products, as well as trying to avoid possible pitfalls of this process.

ESTABLISHING CRITERIA

The first step in establishing criteria to evaluate systems is to create a team where every discipline and every stakeholder is represented for all study activities. This core team will incorporate the knowledge of their individual departments, but they will also be responsible for representing their areas. The team should set up the overall objectives of what they are trying to accomplish which includes the major steps of clinical trial management; establish timelines, needs versus wants and technical criteria. In addition, it might be necessary to establish any overriding constraints or parameters that the organization might have imposed.

Overall Objectives

Some of these major steps are identified below:

- Obtain valid patient data via Case Record Forms (CRFs) as required by the protocol
- Ensure immediate availability of data in the company (the time gap from site to database should be minimal)
- Ensure immediate processing of incoming data (including plausibility/validity checking/database finalization)
- Provide validated databases, both the initial application and upgrades, for product registration and other company needs
- Enable compilation of global and project databases composed from local databases (international clinical trial) for statistical reporting and tabulations

- Provide necessary access to the data of an ongoing trial to satisfy drug safety aspects, ethical and legal requirements
- Fulfill GCP requirements with respect to clinical data processing

In addition to overall objectives there are some other issues that should be considered.

- Will the establishment of standards within the company, and at the project level, for CRF design, database design and report generation lead to an improvement in quality, efficiency and data validity?
- Will plausibility checking for the data of one trial be performed with one globally agreed set of core plausibility checks?
- Will CRF books composed of standard CRFs be stored in a CRF library?
- Randomization, blinding and unblinding, has to follow strict rules to enable integrity of the data of a study; will this be part of the integrated database?
- Does the system allow granting database access for locking databases prior to final data analysis?
- Will reporting needs be internationally consistent?
- Will the entire DM process be integrated, implementing automatic workflow and tracking systems with integrated status documentation?
- The DM process is based technologically on a distributed computer system in a network environment. This system has to be supported by IT specialists in routine operation and maintained by an IT development group
- Will the system allow for the complete DM operation? Will it be subject to regulatory and internal audits?
- Training of monitors and clinical data managers in data management procedures must be conducted regularly at both the global and project levels
- Resources and budgets for the proposed programs should be allocated
- Consideration of the import and export of all data from various sources, both internally and externally, to the company project and how it will be integrated with the clinical database system?
- Will the system need to integrate with other systems as part of an overall IT systems plan?

Technical Criteria

Once your overall user objectives have been set, criteria for the needs of a system should be evaluated. This should include the technical architecture analysis of the system, including the definitions of hardware, software configuration, network configuration, source code control, development tools and back-up and recovery management.

Technical criteria should include, but are not limited to, the following general requirements:

- Distribution of data to multiple sites
- User-friendly system
- Graphical User Interface (GUI)
- Planning, development and validation according to GCPs
- Versatile report facilities
- Language requirements
- Standardization, including support of in-house dictionaries and code lists
- Labs, reference ranges, transformation of units
- Access and Security Rights (these should be flexible)
- Generation of randomization with appropriate security
- Locking of database at various levels (study, patient, visits, items)
- Generation of database structures including data entry screens and CRFs
- Copy Database design features
- Flexibility to handle complex study designs and the storage of these
- User-friendly screens and double key data entry (if necessary)
- Plausibility checking within the system (you may want this to be an easy to use language and be stored within the database with a complete audit trail)
- Easy ways of correcting data with audit trails, electronic and paper, for all corrections at all levels of data
- Flexibility to enter metadata after database is designed and ongoing (protocol amendments may cause changes to data)
- Support of autoencoding
- Interfaces with other reporting systems, SAS or other reporting tools
- Interface with drug safety if not part of the clinical database

Other issues to consider are the ease of use of a system, documentation and training, operational performance, vendor characteristics, vendor support at all locations, and audit of the system and vendor, cost, environment and hardware constraints. Please refer to the first edition of *Clinical Data Management* for further details.

SYSTEM ANALYSIS AND TESTING

Once the criteria are set and agreed upon, the list should be grouped according to needs versus nice to have features, and then prioritized.

This list will help focus the overall evaluation. Each system should be evaluated by a team representing all the areas involved. A gap analysis, to identify the differences between the needs and wants criteria versus the system capacity, should be performed so that the group can identify how the missing criteria can be resolved. A list of criteria separating the needs and wants may help assist the evaluation team. The aim of this analysis should be to identify what changes to the process are necessary, what customization will be needed to the system for integration to other systems, what additional software is necessary, and implementation and training plans. An evaluation of systems and the gap analysis should be completed prior to securing a contract with a vendor, if possible. This will allow you to have a complete understanding of the global scope of the project.

After the evaluation phase is complete, it is always good to conduct a test of the new system as part of your implementation. Design, test and set up a pilot study that is representative of most of your studies. Testing should ensure that the system provides everything specified in the needs criteria and contract. This will be your first assessment of the system in actual use. Testing wherever possible should include as many people, both technical and end users, as is feasible to cover the various stakeholders by job function and geographical location.

The following data structures are recommended to be tested. However, depending upon the types of clinical trials, there will always be additional areas that you may want to cover.

- Subject data/Demography, End of study evaluation
- Visit-related data/vital signs
- Repeated, coded items such as a physical exam
- Adverse events and concomitant medications
- Labs/lab values, blood samples, rating scales
- Patient diary

Upon the completion of testing, the team should make recommendations on possible improvements to the design of the system, and changes that may be required to optimize the implementation. A complete implementation plan should be developed which should include what projects will be used in the new system. Also include which projects will be migrated to the new system versus those which will be maintained on the old system. A timeframe should be developed for migration, and appropriate resources will need to be allocated to work on all of these systems.

Successful implementation will also require technical and procedural training and documentation.

DEVELOPMENT OF CLINICAL SYSTEMS

The development of in-house systems, documentation and training was covered under the system development life cycle in the first edition of *Clinical Data Management.* Much of the process for this development has remained the same. The information listed above for evaluating a commercial system could be applied when developing your own. However, it appears that the trend seems to be more in the direction of purchasing a system and working with the vendor to achieve enhancements and necessary upgrades.

EVALUATION OF COMMERCIAL SYSTEMS

There are new releases of database systems such as Clintrial version 4 from Domain Solutions[1], DLB's Recorder[2], and Oracle's Oracle Clinical[3] that show improvements with interfacing and usability.

New Document Management Systems are now available that provide the tools to allow the study team to integrate and coordinate their activities, increase workflow efficiency, provide tracking of Case Report Forms (CRFs) and aid with electronic submissions. There are now links from the sponsors to the sites and to CROs who may be involved in conducting the trials, and products that offer an efficient alternative to collecting data such as:

- Electronic patient diaries
- Interactive Voice Response Systems (IVRS)
- Remote Data Entry
- Optical Character Recognition (OCR) / Intelligent Character Recognition (ICR)

This chapter will summarize some of the more common systems currently being used in data management. It is not possible to cover the entire scope of everything available so only major systems will be discussed. Before purchasing a commercial system it makes good business sense to check out the company thoroughly as there may be changes in some of the companies that own the software.

Clinical Database Systems

Clintrial Version 4

Clintrial is a clinical trials data management software product line from Domain Solutions Corporation designed to support clinical studies' data management in all phases of drug research. Clintrial software is one of the most commonly used database systems in the pharmaceutical industry. It has been on the market for over 10 years. Clintrial version 4 facilitates the entire process from design of the clinical protocol and database through data entry, validation, data analysis and reporting of data. The system supports, but is not restricted to, standard structures, allowing the company to set up its own SOPs that would then need to be adhered to through established procedures.

Clintrial 4 is a user-friendly Client Server Application System that utilizes a Graphical User Interface (GUI) Client server application. Clintrial version 4 is very different from earlier versions of the software because of this client-server architecture.

Clintrial ENTER supports direct data entry into the database. Second data entry will overwrite during the on-line data entry. Range checking is supported during data entry. Look-up and decode capabilities are available for data entry, data review and validation, as well as, reporting purposes.

Clintrial MANAGE is integrated with ENTER and provides facilities for cleaning, validating, and performing global changes. Clintrial supports multiple language definitions for each of the thesauri, by storing various language terms as different fields in a record. Currently English and Kanji are supported. Adding forms or code lists in different languages can be done within the framework of standard Clintrial functionality. Adding new languages can be done by direct manipulations of the Oracle software database tables. Storing clinical data in different languages is not directly supported by the system but can be implemented by the user on the panel level during design. There is no limit to the number of different coding thesauri used in a Clintrial database. Coding thesauri can be loaded using the standard Clintrial data loading facilities and modified using the editing capabilities. Different versions of a thesaurus can be seen using the Clintrial View facility, which makes it possible to have several versions on-line together with the current version without having to duplicate the full thesaurus. Storage of both code and original text data are standard in Clintrial.

Clintrial DESIGN is a core module used to define and maintain metadata, such as database schemas, data entry screens, field definitions, code lists, validations; including creating, modifying and deleting data. An autoencoding application is provided in Clintrial 4.

The Clintrial RESOLVE module provides a complete query management and tracking application, allowing entry and processing of additional data queries. Plausibility checks, which are stored in the Oracle database, can be defined prior to entering data. Data checking and corrections are defined and programmed using PL/SQL, and can be defined across any data grouping. The system has automatic documentation of all transactions with data. This audit trail displays changes on an individual item basis consisting of the old and new values together with the patient and time point identification, date and time of the change and the user account that made the change.

Clintrial RETRIEVE is a core module used for flexible data access and extraction. Data are stored and retrieved in the database as normal Oracle data items. Clinical study definition is supported as a combination of database structure and information stored in the database. When designing a database it is possible to copy a study definition from another study, modifying, deleting or adding items as necessary. It is also possible to add new data items or modify existing ones after a study has started, using the Clintrial REVISE functionality.

The Clintrial MERGE facility allows for data locking at the individual record level. After cleaning the data, the clean data records are moved to another Oracle table with different access controls. Through the Clintrial VIEW facility, data can be locked retrospectively at the study level.

Clintrial REVIEW is an extended module that provides ad hoc data review and query tools for tabular data browsing and graphs without needing to have technical expertise in SAS or SQL programming.

There is no support of transformation of lab units into preferred units. Unit transformations need to be done in PL/SQL language. The Clintrial LAB LOADER extended module offers extended functionality for managing, validating and storing data collected by central laboratories. There are batch load capabilities for loading external data.

Access and Security Control are implemented in Clintrial at the Oracle database level. Additional security is provided on the application level if required. You have the ability to allow users to see only those options that are available for that user. Access rights for users, depending upon tasks and data status, can be administered by system administration. Access rights can also be granted for specific clinical development projects or single trials.

Clintrace is a comprehensive database software package for tracking and reporting of adverse events to regulatory agencies. It is designed to monitor drug safety reporting for both marketed and clinical trial products and is fully integrated with Clintrial.

An extended module is planned to support randomization schemata for blinded studies.

The extended modules of Clintrial MULTISITE and REMOTE support global replication of both data and metadata, including data item attributes, data entry screen definitions, derived data calculation procedures and data validation checks for corporations which do global product development.

DLB systems

DLB Recorder is a clinical database management system designed by DLB. DLB projects range from standalone PCs to international networks of minicomputers.

DLB's recorder is user friendly with a relatively easy set-up. It has a data entry system that can be interactive or not. Data entry can select which module they want to enter during data entry, allowing flexibility for entry. It is also possible to flag fields or attach notes to a field, then display data and notes through a report. Standardization can be attained through the modular approach to CRF design. There are interfaces with other clinical trial management systems and adverse event reporting and a direct interface to SAS. Recorder provides a unified system for case report form design, data entry screen design, database definition and data quality checking. It can be integrated with DLB MONITOR for the planning and monitoring of clinical trials and DLB ALERT for safety assessments. Recorder allows the application generator to select fields, modules, code lists and plausibility checking from libraries. These are used to develop a complete protocol. The system is flexible enough that the company can define the degree of standardization with the libraries. Recorder supports a hierarchy of standards that can be defined at various levels, world wide, by country, by therapeutic area and by protocol. Once a protocol is generated it can be built and executed on any target machine such as a VAX or IBM PC.

The Library of standard components is the starting point and is used to create a CRF. These components include field and module definitions, code lists, validation rules and checks, and SAS descriptors. These components are selected and can then be modified. The system will then generate database schemata, data entry screens and validation and consistency checks. Libraries of checks can be defined at the module and protocol levels. The results of checks are also stored and can be reported upon. The tracking of these data is linked to DLB MONITOR, if required.

Recorder contains a CRF browse module that allows medical monitors to query their data by patient, by visit, or by module. More advanced reporting capabilities are available through ad hoc query tools such as SQL assist.

Oracle Clinical Version 3

Oracle Clinical is the newest entry into the market. Some of the features of this system are a global library that stores the definitions for standards, both individual and groupings, code lists, thesauri, database validation criteria and standard CRF data entry layouts. The Library is centrally maintained and can be replicated to all global sites using it. This helps ensure that data are poolable, when managed at multiple sites. All data are linked to the global library, providing control and consistency throughout the study. The library can also have study-level components to allow further standardization. Using the global library, CRF definitions, which are mapped to the visit schedules in a spreadsheet-like format, can be set up fairly quickly. This helps to show the expected data at each visit. All data entry screens are automatically generated.

Oracle Clinical has a user-friendly GUI editor, which enables the users to easily create and modify the data entry layout, so that it can mimic the CRF, if desired. The system is flexible to allow multilingual prompts, if desired.

Oracle Clinical has a lab reference range management that allows the users to define labs and their ranges, assign patient CRFs to appropriate labs using a variety of criteria, assess lab values and query lab data. Oracle's validation procedures are stored in a library. These are user-defined in a non-programmatic environment. These definitions are linked to the status of the data, so if a procedure is changed in the middle of your study it will automatically re-execute and identify new problems. The old procedure would then become obsolete. There are also discrepancy reviews on line with the ability to correct or annotate problems. Since the status of the data is linked to the status of the discrepancy, if the data are updated the system will set any discrepancies to obsolete.

Oracle Clinical also has hot links between the discrepancy record and the data. This is a very good feature because it allows the user to see the data while they are cleaning the problem. If you are reviewing the problem and hit the hot link key it will take you to that data and you can make the change and return to the review of problems.

Oracle Clinical has locking features that are defined for the whole study or for a user-defined subset of data, down to an individual patient. Oracle Clinical stores all their data results in a single universal format. One table contains all data instead of multiple tables for each data type.

Oracle Clinical also provides site, patient, and visit tracking, which maintains information on investigators and sites, projected patient enrollments and timelines, detailed visit scheduling and tracking for breaking blind.

Remote Data Entry

There are a few additional issues that should be considered if you are evaluating an RDE system for your company.

- Systems must be validated at the site
- Follow your company's SOPs
- Data changes must be audited
- System should have access security
- Back-up of data on the system and recovery procedures must be established
- Randomization must have high security
- Training should be conducted in-house and at the site

- On-line support at the site is vital
- Ensure staff have the necessary competencies to operate the system selected.

CRF Workflow Systems

Electronic document management systems can offer savings in time for clinical studies, while reducing the physical space needed for storing CRFs. An electronic workflow allows your organization to have access to the data simultaneously within days of receipt of the data, by use of a scanner. It is even faster if the data are received through facsimile. It eliminates excessive copying of paper, allows for easier tracking of data and cuts down on loss of data. With data review and monitoring happening immediately following a patient's visit, errors can be found early on and corrected before they recur at the site. Images are archived and can be used for submissions.

General considerations when evaluating a CRF workflow system:

- Acceptance of usage by Investigator, Monitoring, Data Management, Clinical Development, Medical Writing and Drug Safety Functions
- Use of bar-coding for automatically indexing CRF pages
- Use fax capabilities
- Guaranteed sufficient support from vendor
- Development of an interface to CDBS for study set up and Optical Character Recognition (OCR)/mark-sense definitions
- Development of Intelligent Character Recognition (ICR) features
- Development of an interface to an entry tool, synchronization of entry screens and CRFimage
- Development of an interface to study management tools
- Ease of indexing
- Manpower and increased processing time for imaging data
- Capital Cost of equipment

The setting up and the use and maintenance of the system may need additional manpower, depending upon your clinical database system and how much integration would be required.

CRF-Documetrix[4]

This system is a flexible, user-friendly tool, which defines the workflow of scanned (faxed) and indexed CRFs with sufficient retrieval capabilities. Good tracking facilities exist, however, it does not interface to other systems. The designing of a workflow is very flexible. The validation was done very well. SOPs, documentation and audits are detailed and extensive.

After scanning CRF pages into the system further review of data can be done by patient, CRF page, or data type. CRFs, diaries and Data Clarification Forms (DCFs) are different types of documents and can be handled and retrieved separately. Bar code and FAX facilities are available.

A workflow has to be set up for every study but copying facilities are available for ease of this task. Changes in the defined workflow while studies are ongoing is possible without losing data. Roles and tasks can be defined. At decision points, short SQL-statements have to be added.

Currently there is only an interface to Clintrial version 3.3.1. If possible, an interface could be developed to read this information from your CDBS utilizing SQL.

Due to the lack of an interface, you must define the workflow manually according to the design of your CRF. Copying functionality is not available at this level. The following information has to be entered:

- Page number
- Name of the page (i.e., demo)
- Page type (i.e., CRF, diary, lab, etc.)
- Time structure (i.e., 'baseline', 'visit 1', etc.)
- Assignment of every page to its correspondent time point (e.g., page 1 to 'baseline')
- Repeated pages (i.e., for AEs) and a version control of single pages should exist

Faxing capabilities are available and a fax server would be necessary. Scanning is also an option and the speed depends upon the power of the installed scanner. Once a CRF is scanned or faxed the page is indexed. This can be automated with the use of bar codes. However, additional pages (i.e., lab print out, photographs, etc.) must be indexed manually.

A sample bar-code can be seen below:

STUDYNO / DOCNO / BOOKNO / PAGENO

Different book numbers can be assigned to one patient. By using the bar code facility, 100 pages can be scanned within 20 minutes. Study, book and page number are bar coded, patient number is entered by hand.

USI is developing OCR/mark-sense data entry capabilities, which would help with data entry of data types which could be recognized. However, the interface to your Clinical Database system (CDBS) would need be integrated with the vendor's system.

By using OCR/mark-sense for the first data entry, the second data entry could be done by a data entry person, using the verify mode and adding the free texts from the investigators.

Documetrix could be used as a tool for writing Data Clarification Forms (DCF). DCF can be classified via a user-defined choice list, which are automatically bar coded and can be tracked by the system. Copy capabilities are not available. There are no interfaces to the CDBS checking program to generate DCFs within the workflow. Therefore, all DCFs need to be created within the workflow system by hand. There are DCF reports within the system, as well as missing page reports.

Documentrix supports the use of NT server/client technology. Global use of Documetrix: only Oracle capabilities are available to distribute data.

Planned items:

- Internet CRF and DCF retrieval
- Electronic submission module
- Automated data entry (including mark-sense, Optical Character Recognition and Intelligent Character Recognition
- Remote data entry via Internet
- Documentum integration
- User group meetings

CRFTrack

CRFTrack[5] consists of three main modules for processing CRFs as images. The SCAN or FAX module can be used to capture data from the CRF and index the images. CRFTrack has several ways of automating the indexing process—Forms Recognition, Bar Code Recognition and OCR—all of which help shorten the time it takes to index. Manual indexing is available for the input of unique patient identification. Once the CRFs are indexed, they are part of the workflow and can be routed to any workstation defined in the system. The WORKFLO module uses a flow manager that keeps track of the CRF and creates a history of when and where the CRF has been entered. The workflow can be managed, monitored and changed at anytime during the process. CRFTrack supports dual data entry. The data entry station displays the image side by side to the data entry application. As part of the tracking, there is a tool which tracks and reports missing CRF pages. Version control for the CRF pages is also available. Therefore, if a page comes in with corrections, the most recent version will be on top of the previous version and the user can look through each version of a page. The old versions are tagged so that you always know you are viewing an old version. Bar code recognition is provided. The information is read and inserted into the indexing database. This enhances the accuracy and speed of indexing. Form recognition is used as an alternative to bar coding. This feature identifies unique forms and is used in conjunction with the image enhancement and OCR functions. The image enhancement function includes deskewing the image, removing lines and shading. CRFTrack provides a variety of annotations for tagging data and asking questions about the image; these include: clip notes, redlining, color highlighting. CRFTrack also has other capabilities of browsing data from patient to patient, visit to visit across patients, without going into each CRF book. These save time when reviewing data. Once a selection for review is made, these can be saved in a temporary folder that can hold any other imaged information as well. The import function can be used if you have other image systems with data that need to be brought into this one. The system has storage on a variety of media including network file servers, optical discs, CDs or Jukeboxes. The structure of the database stores images in a directory and uses a pointer to point to the image. Since you are passing pointers and not images the system is fairly fast.

CLINflo Version 2

CLINflo[6] is an integrated system that operates in a client-server environment. It captures CRFs and other related source documents, electronically routing them through the clinical review process, allowing for efficient entry of the information into virtually any existing clinical system. The workflow and routing of CRFs may easily be tailored to meet the needs of a specific protocol, drug or company. Complete audit trails are maintained on all aspects of the document throughout the clinical review and clarification process. CLINflo offers a variety of standard reports for tracking progress of subjects and investigator sites during the trials. A module of CLINflo has been used to support image CANDAs to the FDA and internationally.

CLINflo provides the flexibility of accepting CRFs via fax or traditional paper. CRFs that are faxed are captured 24 hours a day. CRFs which are either faxed or scanned into the system are automatically queued for indexing. Once in the system, the CRFs are indexed with uniquely identifying information. Optionally, this process can be eliminated through the use of bar codes that are preprinted or affixed to the CRF prior to scanning/faxing. CLINflo has a batch split facility which will automatically split a batch of indexed CRFs that contain forms for multiple patients into batches that contain pages for just one patient. The CRF is then routed along its pre-defined route throughout the clinical review process. The workflow component is automated utilizing a FloWare workflow map that can be changed for each study in the system or standardized. The system supports parallel, sequential and bi-directional routing through the workflow. Documents can be simultaneously viewed by any authorized individual. Informational 'post it note' style annotations and correctional annotations can be utilized to provide instructions or seek clarification of information on the documents being routed. The CLINflo system also provides a structured Data Clarification facility that may be used to efficiently resolve any anomalies encountered. When further information is required from a remote investigator site, the CRF, along with the data clarification, can be easily faxed out via CLINFlo's network-based fax gateway. 'Clean' documents are ultimately routed to the data entry activities where the clinical information is keyed into the clinical data systems. Data Entry can be linked into your database system so that the image and the data entry screens can be side by side for data entry.

CLINflo reporting has a variety of standard reports that will track the progress of the study by patient and investigator site. Users can quickly discern missing pages and the status of reviewed and non-reviewed CRFs. Reports may be viewed on screen, printed or directly accessed or loaded in Microsoft Windows application (MS Excel/Access, etc.) or statistical packages (SAS).

CRF Query is a powerful tool that allows users to query the CLINflo system. Multiple documents may be viewed concurrently allowing Reviewers and Data Managers to discern trends and patterns. Users of the CLINflo query facility may easily define queries to select documents by date, protocol, investigator or a variety of other indexed attributes. The batch routing queue displays flags indicating whether a batch contains annotations, notes, DCQs (data clarification queries) or replacement pages. You can view the batch history of each batch.

CLINflo activity selection windows provide the user with a work pending count prior to the user entering into an activity. This is a quick way to identify if there are batches waiting to be processed for a particular activity.

The CRF review application provides a consistent user interface across all workflow activities, from indexing, clinician, CRA review, data manager, data coding, and data verification. All viewing and reviewing activities are included in a work overview menu selection which displays the number of outstanding DCQs assigned to the user for resolution, the number of informal questions waiting to be read, the number of internal messages and the number of batches in the current activity. CLINflo also has a 'go to' page option in all viewing activities which allows you to quickly navigate through the CRF images. When DCQs are created they are 'attached' to the CRF page being questioned. Both the query and the image may be faxed to the site for resolution.

CLINflo has a query library allowing the user to keep language consistent in queries to the investigator site.

In CLINflo it is possible to access questionable pages directly (CRF query function). A magnify function helps reviewers with illegible data.

CLINflo has a role functionality which allows users to be defined as members of particular work groups. The role defines the permission level a user has within the system. It also determines what activities a certain role will have, such as the ability to create annotations or sign off on DCQs. CLINflo has on-line help as part of the system.

AlmediFAX

AlmediFAX[7] provides imaging, cataloging, electronic review, data entry and workflow reporting for Case Report Forms from a Microsoft Windows based PC workstation communicating to network servers. CRFs are completed and faxed into the system. They are indexed, reviewed and sent to data entry. The interesting component to this system is that they have templates which are created for each unique page of the CRF. These templates serve as an overlay of the image enabling data entry. Data can be stored in any ODBC-compliant database. Optical recognition, intelligent character recognition and mark-sense facilities support data entry. Template creation triggers the database table creation, the image data are saved to the corresponding database table at data entry time, this automates check box data entry via Optical Mark Recognition. CRF design is a key element when utilizing this type of system. You want to design your CRF with boxes that 'drop out' when faxed so that the template can work as efficiently as possible for OCR/ICR/MS. The OCR feature in AlmediFAX recognizes printed handwriting and is trained to handle both European numbers and US numbers. You also want to carefully choose your fonts to optimize indexing. Internal confidence of reading the image can be set. AlmediFAX uses a dictionary-driven approach so that they can ensure that proper values exist, reduce the number of false positives and enable simultaneous indexing for multiple studies. The workflow component in this system is procedural-driven and is not automated. AlmediFAX tracks inbound and outbound CRF activity through the clinical process. Multiple studies can share the same tracking information. Management and audit reports can be generated and additional reports can be written using SQL. During review you can annotate a CRF page. Each annotation is connected to its corresponding annotated page area with a line marker and faxed directly to the site showing the CRF image and the problem.

IRIS Clinical

Although *IRIS Clinical* does contain CRF imaging and workflow components, it is actually an integrated system for the planning and execution of the entire data acquisition process, including the tracking of patient enrollment and generation of investigator payments. IRIS is a good (semi-automatic) data entry tool with limited tracking and reviewing features. This tool is developed for CRF designing and data capture and is not a workflow system by itself, but can serve as such, at least for CRF tracking. All scanned batches are available within the system (by network), eligible and accessible for viewing, wherever they were scanned worldwide. An additional FAX facility is not available.

The batches which were indexed or named, include the date of scanning. After scanning/reading is performed, the CRF pages are indexed, with the patient number being included in the index. Further access can be done by CRF module or by patient. During the reading function all numerical data are 'read'(OMR/OCR/ICR) and entered automatically. During the validation step all (numerical) characters are shown sorted by categories in ascending order. In case of wrong assignment or an 'unreadable' character, the data technician can correct the character. In the course of this the character will be marked and put into the right category automatically. During the validation process the scanned text is displayed and can be entered into the text field, which is also given automatically. If a thesaurus is available as a pop-up list, the coding can be done 'automatically' during this process.

During all process steps the corresponding sector (field) of the scanned CRF is shown in parallel by an access to a character. Additionally, the whole image of the CRF page can be viewed by soft key function at each time.

PAREXEL estimates that the entire procedure—indexing, data entry and validation including coding and text entry—takes about one minute per page.

PAREXEL uses neither the plausibility facilities nor the review function, because this part can be handled much more elegantly and faster in their database system (FOXPRO).

The system is user friendly in handling and good documentation is available. There is no interface to project/study management.

SUMMARY

There are a great number of systems out there to select from when trying to improve the clinical data management process. It is extremely important that prior to starting the process of evaluation, you need to understand what direction you are heading in and how much evaluation you wish to undertake. You want to know the entire scope of the project and define your needs and prioritize them before evaluating the system to maintain objectivity. Data management systems should be integrated with workflow systems and document management systems, if at all possible, to avoid duplication of work. Interactive diary data need to be integrated into your database system or imported with minimal effort. It is key to set up your criteria and evaluate each system with the same criteria. Clinical

Workflow table

Table 12.1   Workflow systems table

	Documetrix CRF	CRFtrack image solutions	CLINflo Version 2	AlmediFAX
Indexing tools	Automated bar code and/or assisted manual	Automated OCR and/or bar codes and/or assisted manual	Assisted manual	Automated OCR/ ICR; Vendor claims 70–80% hit rate
Workflow control	Automated via Documetrix workflow engine	Manual; Status checked via reports	Automated via Plexus workflow engine	Manual; Status checked via reports
Image storage and management	Each CRF page is stored as individual files in network file server directory tree. Pointers and status information are in an Oracle DB	Each page is stored as individual files in network file server tree. Pointers and status information are in an Oracle DB	Images are stored as BLOBs in an Informix database. Status information stored in an Informix database	Each page is stored as an individual file in network file server directory tree. Pointers and status information are in an MS access database or Oracle via ODBC
CDBMS	Current integration with Clintrial Version 3.3 and Recorder DCSs can be imported from a CDBMS	Data Entry screens and images can be linked	Data Entry screens and images can be linked	Data Entry screens and images can be linked
European support		Office in Switzerland	From the US	Offices in Switzerland and UK
Validated	Yes, in accordance with FDA guidelines	No	No	No
Extra features		Automated conversion to PDF for FDA submissions		
Future plans	Integration with Clintrial Version 4 and Documentum; Enablement of image management and RDE; Automated conversion to PDF for FDA submissions	Automated Workflow	OCR/ICR indexing	Automated Workflow

systems are very complex and should be given the time necessary for a complete evaluation, including testing and validation by both end users and developers. You want to ensure that the product that you have selected can perform all of the necessary functions and that you purchase a high-quality product from a company in a sound financial position with a long-term commitment to the project. Ensure during the discussions with the vendor that you really understand what is available today and, if future functionality is important to you and your company, that you include appropriate clauses in the contract. The contract between you and the vendor is an important part of any purchase to help avoid any misunderstandings that can affect relations at a later date. Sufficient time and expertise must be assigned to this key step. Once this has been verified, it is essential to have good training for all those who will be using the system and proper communication for working out any bugs or needed enhancements. Implementation plans will be key to making sure that the system you selected is properly put into place. The success of all of the above require appropriate resources to be allocated, both monetary and staffing, together with a good project plan and project management.

REFERENCES

1. Clintrial: Domain Solutions Corporation, 150 Cambridge Park Drive, Cambridge, MA 02140, USA.
2. DLB Recorder: DLB Systems Inc., Bernards/78, 110 Allen Road, Liberty Corner, NJ 07938, USA.
3. Oracle Clinical: Oracle Corporation, World Headquarters, 500 Oracle Parkway, Redwood Shores, CA 94065, USA.
4. CRF-Documetrix: Universal Systems Inc., 14 Avion Parkway, Chantilly, VA 20151, USA.
5. CRFTRack: Image Solutions, Inc., 1280 Route 46, Parsippany, NJ 07054, USA.
6. CLINflo: Trion Technologies, Inc., 760 Beta Drive, Suite F, Mayfield Village, Ohio 44143, USA.
7. AlmediFAX: Almedica Technology Group Inc., 900 Lanidex Plaza Suite 202, Parsippany, NJ 07054, USA.

13 Systems Software Validation Issues—Clinical Trials Database Environment

STEVE HUTSON

Barnett International, a company of Parexel International, Denham, Middlesex, UK

INTRODUCTION

Anyone who has been associated with the pharmaceutical industry during the last few years will be in no doubt as to the consequences of failing to satisfy the requirements of regulators such as the Food and Drug Administration (FDA). Loss of approval of a drug can cost a company millions and even put the company's viability at risk. Yet the cost, in money, time and resources, of gaining and maintaining regulatory approval appears to be spiralling.

It is not so much that regulatory requirements have changed, more that the environment in which they have to be applied has evolved. Guidelines such as Good Manufacturing Practice (GMP) were conceived in a world of data-loggers, chart recorders and lab notebooks. Today they must be applied in the world of the microchip where vast amounts of electronic data are generated and moved around complex computer networks. Despite the increase in complexity the basic requirement of the regulators has remained the same. The pharmaceutical industry must be able to demonstrate the quality, reliability and integrity of all safety and efficacy data.

Increasingly these requirements are not only being applied to the results generated but also to the entire process by which they are obtained. Indeed this now includes the design and manufacture of the plant, equipment and software used in that process. This means that pharmaceutical companies not only need to fully understand their own processes but also must know far more about their suppliers than has previously been the case.

New guidelines, such as Good Automated Laboratory Practice (GALP) and Good Automated Manufacturing Practice (GAMP), acknowledge the importance of computerised systems within the pharmaceutical process

Clinical Data Management. Second Edition. Edited by R.K. Rondel, S.A. Varley and C.F. Webb.
© 2000 John Wiley & Sons, Ltd

and heighten awareness amongst all interested parties, particularly the regulators, of the unique issues such systems raise.

All this has meant that validation, ensuring compliance with regulatory requirements, is making ever increasing demands upon the resources of both the pharmaceutical company and its suppliers.

VALIDATION OF CLINICAL COMPUTER SYSTEMS

Until the introduction of the EC Good Clinical Practice (GCP) regulations in 1991[1], the validation of clinical computer systems was not a serious topic for many clinical managers. This was in marked contrast to their colleagues in areas governed by Good Laboratory Practice (GLP) and GMP where computer validation had been introduced by the FDA in the early 1980s. Clinical managers were further handicapped by:

- A poor understanding of computerised systems and applications coupled with limited regulatory guidance on validation
- An emphasis on developing systems to manage the increasing volumes of clinical data with little or no time allowed for validation
- The move from the corporate mainframe environment to departmental minis and desktop architectures, which encouraged local rather than centralised development of systems and applications. Often these would be poorly planned and managed
- A poor understanding of software engineering principles resulting in inefficient and in some cases ineffective applications being built

Despite these problems, systems and applications were built to manage clinical trials and handle safety and efficacy data and they gave every appearance of working—unfortunately for many this was not the reality and much resource was used to continuously improve functionality and cure problems.

Many of the above problems still exist but the crucial difference now is that regulators have developed better guidance on the validation of computerised systems and applications (see European GCP[1], ICH GCP [ICH:E6][2] and Statistical Principles for Clinical Trials [ICH:E9 Step 2])[3]. As a result all new developments and existing systems have to be validated.

WHAT IS VALIDATION?

Numerous definitions exist depending on your perspective (retrospective, prospective, concurrent and retroactive) and which regulations you consult. The GMP Guide to Computerised Systems[4] describes validation as:

Validation should be considered as part of the complete life cycle of a computer system. This cycle includes the stages of planning, commissioning, documentation, operation, monitoring and changing.

Validation has also been defined as:

Establishing documented evidence which provides a high degree of assurance that a specific process will consistently produce a product meeting its pre-defined specifications and quality attributes (FDA 1987).[5]

and

The demonstration that a computerised system is suitable for its intended purpose.

A definition which seems to combine these has been put forward by the Association for Clinical Data Management (ACDM)[6]:

The establishment of documentary evidence which:

a) demonstrates that the system was developed and implemented, and is operated and maintained, in a controlled manner throughout its life-time up to and including decommissioning,

b) results in a high degree of assurance that the system consistently meets its specification, and is therefore suitable for its intended purpose

WHY VALIDATE?

A formalised validation process has in the past been seen as a chore and a delay in implementing any system and as a consequence has tended to be ignored or at best left until the last possible moment. However, evidence would suggest that not allocating sufficient resource to validation early, leads to a much bigger overhead supporting systems later[7]. In fact building validation into your system development provides a number of benefits over and above the potential cost savings including:

- The opportunity for ongoing testing and reviewing allowing user requirements and functional specifications to be better met
- A formalised validation process with active user participation is a better quality test for a system or application. It also gives the users a greater degree of confidence in the final product
- Validation can indicate where further improvements in quality are possible
- A validated system/application will be a much more efficient and effective one

However, the overriding reason for incorporating validation into your system development is to ensure compliance with GCP regulations. Today, reliable entry, verification, storage, transfer, manipulation and retrieval of data generated in state-of-the-art clinical research has become a strategic factor in successful clinical development. The level of documented control over a clinical data system determines the confidence one can have in the reliability of databases, and availability of correct data.

Computerised Systems—a Definition for Validation Purposes

The term 'computerised system' occurs throughout the EC GCP regulations—for example, 'Entry to a computerised system is acceptable when controlled as recommended in the EEC guide to GMP'—and is used to describe the combination of hardware (PCs, file servers, workstations and the local/wide area network), software (operating system, and software applications) and the associated people and procedures. Computerised systems within the clinical trials area that need to be validated include all those systems deployed by a company in handling, manipulating and transferring patient data. In addition, applications and systems used by local/core labs, Contract Research Organisations (CROs) and subsidiaries who handle trials data should also be included in the validation plan.

Often clinical systems will have been developed over a long period of time and information on their numbers and functionality may be limited. In these circumstances a useful starting point might be to carry out an audit of the systems within the clinical environment to scale the problem (resource and time requirements), prioritise the work and determine what does and does not need to be validated.

Examples of clinical systems include: Randomisation Systems, Data Capture Systems (manual systems—in-house data entry, remote data entry, automated systems—bar codes, Optical Character Recognition [OCR] etc.), Electronic Transfer of Data, Clinical Trials Databases, Drug Safety Databases, Data Derivations, Statistical Software. (NB this list is not comprehensive.)

Regulations

The publication of GCP regulations by different countries incorporating specific sections on computers reflects the growing need to ensure the integrity of computerised data. The EC, The Nordic Council on Medicines, The Australian Therapeutic Goods Administration and the FDA very specifically talk about computer use in clinical trials. Such statements have helped to raise the level of awareness about validation within the clinical development community and brought GCP into line with GLP and GMP regulations for computer systems which were first established by the FDA in the late 1970s and early 1980s.

Below are some extracts from the Notes for Guidance on Good Clinical Practice (GCP) for Trials on Medicinal Products in the EC[1] and The ICH Guideline for Good Clinical Practice (ICH:E6)[2] relating specifically to the validation of computerised systems.

European GCP

3.2 Entry to a computerized system is acceptable when controlled as recommended in the EEC guide to GMP (Good Manufacturing Practice).

3.3 If trial data are entered directly into a computer there must always be adequate safeguard to ensure VALIDATION . . . Computerized systems should be VALIDATED and a detailed description for their use be produced and kept up-to-date.

3.4 . . . For electronic data processing only authorized persons should be able to enter or modify data in the computer and there should be a record of changes and deletions.

3.5 If data are altered during processing, the alteration must be documented and the system VALIDATED.

3.10 The sponsors must use VALIDATED, error free data processing programs with adequate user documentation.

3.12 When electronic data handling systems or remote electronic data entry are employed, Standard Operating Procedures (SOPs) for such systems must be available.

3.15 If data are transformed during processing, the transformations must be documented and the method VALIDATED.

3.16 The sponsors must maintain a list of persons authorized to make corrections and protect access to the data by appropriate security systems.

ICH GCP (ICH:E6)

5.5.3 When using electronic trial data handling and/or remote electronic trial data systems, the sponsor would:

a) Ensure and document that the electronic data processing system(s) conforms to the sponsor's established requirements for completeness, accuracy, reliability and consistent intended performance (i.e. validation).

b) Maintain SOPs for using these systems.

c) Maintain a security system that prevents unauthorized access to the data.

d) Maintain adequate back-up of the data.

Clearly, from the above extracts and by examining similar documents from other countries some common themes begin to emerge:

• Documented physical and logical security of hardware and software systems

• Audit trails for data entry changes

- SOPs for system maintenance and database back-ups
- During data entry consistency and validity checks should be conducted. These should be both computerised checks and original source document verification
- The ability to retrieve the hard copy of archived data
- The use of validated, error-free software programs with adequate user documentation
- Where computerised remote data entry systems are used they should be supported by user documentation and SOPs

Such themes for computerised systems not only run through the GCP regulations but also through GLP and GMP alike. Whilst many regard these guidelines as yet another burden necessary to ensure compliance, they do provide a structure for maintaining control of the computer environment, ensuring efficient and effective use of that resource.

VALIDATING A CLINICAL SYSTEM

Whether or not your computerised clinical system satisfies a regulatory inspection will depend on the level of validation undertaken. This may in turn depend on a number of factors including who developed it (in-house, vendor), when it was developed and whether or not good software/system development procedures were employed.

The Audit

Consider the situation where a company receives a visit from a regulatory authority and the inspectors want to audit the clinical trials computer system. What would the inspectors want to see? In order to adequately answer this question it is recommended that an audit SOP be developed covering responsibilities, policy statements, conduct of meetings and materials that should be made available:

1. Documentation relating to the software development such as the requirements, functional and design specifications, the test plan together with results, change/version control, user manuals, training materials and programming standards.
2. User acceptance testing, including the test strategy, methodology, and results report.
3. Evidence that people are suitably qualified and trained to undertake the procedures allocated to them, for example CVs, training records, user guide and training materials.

4. Security, including physical security, password assignment and changes, access authority and virus checking.
5. System use and maintenance. Will cover user and technical support manuals, standards and procedures along with software and hardware maintenance procedures and records.
6. User support—will detail support/help for problems, manuals and training.
7. Problem management—including the logging of problems and their resolution.
8. System back-up and restoration—back-up (routine incremental and full) and disaster recovery arrangements.
9. Business continuity—arrangements for system and data recovery in the event of a major disaster.
10. Change management—documentation (development, testing and authorisation materials) summarising the major computer system (hardware, software, procedures and people) changes since the last inspection, planned changes, installation and training provisions and revalidation requirements.
11. Decommissioning plan.
12. Archiving—including policy on validation documents, software, hardware and legacy data.
13. Audit arrangements for in-house software development, vendors and CROs together with details on arrangements for maintaining compliance.

A comprehensive documentation checklist is included in the joint ACDM/PSI Guideline on Computer Systems Validation in Clinical Research and is reproduced in Appendix 13.1.

Approach to Validation

By far the best way to approach a large, complex task such as validation is through a well-developed plan and the first part of any plan should be to ensure that the validation of computerised systems is a strategic business issue and as such is part of company policy.

Validation Policy—Does Your Company Have One?

One of senior management's principal responsibilities in a pharmaceutical company is to ensure the integrity of data submitted to authorities in order to prove the safety, efficacy and quality of the product. As most of this data is held in digital form in corporate databases, how do senior management meet this obligation? Without the assurance of a validated computer system they can't.

Therefore the first action that needs to take place is for senior management to create and enforce a corporate policy for validating computerised systems. As such a policy will affect the whole organisation, its development should be funded and staffed appropriately.

The contents of the Validation Policy will need to cover:

- The objectives, scope and company commitment.
  This section will outline the aims of validation together with the general approach including the method used to determine which systems will be validated and which will not. The identification of senior managers as the major sponsors will demonstrate how seriously the company takes this issue and their commitment to see it through.
- Roles and responsibilities.
  For those involved in the validation work, all roles and responsibilities need to be defined in a job description. This section should also re-emphasise senior management's support for system validation and clearly define other critical functions such as who has day-to-day responsibility for demonstrating a system's validity.
- Personnel.
  In accordance with the principles outlined in the GCP guidelines, personnel records for those involved in validation should contain: a curriculum vitae, a record of relevant training and experience and a job description.
- Awareness and training programme.
  Develop an awareness and training programme for delivering the corporate validation policy to all senior managers and staff using the computerised systems.
- Documentation.
  A common deficiency found by regulatory authorities conducting inspections is poor or inadequate documentation, particularly in the area of systems definition, i.e. what is its intended purpose. The validation process needs to be supported by: written policies; SOPs and instructions; the validation plan; software development; user acceptance testing; validation report; operational use; and decommissioning.
- Management of validation
  Ideally the validation exercise should be structured and managed as part of a quality process. How the validated state is maintained during active use of the system and what action is required in the event of system changes should also be documented.
- Decommissioning.
  Access to legacy data will always be a major issue. How clinical systems are decommissioned and what happens to the archived data are critical concerns and need to be documented.

- Quality assurance.
  To ensure compliance with regulations, a formal Quality Assurance (QA) programme should be implemented. This should endeavour to audit the validation activities against SOPs. Audits should be performed on systems: developed in-house; purchased from vendors; developed by third parties; and those used by CROs.

When completed and accepted the document should be endorsed as company policy and implemented throughout the organisation. To ensure success it will also need the active support of top management.

Validation Plan

A validation plan is a document that identifies all systems and subsystems involved in a specific validation exercise and the approach by which they will be qualified and the total system validated. The plan will differ depending on whether it is an existing computer system (sometimes referred to as retrospective validation) or a new development (prospective validation), that is to be validated.

Retrospective computer validation

Many organisations adopt the approach, 'if it ain't broke don't fix it', and as a consequence many are still using computerised systems developed several years ago, possibly even before the incorporation of validation into GCP. Under these circumstances, it is quite feasible that an audit would reveal missing documentation, tests, and so forth. Despite this, management may decide to retain the system and instigate a retrospective validation of the system to plug the gaps. In contrast, because a retrospective validation can be a costly endeavour in terms of resource, time and funds, management may take this opportunity to replace the system rather than repair it.

Also, depending on what your policy is for handling legacy data (leave in existing system, archive or transfer to new system), replacement is not always as straightforward as you would imagine as products already on the market will be supported by data held on these older systems and the company and regulatory authorities need to be assured of the validity of those data. The authorities expect every computer system used to be validated—nowhere does it state that old systems are excused. Figure 13.1 gives an indication of the steps involved in a retrospective validation.

Validation team. To conduct a validation exercise (retrospective or prospective) within the clinical environment a validation team resourced and supported by senior management (Medical Director and heads of relevant

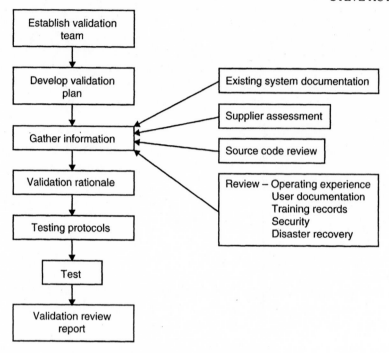

Figure 13.1 Steps involved in a retrospective validation

departments) will need to be set up. Because many of the clinical systems are interconnected and support more than one functional area, the team will need to reflect this. For example, for the validation of a clinical data management system the team should have representatives from: Statistics, Data Management, Clinical QA, IT managers (software and hardware), CRAs, Monitors, Database Administrators as well as a Project Manager.

Validation team responsibilities. The principal role of the validation team is to develop a validation plan that will identify all the activities required to determine compliance with GCP and rectify any deficiencies. For an existing computerised system handling clinical trials data, the team would need to produce:

- An inventory of existing computer systems and subsystems including hardware (make and model of computer, machine architecture, data storage, etc.), software (including operating systems, applications being used, e.g., the clinical database management system, communications and security), network configuration and security management, and other software such as remote transmissions, data entry, etc.

- An inventory of all documentation associated with the systems, e.g. the system specification, the system design manual, source code, installation manual, user manual, service contracts, system logbooks, upgrade and new version installation records, policies and procedures covering back-up, data recovery, archiving, training and security policies.
- Changes that have occurred to the hardware, software, documentation and personnel need to be documented. Ideally this will have been done at the time and captured in the Change Control Documents.
- A written history of past and present system experience compiled by those with the greatest knowledge of the system. This should give a description of the system (functional specification) and refer to documents linking the proposal, acceptance testing, systems and user manuals, maintenance, upgrades, code changes and audit reports. The history should also document all experience with the software since it was first installed and cover who owns it, uses it, the current configuration, the support for version control, back-up and disaster recovery, security, training, vendor contractual arrangements for software support and upgrades along with recent audit findings. The history should be supported by reference to maintenance logs, and other system documents.

Having identified all the systems/subsystems and assessed their maturity and stability together with the quality and completeness of the documentation, the team will be in a good position to prioritise the work required and assess the resource implications. Ideally, in a retrospective validation all functions of a system should be validated in detail. Unfortunately this would not be cost-effective and a pragmatic approach needs to be adopted. Risk analysis will aid the prioritisation process by identifying those components of a system that are not critical, and for which a simple validation will have to suffice, and those components that are deemed critical to the system, where a more detailed validation will be required.

Armed with this information the team will then need to write:

- The validation plan, which should describe all roles, responsibilities and activities involved in the validation exercise
- The test plan, describing the approach to be taken under the validation plan. This should include items to be tested, the tests, personnel needed, reporting requirements, evaluation criteria and any risks
- The test procedure script, which details the set-up, operation and evaluation of the results for a particular test
- The test report which captures the results and compares them to those expected

Clearly, for existing systems, retrospective validation is a distinct and separate operation from the development activities. In most instances the system will already be in use and hold data. As we have already seen, under these circumstances the validation proceeds in distinct stages. First, the validation exercise must be carefully planned, identifying the appropriate tests. It may be necessary to take the system out of use temporarily. Second, the system is examined and a report produced which identifies areas in which the system is deficient. Finally, the defects are corrected and the system is revalidated.

In contrast, for new computer systems, validation should be an integral part of the process of designing and building a computer system according to good professional practice. In other words, it becomes part of the quality control process. This is what is known as prospective validation.

Prospective computer validation

As with retrospective validation you will need a validation team who will be responsible for developing a validation plan.

The validation plan/strategy. To design, develop, coordinate, install, implement and use successfully any new computer system, whether developed in-house or purchased, requires effective project management. This will require sound plans and procedures together with mechanisms for controlling and monitoring the project. To control and manage a software and systems project you need to adopt a system development life cycle model (SDLC) such as the PMAs validation life cycle approach[8] or the V model (STARTS)[9]. Furthermore, if you want your new clinical computer system to be more efficient and effective and readily accepted by the users, then validation should be part of the SDLC model.

An SDLC model is a general framework or outline of tasks to accomplish the development of a computer system. It typically includes the stages of planning, specification, programming, testing, commissioning, documentation, operation, monitoring and changing and the V model (see Figure 13.2) represents the current best practice for building quality systems. This model describes a project in terms of a progression of stages that define what the system should do (left-hand side of the V), together with associated processes that provide the assurance that a system actually does what it should (right-hand side of the V).

At each definition stage there are three activities that provide this assurance:

1. *Verification* (am I building the right system?) Verification will establish that any functionality defined in the specification is attributable to at least one requirement, and that each requirement is covered in the specifica-

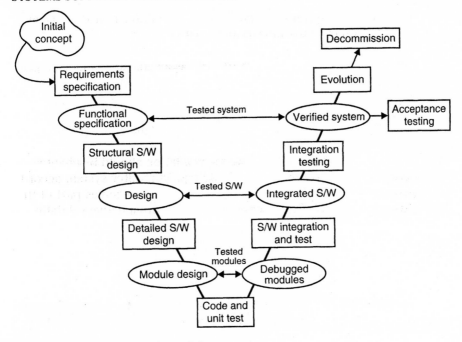

Figure 13.2   The V process model

tion. This is usually established through document reviews, prototyping and code inspection.

2.   *Validation* (am I building the system right?) Validation establishes that deliverables are complete and consistent. Standard methodologies and tools (PRINCE, SSADM, CASE tools, TickIT) force developers to adopt controlled techniques and disciplines and provide the purchaser with the assurance of functional accuracy, completeness and reliability of the system.

3.   *Testing* (does the system do what it should?) A test plan to demonstrate that inputs, processing and outputs are handled correctly should encompass data precision, maintenance of raw data, security and audit trails. Results should be recorded and any changes to the system should be formally documented. The plan should also cover how to test, test case definitions and preparation of test data. Functional testing is performed to demonstrate that the system functions correctly according to its specifications. Stress testing is carried out to ensure that the system rejects erroneous input in the proper ways.

Documentation from the development life cycle process (Table 13.1) provides validation evidence of the quality assurance of the system.

Table 13.1   Documents associated with the SDLC

Software life cycle phases	Software life cycle documents
Initial phase	Initial concept
Requirements phase	Requirements specification
	Functional specification
Design phase	Design specification
Implementation phase	Source code
	Module test results
Integration phase	Integrated test results
	System test results
Install and verification phase	Installation qualification
	User and system manuals
	Acceptance/validation test results
	Review and release
	Training documentation
Operation & maintenance phase	Change & problem mgt documentation
Decommissioning phase	Decommissioning documentation

The V model is also relevant to off-the-shelf packages. Vendors of such systems generally provide those parts of the model associated with:

- Software development methods
- Software fault management
- Documentation management
- Configuration control
- Development personnel
- User manuals
- Release notes
- Training and support
- Upgrade mechanisms

The user will be responsible for:

- System installation
- The operating environment
- User acceptance testing
- User training
- Change control procedures
- Disaster recovery and reporting of software faults

Quality plan. Because of the iterative nature of software development and the interdependence of programs and modules, it is not always possible to demonstrate software quality assurance (QA) simply by testing the functionality of a particular deliverable. Quality has to be built into the development of such systems through the adoption of formal methods, project controls and quality plans. A quality plan will:

- List all the deliverables
- Define how their quality features will be defined (specification and standards)
- Define how those features will be checked for (i.e., define how the Quality Control will be done)

The contents list for a Quality Plan may include:

The system specification

- The acceptance criteria
- A list of deliverables that will be produced during development
- A definition of each deliverable's quality features with reference to a specification and appropriate standards
- A definition of how each deliverable's quality features will be verified and what records will be kept of the verification
- Indications in all cases of the levels of authorisation that will be required for approval of specifications, approval of verification and approval of outcome

Your quality plan might also be an appropriate place to describe:

- Change control procedures
- Fault management procedures
- Purchasing procedures
- Project reporting and debriefing procedures
- Training requirements
- Security considerations

CASE STUDY—VALIDATION OF A GLOBAL CLINICAL TRIALS DATABASE

To demonstrate the potential range and complexity of a validation exercise in the clinical environment a synopsis of a project undertaken on behalf of a global pharmaceutical company is outlined below.

Background

The company wished to validate their clinical trials database used to hold patient data from Phase II and Phase III clinical trials. However, the validation had to cope with a number of complications:

1. The database had a number of different instances:

   - UK Patients
   - UK Volunteers
   - US Patients
   - US Volunteers
   - Training

Each with its own set of data.

2. The five databases were installed on two separate machines:

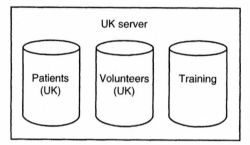

3. The company had configured the clinical trials package:

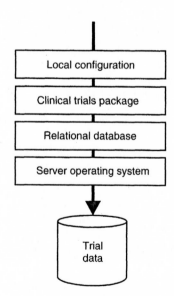

4. The company had written other software to access and manipulate the data:

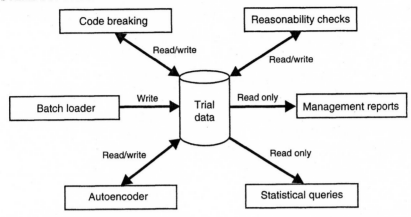

The problem

The problem was how to validate this very complex environment in a pragmatic and timely fashion? The complexities included such issues as:

- Multiple departments within the company responsible for areas such as the servers, the software installations, the networks, code developed by the statisticians, etc.
- Varying procedures, for example it was acceptable to delete patient data on the training database, but not on the 'live' US patients database
- Many existing company SOPs covering areas such as software development, validation, use of the Clinical Trials database, training, etc.

The Solution

1. *The company's own standards were used to drive the validation:*
   From the company's own SOPs for validation, a checklist was prepared for each area (e.g., user training, backups, change control, etc.).
2. *The following were excluded from the scope of the validation:*
   - System level software, including operating systems, the relational database, the network, and the standard PC client. It was argued that the correct functionality of all such software was adequately demonstrated by the testing performed on the software which sat 'on top of' this base software.
   - The underlying data. It was argued that the validity of the data was checked on a protocol-by-protocol basis in accordance with existing SOPs.
   - All of the software which accessed the data, with the exception of the reasonability checks and the autoencoder. It was argued that the validation of all other software systems was the responsibility

of the owner of the software, but that these two were sufficiently critical to require special attention.

● Compliance with existing SOPs. It was argued that this was checked by the routine internal quality audits.

3. *The overall system was broken down into a number of separate validations (see Figure 13.3):*
    1. The *use* of the patients database (whether US or UK)
    2. The *use* of the volunteers database (whether US or UK)
    3. The *use* of the training database
    4. The US machine, particularly the installation of the software
    5. The UK machine, particularly the installation of the software
    6. The reasonability checks software
    7. The autoencoder software
    8. The clinical trials package

By defining the scope of the work, breaking it down into well-defined subprojects, and listing all identifiable risks to system validity, what appeared initially to be a monstrous task began to take on more manageable proportions. Next, as part of the global validation programme, validation plans were developed and agreed for each subproject, describing the

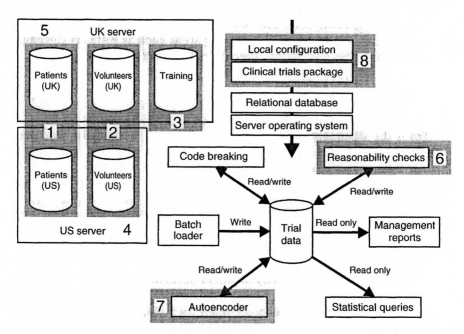

Figure 13.3 Diagrammatic representation of the separate validations

measures to be taken and who was responsible for delivery. To avoid duplication of effort the boundaries for each subproject were clearly defined and documented as was the extent of the validation to be conducted. Good project management practices were employed to keep all activities on track and the final validation report, confirming that all the measures and documentation identified in the plans had been produced, was delivered on time.

CONCLUSION

Today most industries, including pharmaceuticals, are developing computer systems to provide enterprise or businesswide functionality. As a consequence the landscape is changing and the islands of technology that existed in the 1980s, supporting small business units such as clinical data management, are being integrated into systems that better support the wider business needs.

Such computer systems are complicated and expensive to develop and although the principal focus for systems validation remains satisfying the regulatory requirements, it has also become a good business practice that enhances system reliability, minimises development costs and increases quality.

Appendix 1—Validation Documentation

The following list suggests documents for inclusion in the validation document set of a project or for inspection during an audit, and is taken from the Joint ACDM/PSI Guideline on Computer Systems Validation in Clinical Research.

While common core documents are listed, it is recommended that the validation document set requirement be assessed for each project individually, since each project may incur special risks, necessitating additional documentation.

Category of deliverable	Document	Source	System validation	Audit of CRO	Audit of vendor
Validation	Validation Policy	Corporate Management		X	X
	Validation Plan	Validation Manager	X	X	X
	Validation Report	Validation Manager	X	X	
QA	SOPs (see above)	QA	X	X	X
	System Analysis Standards	Senior System Analyst	X	X	X
	Programming Standards	Senior Developer	X	X	X
System design	Requirements of System Spec.	Systems Analyst	X	X	X
	Hardware & Operating Environment Spec.	System Analyst	X	X	X
	Database Design Spec.	Systems Analyst/DBA	X	X	X
	Technical Spec.	Developer	X	X	X
	Installation Instructions	Development Team	X	X	X
Impact assessment	Impact on SOPs, Working Practices and Guidelines	User	X		
	Impact on other Computer Systems	Senior Developer with owners of other systems	X		
	Security Implications	Senior Developer, DBA, User, Systems Management	X	X	
Test strategy	System Test Strategy	System Test Manager	X	X	X
	User Acceptance Test	User Test Manager	X	X	
Test	Source Code Review	System Test Manager	X	X	X
	Module Test Plans	Developer or Tester	X	X	X
	Module Test Results	Developer or Tester	X	X	X
	System Test Plans	System Tester	X	X	X
	System Test Results	System TesterX	X	X	

Category of deliverable	Document	Source	System validation	Audit of CRO	Audit of vendor
	Database Integrity Test Plans	DBA	X	X	X
	Database Integrity Test Results	DBA	X	X	X
	User Acceptance Test Plans	User Tester	X	X	
	User Acceptance Test Reports	User Tester	X	X	
Problem tracking & management	Pre-release Incident Reports	Developer, Tester, User, DBA	X	X	X
	Pre-release Incident Management	Senior Developer	X	X	X
	Post-production Release Incident Reports	Users	X	X	
	Post-production Release Incident Management	Maintenance Team	X	X	
Process control	Authorisation for Release to Test Environment	User Test Manager	X	X	X
	Ratification of Validation Report	Senior Manager(s), User Department(s)	X	X	X
	Authorisation for Release to Production	Project Manager	X	X	X
	Release Notes	Senior Developer	X	X	X
	Evidence of Document Review and Approval	Designated Reviewers and Approvers	X	X	X
Personnel	CV	All Project Staff, Maintenance Staff and System Users	X	X	X
	Record of Training and Experience	All Project Staff, Maintenance Staff and System Users	X	X	X
	Competency Records	All Project Staff, Maintenance Staff and System Users	X	X	X
Training	User Guide	Technical Author	X	X	X
	Training Materials	Training Manager	X	X	
	User Training Log	Training Manager	X	X	
System maintenance	Service Level Agreement for System Maintenance	Maintenance Team, Vendor	X	X	X

REFERENCES

1. EC CPMP (1991) Good Clinical Practice for Trials on Medicinal Products in the European Community, Brussels, Commission of the European Communities.
2. ICH:E6, GCP Consolidated Guideline. http://www.ifpma.org/pdfifpma/e6.pdf
3. ICH:E9. Statistical Considerations in the Design of Clinical Trials. http://www.ifpma.org/pdfifpma/e6.pdf
4. EC Commission (1992) Good Manufacturing Practice for Medicinal Products in the European Community, Brussels, Commission of the European Communities, January.
5. FDA (1987) Guidelines on General Principles of Process Validation.
6. Joint ACDM/PSI (1997) Guideline on Computer Systems Validation in Clinical Research (Draft).
7. Validation key practices for computer systems used in regulated operations (1997) *Pharm. Technol.*, June, 74–98.
8. PMA Computer Systems Validation Committee (1986) Validation concepts for computer systems used in the manufacture of drug products. *Pharm. Technol.*, **10**(5), 24–334.
9. *The IT STARTS Developers' Guide* (1988) ISBN: 0-85012-733-5. NCC Publications, The National Computer Centre, Oxford Road, Manchester, M1 7ED, England.

14 Re-engineering the Clinical Data Management Process

STEVE ARLINGTON, PAUL ATHEY, JOHN CARROLL and ALISTAIR SHEARIN

PricewaterhouseCoopers, London, UK

THE NEED FOR RE-ENGINEERING

Pharmaceutical companies are under heavy pressure; fundamental change in the world of healthcare is creating a 'financial squeeze' which is set to intensify (see Figure 14.1). With government initiatives to contain the soaring cost of healthcare, due in part to an ageing population and ferocious competition from generic manufacturers, many companies are experiencing a reduction in their margins.

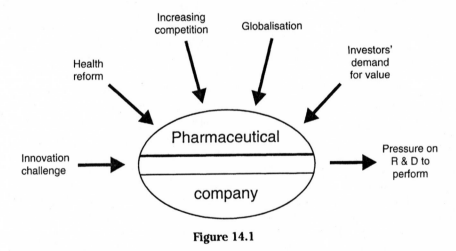

Figure 14.1

The increasingly toughening market climate has resulted in many acquisitions, mergers and cooperation agreements. In addition to this, efforts are being seen to be made to cut costs wherever possible. The cost

Clinical Data Management. Second Edition. Edited by R.K. Rondel, S.A. Varley and C.F. Webb.
© 2000 John Wiley & Sons, Ltd

cutting has been seen primarily through personnel reduction, but cutting costs indiscriminately, without regard for those activities which add real value, jeopardises companies' lifeblood.

Leading analysts are clear that the organisations most likely to succeed will be those which can discover and develop truly innovative products and thus command premium prices. Indeed, given the consolidation of the industry, as shown by the stream of mega-mergers, the ability to deliver a steady supply of new products through highly efficient and effective R&D processes will be critical to survival.

The drive to speed up the discovery process has produced new technologies such as combinational chemistry and high-throughput screening. These have revolutionised the way in which some aspects of research are conducted. However, they have put strain on other parts of the pipeline: *in vitro* and *in vivo* screening to optimise the leads.

Once the elusive new compound has been found, the race is on to ensure that it is first to market. With a blockbuster, the benefits of a two-year reduction in time to market are worth as much as $1.6bn. Thus, for every day's delay the company loses about $1m in sales.

The best practitioners have whittled the gap between developing a drug and launching it from 11–12 years down to just 5–6 years. However, increasing regulatory pressures may limit further progress. Today, regulatory review is seen to account for about 20% of the time the industry has traditionally taken to develop a new drug. While review times are reducing in the US, the initial impact of the EMEA has resulted in a small decrease in overall time.

In short, R&D must contend with a host of challenges, including intense competition, greater difficulty in discovering breakthrough drugs, new types of drugs from technologies such as protomics and genomics, spiralling development costs and the growing regulatory burden.

The need to re-engineer is clear; costs must be brought under control and output increased. The numbers are compelling: it takes up to $600m to bring a single drug to market and this cost is likely to rise; the market is growing or set to grow at a maximum 7% p.a.; and the major pharmaceutical companies are setting new product launch targets some three- to four-fold higher than today.

R&D is therefore under unprecedented pressure to perform and 10% improvements will not achieve this. Process redesign or re-engineering must achieve significant productivity improvement.

Development Processes

New product development timelines for projects initiated in a re-engineered environment are now expected to take between five to seven years from candidate nomination to launch in key territories. Very few products have reached these impressive targets and many organisations are reviewing their processes for the second time.

The development process faces both internal and external pressures, which affect productivity. Our focus on clinical data management cannot ignore the interfaces upstream and downstream which both affect and are affected by clinical data management and the trends towards outsourcing the use of HMOs, SMOs and CROs.

Clinical Research, Issues for the 90s

Clinical research faces a number of pressures. These can be viewed as within-company and external pressures (Table 14.1). The drive for an increase in output at reduced cost and time, yet at the appropriate quality, has put all of the elements of clinical departments under stress. Add to this the resource-constrained environment many companies are now facing and the need for global trials, and it is relatively easy to predict that today's process is under threat. New technologies also have a part to play in this scene.

Table 14.1

Internal	External
Cost	CROs, HMOs, SMOs
Time	Regulatory
Quality	Investigators
Consistency	Patients
Resources	Health Economics
Geography	Safety
Technology	

Small improvements in clinical trial management, data acquisition and data transfer systems have resulted in mixed reviews and varying success rates. Remote data entry, global databases, knowledge sharing, trial tracking, and so on are all buzzwords often associated with the latest technology updates.

The trend towards outsourcing continues unabated with many organisations increasing the percentage of trials performed by the CRO or similar organisations. Indeed in their quest for cost containment, headcount freezes have resulted in lucrative 'rent a CRA' or 'data manager' businesses as well as the more traditional CRO work. When outsourcing, care does need to be taken to ensure that all costs are taken into account and that the contracting organisation has a clear understanding of management time requirements, otherwise CROs may look artificially attractive.

Re-engineering has delivered quite substantial time improvement in a number of areas within the clinical development process (Table 14.2). These improvements have been achieved by gaining a clear understanding of the present process and identifying improvements that can be achieved through estimation of non-value adding tasks and the application of automation, and so forth.

Table 14.2

Process component	Industry average	Emerging best practice
Protocols	7.5 m	3.0 m
Investigator recruitment	6.0 m	3.0 m
CTx preparation	5.0 m	1.0 m
First to last site initiation	6.0 m	0.5 m
Clinical trial supply	6.0 m	2.0 m
Last patient out to database locked	10.0 m	3 days
Data analysis (includes statistical analysis and statistical report)	11.0 m	2.0 m

m = months

A radical review of the development process may conclude that whilst substantial opportunity exists to improve the processes as they stand today, our targets as stated by industry leaders of launching three NCEs every year valued at greater than $500m revenues p.a. will not be achieved without some significant re-engineering and a new approach to the problems we are facing.

The regulators are not standing still, they too demand more relevant trials, better data, and moves closer to 'real life'. The need to show benefits in terms of improvement over present therapy and economic superiority is now here too.

Patient pressure groups are keen to get involved in trials where life-saving innovations are under test; this too adds to the complexities companies face with highly sophisticated patients 'surfing the net' and exchanging information about trials and potential medicines in development.

Safety data are critical and a highly efficient pharmacovigilance process is demanded. Authorities are aware of adverse events as soon as companies are, and in some cases even earlier. The pressure is thus increased for timely and accurate adverse event reporting.

One could be forgiven for thinking that life in clinical development, including data management, is definitely far less than comfortable. Never before has the clinical data management process been subjected to these degrees of change in a cost-contained and productivity-focused environment. A new process must be designed to meet the continued challenge.

WHAT IS RE-ENGINEERING?

Is re-engineering a philosophy, a management tool, a methodology, a technique, a fad or even as some might venture to suggest, a myth? Over the past 10–15 years, re-engineering or its forerunners has rightly and, at times unjustly, carried each of these labels. With up to 40% of re-engineering projects failing to deliver meaningful results while only 33% of companies claim their re-engineering efforts are successful, the scepticism and confusion are understandable (Table 14.3). However, statistics without understanding are dangerous. Is how we define re-engineering part of the problem or part of the solution?

Table 14.3

Why projects fail?	What is success?
Not managing the human and organisational aspects of change	*Time:* 50–60% reduction in clinical development process duration
Poor project management and communications	*Quality:* zero data inconsistencies in a central study database
Lack of senior management commitment and leadership	*Cost:* 20–30% reduction in ongoing clinical trial costs
Poorly clarified needs and goals	*Service:* 'one call' problem resolution for Investigators

As re-engineering has matured over the years, we have seen a number of definitions emerge—from the very broad and general, such as James Champy's 're-engineering is the fundamental rethinking and radical redesign of business processes to achieve dramatic improvements in critical, contemporary measures of performance, such as cost, quality, service and speed', to the very narrow and specific, such as a clinical project leader's 're-engineering is about getting that last case report form into this study database in less than 2 days, so we can get on with analysis'.

We often struggle to adequately define re-engineering as it is different from other types of business improvement initiatives, such as Total Quality Management, Right-sizing, Just-in-Time, in that re-engineering is not prescriptive, for example, 'do this, that way and you will get this benefit'; it is just the opposite, for example, 'If I want this benefit, I should do things this way which means I'll have to start doing this differently'.

Re-engineering has also been described by some as a journey, not being able to predict what lies ahead yet still drawn by the quest for something different. The bottom line? Discard the text book definitions since an explicit definition of re-engineering will not help you decide what to do or influence your success. You must, however, accept that your approach to embracing re-engineering-driven change will be critically dependent on and linked to the level of ambition within your organisation. This in turn determines the scope of the re-engineering initiative, the potential scale of improvements, and likely resultant commercial impact—all offset by the capacity of your people to embrace and assimilate the required changes. You, not others, decide how to define re-engineering!

Getting Re-engineering Right, First Time

Getting re-engineering right, first time, depends on adopting an approach that will help you to:

- set targets for where you want to be;
- communicate targets early and regularly in a language common to all personnel;
- prioritise and develop ways for achieving required changes, keeping a focus on real customer needs (internal as well as external);
- clarify what the changes mean, dealing openly with people's fear and anxiety;
- demonstrate clear sponsorship and leadership, reinforcing this throughout;
- balance 'quick wins' with longer term development initiatives;
- achieve and communicate measurable results and benefits appropriately throughout the re-engineering process.

In our experience, a well-structured and phased approach (Figure 14.2) to re-engineering provides the framework for incorporating all these important aspects and for getting re-engineering right, first time.

Setting and communicating re-engineering targets (Process Diagnostic)

How do you set targets for where you want to be and communicate this early and regularly? This critical step requires you to understand where you are now through a detailed assessment of current operations, using appropriate comparative measures to understand the critical gaps in current performance relative to the level of your organisation's ambition. The best comparative measures are those that allow you to compare your organisation's performance against those best at doing something you need to do, regardless of industry; the worst measures are internally oriented, focusing on how you are performing now compared with the past. The assessment, comparative positioning and target setting should create the compelling need to change (Table 14.4).

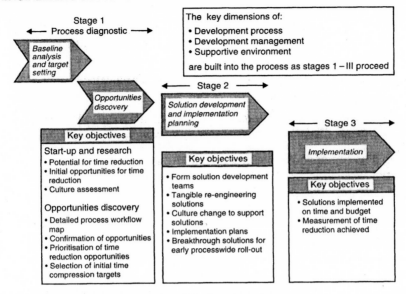

Figure 14.2 ICH administrative steps

Table 14.4

Performance measure	Achievement
1. Protocol design to database set-up	2 weeks
2. Number of queries generated per completed patient	0.7
3. Protocol approval to first patient enrolled (can vary due to specific ethics committee country regulations)	3 weeks
4. Last patient last visit to database lock	3 days
5. Database lock to completion of study report	1 month

The figures in Table 14.4 represent best case scenarios achieved through elements of re-engineering within the biometrics groups of large pharmaceutical companies. However, the figures will naturally vary depending upon the size and complexity of the trials conducted. These figures simply reflect some of the best performances of each component regardless of the specific trial dynamics and company.

Having established your targets, communicating them in clear, common and compelling language is critical. For example, as in the case of Company 1, the target is stretching yet not necessarily compelling as it has a strong internal focus. On the other hand, Company 2's message is as clear, commercially oriented, and more compelling in that people are likely to imagine what achieving this target might mean to them personally in terms of status, opportunities, rewards, growth and so on.

Company 1

The core goal of R&D is to shorten the mean development times—2000 in 2000—
reducing the mean development cycle time to 2000 days by the year 2000.

Company 2

Produce the equivalent of three £400 million products per annum.

*Developing and prioritising required changes while focusing on
customer needs (Solution Development and Implementation Planning)*

Having developed some insights during the assessment and target setting
activities you need to commit the appropriate resources, giving them
ample time and support to work through and formulate the changes that
will be needed to achieve your targets while managing the impact on
current operations.

The teams should be cross-functional in nature, having adequate representation from all R&D groups and structured such that a holistic approach to formulating the necessary changes is taken. The teams should
be prepared to involve others to ensure all aspects of the needed changes,
including business strategy, ways of working, organisation, competencies,
behaviours and information technology, are addressed and the proposed
changes validated with those who will need to change. The best solutions
address and balance and, where possible, integrate both the technical and
the behavioural aspects of change, for example:

Technical change

Data is captured closest to source and cleaned on a visit by visit basis.

↓

balanced and/or integrated with

↓

Behavioural change

As the CRA and the person closest to the investigator, I have the attitude, skills and
tools necessary to proactively and continuously improve data quality working in
collaboration with clinical development and data management.

Proposed changes should be prioritised, based on a combination of how
difficult they are to implement and what potential performance improvement they offer. Those that are easy to implement and deliver some but
not significant performance improvement, for example, Global Project Reporting, should be your top priority in order to keep up momentum
through demonstrable 'quick wins'. The changes that are difficult to implement and have little potential to improve your performance should be
discarded. All other changes should be prioritised and phased in two or
more implementation waves depending on the scope and impact of the
total programme for change.

Structuring for implementation to achieve measurable results, quick wins and longer term initiatives (Implementation)

Implementation begins in solution development; to ensure the quality and acceptability of the changes, the teams must regularly assess the approach to and feasibility of implementation, again involving those who will need to change and striking an appropriate balance between ease of implementing the changes and potential to improve performance for each solution under development. Your priorities will emerge from this process. You should then focus your efforts first on the changes that are easy to implement yet carry a lower potential to improve performance ('quick wins') while developing plans and appropriate phasing of those changes that have significant potential for improved performance in line with your targets.

GETTING STARTED: THE DIAGNOSTIC

Success is dependent on the quality of the preparations this is particularly true of a major re-engineering project, which will require the concerted efforts of many people within both the Data Management function and other organisational units. Pressures from management and enthusiasm from within the team should not allow your implementation of change to get off to a premature start.

For any re-engineering project, the basis of sound preparation is the Diagnostic stage, in which the initial project team will establish:

- The scope of your re-engineering project, including the business processes which will be addressed and the organisations which will be involved
- The targets which you aim to reach. These should be ambitious enough to stretch and challenge the organisation, but within the bounds of reality
- The approach which the project will take to communication and involvement, to ensure that the project has the understanding and acceptance of all who will be affected by it.

At this stage, the project team will consist of a small core team, who will go on to become key members of the full development and implementation team. Selection of team members is important. They must have a sound understanding of the way in which the organisation operates, and should include your opinion-formers. It is essential that team members are open-minded and sensitive to the position of staff outside the team. The way you approach the diagnostic strongly affects the way in which the project is perceived since recovery from a bad start is almost impossible.

The principal elements of the diagnostic stage are summarised in Figure 14.3. Mobilisation includes the formation of the project team, and a plan for its activities, together with a workshop and interview plan identifying participants outside the core team. Availability of these participants is often the key factor in determining the duration of this stage. It is also important to set out clear communications about the project from the outset. The need for re-engineering must be established both for participants within the data management function, and for those closely involved such as CRAs or Monitors who will be involved, but who may not feel they are part of the area.

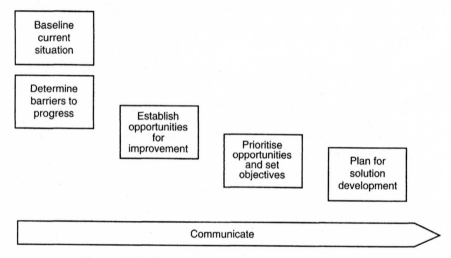

Figure 14.3 Principal elements of the diagnostic stage

During mobilisation, it is necessary to plan for training of the project team, to obtain specialist skills such as behavioural science and informatics.

For the team to work effectively at this stage, a clear definition of the information to be gathered, its format, and a formal repository for this information must be established and communicated to all those involved. Finally, project control mechanisms and a steering committee covering all sponsors and stakeholders should be established.

Baselining and analysis of barriers will proceed in parallel; indeed the tasks of gathering information for these two elements will often be conducted as one activity, with the results feeding into the two streams. It is often convenient to consider the information which you are developing at this stage under the broad categories of Process, People and Systems. This can be especially valuable when preparing interviews and workshops, and documenting the results.

Baseline the Current Situation

Baselining the current situation involves the team in developing an agreed and easily communicated view of the way in which data management currently operates, and of the efficiency and effectiveness it achieves. The basis of this work will be the creation of a clear definition of the processes, tasks and activities of data management. These will be represented diagrammatically in a Process Model. Since this represents the current situation, it is known as the 'as-is' Process Model. It is often most effective for two or three people experienced in process modelling to quickly develop an initial draft of the model, which can then be refined, developed and confirmed by wider involvement in a series of structured workshops. The model covers all tasks within the clinical development process in which data management is involved.

In addition the model needs to include decision and coordination steps, information flows, and boundaries between organisational units, plus, where they are a regular feature of your operations, rework loops such as query handling.

The model provides a tool allowing you to analyse the effectiveness and efficiency of each activity, and of the overall process. To do this it is usual to consider Achieved Performance, and External Benchmarks and Best Practice.

Achieved performance will include metrics where available—it may be necessary to establish these if this is not a regular occurrence, together with issues identified in workshops and interviews. Metrics will include the parameters of time (duration), resource utilisation, cost and quality.

Information available on the performance of the data management functions in other companies (external benchmarks) and from the growing body of best practice will provide the team with a useful basis on which to challenge current performance—are you achieving results alongside the best of the best? Of course you will use such information with discretion. Although it is useful in identifying performance gaps, care must be taken since organisations are not always comparable, and this project is specific to your company.

Barriers to Progress

For change to occur and the project be deemed to be successful, the team must identify and address the factors which have given rise to the current ways of working, and those which may inhibit progress in the future. Whilst many of these factors may be common knowledge within your organisation, they may become lost in the need to get the job done. It is therefore important when attempting to identify barriers to progress, that the team and their management are able to bring an open mind, and an objective approach. Areas to be analysed will include:

- Culture
- Management style (e.g. decision making)
- Organisation
- Skills
- Information systems

The first four of these areas are particularly emotive in most organisations. It will require considerable tact to conduct the analysis without antagonising management and staff, whose active cooperation will be needed to implement changes. It is, however, equally important not to use this as an excuse to avoid addressing the barriers to progress. If not tackled, they can negate the value of the re-engineering project.

The inclusion of information systems as a barrier may be surprising; however, they condition strongly the way in which an organisation goes about doing its job, and can be very difficult to change in the short term. A comprehensive review both of operational systems (such as the clinical data management system) and of management systems (such as project control, trial management, MIS and others) should be included.

Finally, it must be remembered that this work traverses a number of organisational silos and customer–supplier relationships must be borne in mind throughout the project.

Establish Opportunities

Following 'as–is' analysis you will have a clear understanding of how the process operates today, and with what success. You will also understand, from the external benchmarks, what is being achieved elsewhere in the industry. Armed with this knowledge, you can identify areas in which to develop opportunities for improvement.

For these areas, the root causes of performance gaps require analysis. This is particularly important as problems are frequently caused much earlier in the process than the point at which their effects are seen.

Having identified the areas within the process which offer opportunities for improvement, it is necessary to outline how this is to be achieved. This is a creative process which should be open and unconstrained. Once a set of opportunities has been created, they should be subjected to further analysis, including quantification of the benefit expected, tasks involved in delivering the benefit, effort, cost and time involved, and any risks identified.

An important point to note at this stage is the need to build consensus outside the core team, this is delivered through workshops and communication to ensure that the stakeholders have been both involved and consulted.

During the development of opportunities, it is tempting to focus only on individual activities within the process, at the expense of the bigger picture. The result would be suboptimisation within the process, and is best avoided by looking for overall improvement opportunities, rather than looking at smaller and smaller activities. As an example, if excessive numbers of discrepancies are being handled on a regular basis, the cause may be found in CRF or Protocol design, and needs to be addressed there rather than looking for a better process to handle queries.

Quick Wins

At any stage from the completion of the baselining of the current situation, opportunities may be identified which could result in a 'quick win'. These will have the characteristics of being widely accepted, a high benefits to cost ratio, little risk and no dependency on other actions.

It is not always necessary to wait for the completion of the planning of the diagnostic and development stages before proceeding with them, especially if the steering group has the authority to approve them. In some cases quick wins have been seen to pay for the rest of the re-engineering programme!

Prioritise Opportunities

Identification of opportunities should generate a rich set of possibilities, of varying effectiveness, risk and feasibility. It is likely that not all of these can be addressed at once and a prioritisation must take place. This is a straightforward activity, which should nevertheless follow a structured approach to avoid conflicts of individual preference.

Initially, the team should establish, in conjunction with senior managers, the goals and criteria for assessing opportunities, and these should be agreed by the Steering Committee in advance. The criteria can then be applied to produce a prioritised set of opportunities which fit the constraints of cost, resource and time, and which collectively achieve the proposed improvements in performance. The steering committee then approves the targets for improvement, and the opportunities which support them.

Plan for Solution Development

Once the targets and opportunities have been approved, a plan for the Solution Development stage is required. This stage is described below, and it is these activities that will be planned at this point. Also at this point, the team will begin to grow beyond the initial core, as a wider set of skills and greater involvement by stakeholders including those outside data management will be required; this expansion should be planned and care must be taken to train the new team members and welcome them to their new project.

SOLUTION DEVELOPMENT

The diagnostic phase has identified and prioritised your opportunities for improvement within data management and established specific improvement targets. In this phase your initial project team needs to be expanded to form solution development teams. They are responsible for developing tangible re-engineering solutions to meet the performance improvement targets, assess the level of cultural change needed to support the solutions, and provide plans for their implementation.

The impetus generated during the diagnostic phase must be maintained with your solution development teams working to establish:

- The ratification of the performance improvement targets which will form the basis for the performance measurement aspects of your re-engineering effort
- Re-engineered solutions for your selected data management activities in order to achieve the performance improvement targets set by the steering committee, e.g., reducing the time from Last Patient Last Visit (LPLV) to Database Lock from three weeks to three days
- Preparation for organisational and cultural change by communicating the likely impact to all affected organisational units at the earliest possible stage
- Implementation plans for your data management improvement solutions

It is important that the priority and sequence of your solution development projects are clearly defined. In our opinion three to five of your high opportunity areas should be launched first, and subsequent solution development teams should then target the remaining areas.

As solution development is concerned with developing improvements and therefore changes to the data management function, the factoring of change principles into the project at an early stage will ease the transition to and sustainability of your solutions. Therefore in the expansion of your solution development teams their role and potential to act as change leaders for the proposed solutions cannot be overlooked.

Expanding Your Team

High performance teams require your very best people, capable of bringing operational skills and the ability to work outside their comfort zones. It is also important to be realistic about team members' workload before committing them. In our experience almost all organisations underestimate the effort required by the project team.

A well-balanced multidisciplinary team must be selected in order to provide you with a truly effective solution. Therefore the method of team selection should be given some considerable thought and the use of approaches such as Belbin to highlight the characteristics of your team members will increase your chances for success.

Change aspects from the project must be supported, responsibilities will include counselling project sponsors, running team-building activities, identifying development needs within the affected areas and identifying issues related to recognition and reward. A separate team is often required for this.

Building Your Team

Once the team has been selected, bring them together for a training and development workshop. This workshop should be used as a start-up or 'kick off' event where the scope and objectives of the re-engineering initiatives are described, the specific tools and techniques that will be used during the project are outlined, and a sense of involvement developed to build the participants into a team.

Remember, however, that a sense of being a team is not created just through activities that take place in the work setting. It is equally important to build-in activities that span the social aspects of your team as well. This again is often seen as unnecessary, extravagant or a waste of time. Our view is that this activity is one of the last that should be sacrificed in your haste to get started.

The Solution Development Approach

As solution development is primarily a team-based approach, it is best undertaken through a series of workshops where each one has a very specific function as shown in Figure 14.4 below; this depicts a cascade of workshops which is used in solution development.

In generating the potential solutions or options your solution development teams must be encouraged to begin with the performance improvement targets and then to look for innovative approaches which may provide a different perspective. This divergent approach is used to identify a range of fresh alternatives to a problem that can then be analysed and refined through a convergent approach to hone down the options by rationally defining and evaluating the different solutions.

Solution development teams are charged with focusing on improving the value adding activities within data management that directly impact the targets identified in the diagnostic phase. For example, to reduce the data cleaning cycles (queries) from four per patient down to one may involve the development of solutions focusing on periodic monitoring,

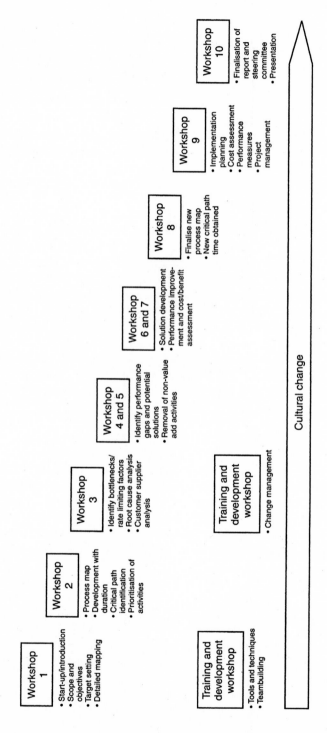

Figure 14.4 Solution development workshops

fully trained data entry operators and clearer CRF books (e.g., reduce the need for volumes of handwritten comments).

To communicate the emerging solutions and identify the potential impact of changes to the organisation structure we recommend that the team develops process-level views of the solutions as a process model. This reflects the future view of the process; they are known as to-be process models. They should be used as a vehicle for gaining consensus and agreement which is brought about by listening to the wider organisation's views and further refining the models during your workshops so that they communicate effectively how your solutions will meet the set performance targets for data management.

At this point in the project it is important to keep the steering committee informed of progress and we recommend an interim report midway through the workshop sessions. In this way the steering committee is given a vehicle to discuss any concerns they may have at an early stage when issues can be more readily resolved.

Bear in mind that often you have numbers of solution development teams running in parallel, each focusing on a different improvement opportunity. It is vital that you take account of the work of the other teams to manage overlaps and ensure that the solutions are supportive of each other. It is also important to remember that your solutions will impact other areas in the organisation and these changes must be well communicated and customer focused.

Before facing the steering committee for approval, you must ensure that detailed plans for solution implementation are drawn up. At this stage details of your solutions must be well defined and include comprehensive details of the costs and associated benefits that they will provide.

One word of caution in using a workshop-based approach to solution development. It is easy for the members of the team to attend a workshop and then drop back into their other commitments, leaving the tasks or 'homework' required to be completed in between each workshop until the last minute. Therefore it is important to focus on the actions arising out of each workshop and to ensure that each team member is clear on what they are expected to deliver before your team meets again. The project team leaders must carry out this task relentlessly.

Presenting Your Solutions to the Steering Committee

Following completion of the workshops your solutions should now be ready for presentation and consideration by the steering committee. In demonstrating the benefits and value of the solutions you must clearly demonstrate the means by which, for example, the inherent quality of the data management process and levels of service will be increased, while at the same time reinforcing the cost-effective nature of your proposed solutions.

Detailed implementation plans, cost–benefit analysis and resource requirements must be presented. Barriers to implementation, for example, cultural obstacles, should be discussed openly and requirements for the management of change fully assessed with the steering committee. Once again care must be taken not to overlook the barriers to change.

This presentation will result in the steering committee either giving approval for implementation ('go decision'), deferring or not approving your proposed solutions ('no go decision'), or requesting that elements of your solutions are reassessed and reworked. The 'go decision' is much more likely to be attained if effective communication with the steering committee has been maintained throughout the workshops.

In summary, the adoption of the most effective solutions results from a recognition, early adoption and encouragement of active communication. Anticipate the issues and communicate your position and progress from day one, communicating success at all levels is an essential part of managing this change.

Typically, some of the re-engineering solutions identified during this phase can be implemented almost as they emerge. Others that require more investment in time and capital are best implemented by the solution teams themselves on the basis of the momentum and internal team leadership built up throughout this phase.

Focus on designing simple, clean and fast processes that are geared towards supporting both your internal and end customers.

Keep the impetus up; move swiftly from the steering committee's 'go decision' into implementation.

Managing the Transition/Implementation

Following the steering committee approval of your solutions, with detailed definitions of each one, and a set of plans for implementation, the teams should move rapidly to implementation of the change projects. The focus of your communication programme will have ensured that the need for these changes has been understood, and that management and staff are committed to their achievement.

Project Teams

Once again, the team structure will need to change. The re-engineering team will be reformed into a series of discrete project teams, although a small group may remain to provide overall coordination of the programme. During this reformation project teams should include members of the re-engineering development team to ensure continuity of vision and objectives. Project teams should have their own goals, and it is essential that through their members, they have both the responsibility and the authority to achieve the quantified benefits targets set for them.

Most project teams will require a balanced set of skills and experience, across all the disciplines involved. It is helpful when structuring each team to consider the nature of the tasks involved and hence the depth of particular skill required. Once again, do not overlook the need to form a balanced team, focusing on the need for individuals who are 'completer finishers'.

Methods

Use of formal methods will assist in providing frameworks for teams to reach their joint activities. Some of the most useful of the formal methods cover Project and Programme Management, Change Management and Systems Delivery. If your projects include any significant systems changes, you will find that a formal method is essential to ensure that the solution can be validated.

Many companies already have a set of formal methods, often tailored to their own requirements. If your company does not have suitable methods available, you would be well advised to obtain them to support these projects resulting from the re-engineering.

IMPLEMENTATION

Most of the changes we are referring to will involve large-scale activities, performed by many people. In most cases it will be necessary to cut-over from the current way of working to a new approach. You will be faced here with a fundamental choice between a gradual roll-out of the new way of working, probably preceded by a trial or pilot implementation to gain experience, and a large-scale ('big bang') cut-over from the old to the new.

In general, a staged roll-out is easier to assimilate, gives time to accumulate experience, and allows the risks to be minimised. It is clearly a slower method of implementation, but if time is not critical, has much to recommend it. The 'big bang' is often the only solution where time is critical, but may also be the chosen approach where the process being changed has many downstream dependencies. This is often true of new systems, where a complete suite of new functions has to be brought into use at once. As this approach has the greater risk, more detailed planning is necessary, and fall-back options need to be prepared should the worst occur and the new solution have to be reviewed.

Many re-engineering projects fade once the implementation phase has been reached. Only too often re-engineering teams believe the hard work is over following solution development; they could not be more wrong. Implementation requires detailed planning, using recognised tools and techniques, project management, change management and, above all, continued sponsorship.

Often the external assistance used in a re-engineering programme leaves the work as implementation begins. This requires the organisation to commit the correct internal skills and level of resource to ensure change is delivered. Alas, all too often short cuts are taken and the initial investments are all but lost. Cynically, it is at this point that re-engineering methods, or the consultants, get the blame.

There are no short cuts to implementing change—up to 70% of the projected time and effort needed for successful re-engineering is implementation. It is necessary to ensure teams are not fatigued and to consider refreshing them with some new members if you feel there is a danger of a loss of momentum.

Senior management sponsorship cannot be seen to wane, nor can the relentless drive for measurement using the key performance indicators developed in the diagnostic and solution development phases be seen to diminish. The targets set at the end of the diagnostic phase need to become the objectives by which data management will be measured and rewarded in the future. Opposition to change during implementation cannot be underestimated and many teams are surprised to find organisational inertia to the proposed changes. A comprehensive set of training events, changes to management actions and almost continual communication are all required during implementation of the various changes. Constant review throughout implementation is recommended. Furthermore, we recommend the appointment of a full-time director for re-engineering throughout implementation.

Communication

Once again, communication is an essential element of managing the transition. Staff and management must be kept aware of changes that will affect them, individual projects teams need to keep each other informed of results and progress, especially on areas of joint interest. Perhaps the most important aspect of communication is celebration of the achievement of milestones and the delivery of proven benefits. This communication helps the morale of the project teams, underlines the utility of the project with staff, and gives management the confidence to continue funding.

CONCLUSION

Re-engineering is a powerful methodology which is capable of delivering step change in the efficiency and effectiveness of areas within R&D such as clinical data management. Our experience shows that a process approach linked to a robust methodology delivers targets deemed impossible to achieve at the outset of the programmes.

Implementation is often overlooked and most programmes fail at this hurdle; over 70% of the resources and effort are expended as the changes are implemented and become the new way of working. These changes cannot be achieved via short cuts nor can they be expected to last without continued sponsorship and monitoring of performance against agreed targets.

15 Working with Contract Research Organizations

KENNETH BUCHHOLZ

INC Research, Charlottesville, VA, USA

INTRODUCTION

The pharmaceutical-biotech industry today is under increasing pressure to accomplish more work in less time with the same or fewer staff. Although technology is heralded by many to be the ultimate savior, we will probably always be expected to do more work than we can with current in-house staff, regardless of how many new technological applications we employ and how efficient we become. Thus we have two options: (i) less critical work simply does not get done, or at least does not get done in a timely fashion; or (ii) we employ Contract Research Organizations (CROs) to supplement our in-house staff to get the work done in a timely manner.

Only a few years ago CROs were viewed by people in the pharmaceutical industry as being staffed by inexperienced or less competent employees who produced low-quality work inexpensively. During the past several years, mergers and acquisitions in the industry have resulted in a large number of staff reductions at pharmaceutical and biotech companies. This has had two major effects: (i) many seasoned professionals with excellent industry credentials found themselves back in the job market and available to CROs; and (ii) the downsizing of staff within companies means there are fewer staff to do an increasing amount of work. Therefore more and more projects are being contracted out to CROs. Similarly, CROs have come to realize that in order to be successful, they must recruit and maintain highly qualified staff and concentrate on providing a higher quality product in a timely manner. The net results have been that: CROs now compensate staff in a manner more commensurate with pharmaceutical and biotechnology companies; CRO staff are much better qualified than in the past; recent consolidations in the CRO sector have yielded fewer but larger and more stable companies with greater staff stability; and the quality of goods and services provided by these companies is now higher than in the past.

Clinical Data Management. Second Edition. Edited by R.K. Rondel, S.A. Varley and C.F. Webb.
© 2000 John Wiley & Sons, Ltd

REASONS FOR WORKING WITH A CRO

There are several excellent reasons for deciding to work with a CRO, all of which are related to inadequate in-house resources. Probably the top three reasons for working with a CRO are:

1. Inadequate internal staff resources.
2. Access to additional sites/patients.
3. Lack of therapeutic, regulatory or functional expertise.

Inadequate Internal Staff Resources

A CRO serves as supplemental staff, enabling the department to perform more work than current in-house staffing will allow, as well as more successfully managing an ever-fluctuating workload. Employing temporary staff to supplement in-house staff is effective, but using a CRO to supplement the workforce saves the time and effort of recruiting, hiring, training, providing office space and managing temporary employees. The savings in management time alone can be considerable over using large numbers of in-house temporaries during peak workflow. Furthermore, CRO staff are full-time employees of that company, receiving full benefits (medical, dental and life insurance, etc.), and represent less risk than temporary employees, who are more likely to leave for another, full-time job offering company benefits. In addition, the onus of training resides with the CRO, further reducing the sponsor's time investment.

A CRO also allows better management of workflow fluctuations. Most projects have peaks and valleys and one of the most difficult things to manage is adequate staffing to ensure coverage during peak workflow on multiple projects. A medium to large CRO is more apt to respond quickly to unexpected workflow peaks because it can balance work peaks across projects *and* across clients. A CRO can also readily move unused resources to another client's project, eliminating the costs of carrying unused resources.

A CRO is also a hedge against internal overstaffing. Should a major project terminate prematurely after your organization has 'staffed up' to meet the expected demand, you are left with more staff than needed and may face the situation of having to lay-off full-time staff. If, on the other hand, CRO staff are used to cover a portion of the projected workload and a project ends early, the distribution of work between CRO and sponsor company can always be shifted to support the internal full-time staff. Most CRO contracts have early termination clauses which may bear a financial penalty, but such penalties are generally far less than the financial and morale costs of terminating good in-house staff.

A CRO may also be used to temporarily free in-house staff for other projects which have significant benefit to the long-term operations of the company, such as development of a new computer system for data management or clinical study monitoring, writing SOPs, and so on. Such projects are temporary in nature and represent excellent opportunities to provide internal staff with additional career opportunities while providing long-term operational benefits in that the staff who will be using the products of these projects are often in the best position to lead the efforts.

Access to Additional Sites/Patients

CROs may provide an excellent means of access to additional investigator sites or specific patient populations. For example, a CRO may have previous experience with sites that your company does not have and thus can assist in the selection of 'productive' sites (that is, sites with proven track records in obtaining evaluable patients and providing high-quality patient data).

Lack of Therapeutic, Regulatory or Functional Expertise

CROs may provide an excellent source of expertise in a therapeutic, regulatory or functional area that is currently lacking within the sponsor company. In all of these scenarios, a CRO may not only provide the staff resources to accomplish the task at hand but may also provide training to the sponsor staff. For example, if the company moves into a new therapeutic area, a CRO with expertise in that therapeutic area may be used initially to conduct the first set of clinical trials while in-house staff gain knowledge in that area. Thus the CRO is not only providing staffing but also serves to train in-house staff in the area. Young, start-up companies typically find that they have significant internal therapeutic expertise but lack regulatory or specific functional expertise, such as computer databases and networks. In these situations, the sponsor may utilize the CRO both to perform critical project work while simultaneously training staff and possibly serving in a consultant capacity for internal systems development.

CRO SELECTION CONSIDERATIONS

Quality

There are many parameters to consider when selecting a CRO. The most important is the CRO's reputation for providing quality goods and services in a timely manner. Just a few years ago, many companies would select a CRO primarily upon a price basis. Most have learned the hard way that basing decisions solely or primarily upon price generally costs more in the long term when the CRO doesn't meet expectations and most or all of the work has to be redone by in-house staff once the study ends. One of the keys to selecting the right CRO is to balance the CRO's reputation for producing quality work on time and within budget.

Requests for Proposals

Most companies today will submit a Request For Proposal (RFP) to several CROs before contracting a study. RFPs need to be clear, concise, and must ensure that the work being requested is mutually understood. For example, if one of the deliverables being requested is a 'data management plan', clearly state what a data management plan contains since the contents of data management plans vary by company.

Returned RFPs which are significantly lower in price from others require further communication with the CRO(s) presenting the lowest price(s) to determine why their proposals are so much lower. Many times you will find that a low bid reflects a misunderstanding between the CRO and client in terms of expectations of what work is to be done.

CRO Size

Another important consideration is the CRO's ability to perform the project without stressing its internal staff resources. It is important to select a CRO which has sufficient staff and which has not overcommitted to other clients; thus you need to question the CRO as to its current work commitments and how it responds to unplanned increases in resource needs. This will help ensure that the work is performed in an expedient and quality manner and is not competing with projects of other, possibly larger and more influential, clients.

Stability of Staff

Question the CRO about handling sudden changes in project priorities and how it would acquire additional staff for projects suddenly requiring more staff than originally planned. Does the CRO compensate staff well enough to recruit and then keep well-qualified staff? What is the staff turnover rate? Frequent staff changes may adversely affect your project in that consistency of work is negatively impacted, communications are constantly disrupted, interpersonal relationships don't mature, the time and cost of training escalate, and so on. The CRO's ability to meet your quality standards in a timely manner is in direct relation to the stability and qualifications of its staff. Determine as best you can that the CRO's staff turnover is not overly high and request a 'guarantee' from the CRO that the staff which is initially assigned to your project will not be pulled off and reassigned to other projects during the course of your project.

Physical Conditions of the Work Environment

What are the conditions of the CRO's work environment? If the environmental conditions are undesirable, staff may be unable to perform their jobs well (which may also contribute to high staff turnover). For example: (i) Are the clinical data reviewers forced to work in a noisy environment which may adversely affect their concentration? (ii) Is the work area neat or will you have to worry about your data being lost amongst the work of your competitors? (iii) Is the work environment secure or will the threat of theft be of concern? (iv) Does the computer system often experience crashes and other downtime? Do not underestimate the importance of a favorable work environment in selecting a CRO. It is beneficial to visit a CRO prior to contracting a study since much can be determined about the company's values from examining their workplace.

Compliance and Validation

Another key element in selecting a CRO is systems validation and compliance. Inquire about: (i) Are the computer systems used by the CRO validated and well documented? (ii) Does the CRO have reasonable SOPs implemented? (iii) How does the CRO assure compliance with its SOPs? (4) Has the CRO obtained all necessary certifications? (5) When was the CRO last audited by a regulatory agency and what were the results of that audit? Whenever possible, it is recommended that your company's internal auditing group conduct a pre-contract inspection to ensure that the CRO would pass a regulatory audit.

Procedures

When selecting a CRO, should you try to select a CRO which matches your internal processes as closely as possible? Should you try to force the CRO to replicate your processes or should the CRO be allowed to operate in its standard environment? As a general rule-of-thumb, it is in the best interest of time and effort to concentrate on the quality and timeliness of the product to be delivered rather than on process. Just as your internal processes are reflective of your staff and internal systems and are tuned to maximize your efficiency, effectiveness and expediency, so too are a CRO's processes. If a CRO is requested to greatly modify its internal processes, its efficiency is being reduced (adding to the costs of its services), its ability to quickly move resources onto the project is reduced, and the possibility of errors increases since the staff are deviating from procedures they are accustomed to. Concentrate on evaluating whether the processes will yield quality work and whether SOPs are followed internally and let the CRO operate, as much as possible, under the processes it has developed to maximize efficiency, effectiveness, expediency and accuracy. Again, consistency plays an important role in determining the quality and timeliness of the product which will be delivered to you.

Disaster Recovery

Most sponsors do not consider disaster recovery (sometimes called business recovery) when selecting a CRO. Disasters include key staff departures, equipment failures, financial failures and natural disasters including fire, floods, earthquakes, and so on. Does the CRO have sufficient disaster recovery plans in place for each of these potential disasters? Are electronic data backed up frequently and consistently? Is original paper stored in a secure, fireproof location? Are all computer systems secure? Do key staff have sufficient back-up in the event of illness, death or departure from the company? Does the CRO have a formal disaster recovery plan in place to restore its normal business operations in a reasonable time following a disaster? Do its staff perform regular drills to ensure that their disaster recovery plan is effective? Consider disaster recovery plans like life insurance: you hope you never have to use it but you know it's only a matter of time before you will.

Disaster recovery plans extend to the client as well as to the CRO. If the CRO conducting the key clinical trial should declare bankruptcy or its facility is destroyed by a natural disaster one or two months prior to the clinical trial ending, what mechanisms are in place internally to allow for a quick recovery and resumption of the project?

There are several simple things you can do to enhance your ability to recover from a disaster at the CRO's facility:

1. Never give the CRO the only copy of data. Always maintain either the original or a copy of any data provided to the CRO in a secure location *in-house*.
2. Develop and maintain excellent and frequent communications with the CRO staff so that you have forewarning of any impending situations which may adversely impact the project, such as key staff re-assignments or leaves-of-absence, negative changes in the work environment, etc.
3. Receive frequent interim data transfers (preferably in electronic format) and status reports from the CRO. Do not wait until a project is completed before receiving a data transfer from the CRO. Interim data transfers provide both the opportunity to check on the quality of work being performed during the course of the project as well as a good basis for in-house recovery in the event of a disaster at the CRO's facility—only the work performed by the CRO since the last data transfer will be lost and thus project recovery is faster. Definition of exactly what will be delivered, and when, should be clearly stated as part of the contract itself.

4. Visit the CRO and meet the staff who will be assigned to the project before signing the contract. Review their SOPs and systems validation documentation applicable to the project. Observe the workplace environment as well as the morale of staff. The last thing you want is staff with morale or attitude problems working on the project.

5. Conduct reference checks of the CRO's recent clients. A reputable CRO will provide references upon request. In addition, professional meetings are excellent opportunities to solicit input from colleagues on their recent experiences with CROs. When conducting reference checks, inquire not only about the performance of the CRO per se but also ask the reference what, in hindsight, they would have done differently to make the experience more successful, as a means to glean important advice on your in-house conduct as well as that of the CRO.

It is important to realize that the cost of converting a CRO study to an in-house study is generally high under the best of conditions and is even greater when done under disaster conditions. As such, a disaster recovery plan prepared *before* disaster strikes is instrumental.

THE CONTRACT

Before entering into a contract with a CRO, it is best to appreciate the fact that, no matter what work you contract to the CRO, you remain ultimately responsible for the quality and timeliness of that work within your company. Therefore the contract should adequately address three primary areas.

Expectations

What expectations do you have of the CRO and vice versa? It is generally beneficial to include, as attachments to the contract, documents such as Data Management Plans, Data Entry Guidelines, database schemata, and so on, which clearly define the deliverables and quality expected. Most Clinical Data Management departments today prepare detailed plans for the data management activities of each study conducted in-house, and these plans state what data will be reviewed, how they will be reviewed, how data will be entered into the database, and so on. Why would you not have the same done for studies conducted on your behalf by a CRO?

Delivery Dates

Before entering into a contract, both parties should clearly define a project plan that includes agreed-upon completion dates for all deliverables. Although it is always best to define precise dates, include elapsed time periods as well since many predecessor events are difficult or impossible to predict (e.g., date the last patient will be enrolled into the trial). For example, rather than specifying that 'the final clinical trial database will be delivered on 4 September', it is generally best to state 'the final clinical trial database will be delivered within 30 business days of the last patient's final visit' since patient enrollment almost never goes as planned. Once dates are defined in the contract, it is critical to maintain excellent communications so that changes to the project plan are communicated and agreed upon by both parties in a timely manner.

Definition of Quality Standards

It is critical to have a mutual understanding about the quality standards you expect along with the metrics on how quality will be measured. For example, if you include a quality parameter which states that 'the database error rate is not to exceed 0.02%', will that be measured as the number of error fields in the database compared to what is recorded on the CRF or to what is recorded in the source documentation at the investigator sites? By clearly stating your expectations upfront you ensure that your quality standards will be met and that the relationship with the CRO will be a good, friendly and constructive one.

Utilizing In-house Staff During Contract Negotiations

Most companies have a 'contract group' of some sort which assists in negotiating the contract. Such groups typically have expertise in legal, financial and contract negotiation skills. It is usually best to involve these internal resources right from the start of the project. Furthermore, such contract groups can usually assist in preparing a primary list of CROs at the start of the CRO selection process, and typically may provide valuable information regarding your company's past experience(s) with specific CROs.

Investing the Time Up-front

One of the most challenging aspects of working successfully with a CRO is that of securing the in-house resources and adequate time commitment upfront to establish an environment of success. All too often, companies' annual goals are weighed heavily on *starting* new programs/trials rather than on successful completion and regulatory submission, and thus the internal pressures to quickly start new programs is extraordinary. Working with CROs can be quite successful, but that success requires an upfront investment of time and resources on the part of both the CRO and the sponsor to develop that environment of success. Companies need to redirect their corporate strategies and annual goals to emphasize completions, not starts, and to concomitantly commit the necessary in-house resources for proper upfront planning and execution.

Other Considerations

It is important to appreciate and respect that a CRO should make a reasonable profit for the work performed. Requests to cut price are usually met with cuts in services, reduction in product quality and/or extensions in delivery time. If expectations are not clearly stated upfront, and the costs of providing those expectations allowed to be built into the initial contract, you will be faced with escalating costs during the trial or the CRO will recover out-of-contract costs by cutting other services and/or by 'cutting corners' so that quality of product is jeopardized. Again, you are ultimately responsible within your company for work performed by the CRO. The failure of the CRO to meet your company's quality standards in a timely fashion will be due in part to a failure to communicate clear expectations up-front. Using a CRO saves time and staff resources only if you do not have to reprocess what they deliver.

Another consideration is whether to enter into a fixed-price or a time-and-materials contract. In the fixed-price contract, the CRO guarantees that it will deliver the specified products for a fixed cost. If the actual cost of providing those goods and services is less than estimated under the terms of the contract, the CRO makes a greater profit but if the actual costs exceed what was estimated under the contract, the CRO makes less profit or even loses money. In contrast, a time-and-materials contract states that the cost will be based upon the actual cost, to the CRO, of providing the goods and services, thus the eventual actual cost of the project is not agreed upon at the time of the contract but is somewhat open-ended. As such, most time-and-materials contracts have a 'not to exceed' cost specified as a protection for the sponsor company. In general, a fixed-price contract requires a great deal more upfront planning and definition of deliverables (goods and services) and takes longer to develop than time-and-materials contracts due to the risk to the CRO. Regardless of which type of contract you develop, it is generally a good idea to specify in the contract how unforeseen events will be handled and paid for. For example, you may plan to have only three interim data transfers conducted but the contract should state that, if additional interim data transfers are required, each data transfer will be billed to the sponsor at some pre-defined cost.

MAKING THE RELATIONSHIP WORK

Although a clear agreement on expectations is critical, it is by no means the only important parameter in making the CRO–sponsor relationship a successful one. Communications extend well beyond the initial contract negotiations, and clear, honest and frequent communications are necessary throughout the duration of the project.

Many in-house projects have a cross-functional project team governing the conduct of the project. How are the decisions made by the project team relayed to the appropriate CRO staff? Is the CRO staff copied on project team meeting minutes or is there a separate communication vehicle to forward pertinent information to them? It is usually very beneficial for a CRO representative to be included in the project team. Depending upon the nature of the project and work contracted, CRO staff may participate in part or all of your project team meetings (depending on the agenda of issues to be covered), either in person or via conference call.

Another good concept to employ is that of a 'point person'. For example, if the CRO will be performing data entry and data review activities, there should be one point person at both the CRO and within your company to address issues about these functions and to take responsibility for disseminating information to the rest of their teams. Although communication among all staff should be encouraged, it is very important to channel communications between point people in order to effectively manage communications. When using point people to coordinate communications, it is important to have the communication pathways from the point people to the rest of their staff well defined. The point people must not become so preoccupied with communications with their counterpoints that they become isolated from the rest of their own staff.

A basic aspect of the CRO–sponsor relationship is trust. Develop a level of trust between CRO staff and in-house staff right from the start. Since we tend to be distrustful of those we don't know well, it is important for the staff to become familiar with one another. Oftentimes, a simple face-to-face meeting of the CRO and sponsor staff is all that it takes. It may be helpful to send your staff to the CRO for a day to become familiar with the CRO's staff, processes and general environment. If financial restrictions prevent this, have at least some of the critical function CRO staff visit your company site to meet staff and review your processes.

Because familiarity is so important in the relationship, it is recommended to work with a small set of CROs whenever possible rather than to try a new CRO for every project. Building long-term relationships with a few CROs maximizes efficiency as well as success in outsourcing. Also, if a CRO understands that a long-term alliance with your company is possible, it will cherish the relationship and do more to make sure that you are a satisfied client. Furthermore, when a CRO becomes familiar with your expectations and business practices, the less likely there will be costly, unexpected requests. As such, the CRO may be able to provide services to you at a lower cost by eliminating some of the cost buffers associated with unexpected situations.

On the other hand, it is important to appreciate the dangers of working with a single CRO exclusively for the same reasons that manufacturers do not typically single-source suppliers of raw materials. If you single-source all of your work to one CRO, you greatly increase your risk that, should a disaster strike that CRO, all of your out-sourced work is jeopardized. In contrast, if you have alliances with several CROs and disaster strikes one, you have an opportunity to have the other CROs assist you in the recovery. There is much truth in the old adage, 'Diversity breeds stability.'

How do you react when the CRO fails to meet an expectation? When one of your in-house staff fails to meet an expectation, you probably communicate immediately with them about the failed expectation in a respectful manner and then work with them to resolve the situation. Since a CRO is your staff, it is best to follow that same strategy of immediate communication in a respectful manner and a willingness to work together to resolve the issue. In short, practice good communications and management skills and be respectful at all times.

NEW APPROACHES

Just as new technologies improve our internal operations, they may also improve our working relationships with CROs. Advances in network security, for example, not only improve our internal intranets but also make available the Internet for data transfers and confidential communications, thus providing an additional tool for CROs and sponsors. It is now easier and less expensive to transfer data between CROs and sponsors, and to allow CRO staff to work directly on sponsors' internal networks and systems without the severe security concerns of just a few years ago. Another novel approach is to allow the sponsor staff access to the CRO's internal systems for such activities as reviewing the progress of the CRO, conducting preliminary analyses or even allowing the sponsor staff to supplement the CRO's staff when urgent situations necessitate such. Several CROs have developed their own remote data entry (RDE) or remote data acquisition (RDA) systems to enhance the services they provide to sponsors and can actually acquire and process data faster than their clients. Today's CROs seem able to develop new technological applications more successfully than their clients and thus their services have become even more valuable.

Another new approach gaining popularity is that of the CRO opening a satellite office in close proximity to the client. Many companies are hesitant to send critical projects to a CRO which is physically distant, but are far less hesitant about sending a critical project to a local CRO due to ease of communications (not having to contend with different time zones and the expense and hassle of travel makes for better communications). An enhancement of this concept has the sponsor extending their internal computer network into the CRO's local office so that the staff work directly on the sponsor's own systems. This eliminates the need for data transformations between CRO and sponsor systems and provides real-time access to the data by the sponsor. This provides all the benefits of doing the study in-house with supplemental temporary staff without the full cost of recruiting, hiring, training, providing office space and managing the staff. Such CRO–sponsor alliances require a significant commitment by the sponsor, usually a guarantee of a certain amount of work for several years. The sponsor reaps all the benefits of a long-term relationship with a CRO that is familiar with the company's procedures and standards of performance. Another potential benefit is that the CRO may more easily locate staff temporarily at your location when such temporary needs arise. Such a commitment, of course, requires that you carefully select the CRO with which you wish to ally.

Another novel approach is a CRO–sponsor partnership in the development of a product. For example, electing to use one CRO exclusively for all clinical trials in the development of a single product may ensure that the CRO has a very vested interest in doing the best job possible. In this approach, the CRO is offered a significant financial incentive associated with approval of the product; that is, if the product is approved, the CRO receives a significant financial (cash or stock) bonus. Such a partnership may be structured so that the CRO provides its services at a reduced fee and upon approval of the product, it recovers the difference plus an additional bonus payment. Both sponsor and CRO share the risk of clinical development but reap the benefits if the product is successful. Management Incentive Programs provided to many top executives are structured in a similar fashion whereby salary is comparatively low but incentive bonuses based upon performance and company success are high. Why not try the same with a CRO?

SUMMARY

Staff reductions within sponsor companies, improvements made in the CRO sector and recognition of the benefits of contracting excess clinical development work guarantee that recent industry trends of outsourcing will most likely continue for several years before leveling off. For many Clinical Data Management departments, the use of CROs is the only option available to accomplish all of the work required of them. Regardless of whether the work is conducted by in-house staff or outsourced, the ultimate responsibility for the quality and timeliness of the work resides with the sponsor. It is therefore in the best interest of the sponsor to make the CRO–sponsor relationship successful. The keys to a successful relationship are: good contracts which clearly specify expectations of both parties; frequent communications throughout the duration of the project; familiarity between the CRO and sponsor of internal systems, process and cultures; an adequate investment of staff and time upfront in planning; and the practice of good interpersonal and management skills at all times. In short, the elements of effective management of internal staff and projects are the same, and need to be applied with equal vigor, to the management of the CRO and CRO-conducted project.

ACKNOWLEDGEMENTS

I wish to thank Diane Ascoli, Marianne Bradley and Paula Chambers (Amgen) and John Seman and Raul Zavaletti (Avantec) for their review and helpful input.

16 Data Management in Epidemiology and Pharmacoeconomics

MICHAEL F. RYAN and ANDREAS M. PLEIL

PharmaNet, Inc., Princeton, NJ, USA and Pharmacia & Upjohn, Stockholm, Sweden

INTRODUCTION

Since the publication of the first edition of this book in 1993, pharmaceutical developers have placed increased emphasis on two types of research: epidemiology, with an emphasis on large-population safety studies (pharmacoepidemiology), and the economics of drug therapy (pharmacoeconomics). The growing importance of these disciplines coincides with a shift in emphasis from the individual patient to the society as a whole. As societies seek to optimize drug utilization, epidemiology contributes to a fuller understanding of disease within populations, and economics quantifies our understanding of limited medical resources. With the power of these disciplines to provide data for therapeutic decisions, the collection and use of both epidemiologic and economic data continue to grow more important. In this environment, the managing of these data is an essential task for data managers. The clinical data manager must be aware of the objectives and designs of epidemiologic and economic studies, the relevant regulatory issues, and the practical aspects of the retrieving, editing, validating and reporting of these data.

This chapter is an overview of these topics. For those who wish a more detailed review, suggested reading is listed at the end of the chapter.

EPIDEMIOLOGY

An early impetus to the use of epidemiology in the study of drug therapy was drug safety. Clinical scientists and regulatory professionals have long recognized that the study of new candidate drugs in small, narrowly

Clinical Data Management. Second Edition. Edited by R.K. Rondel, S.A. Varley and C.F. Webb.
© 2000 John Wiley & Sons, Ltd

selected populations cannot produce sufficient data to assure the safety of
the potential drug. This fact was demonstrated tragically with the introduction of thalidomide in the early 1960s. Numerous birth defects were
discovered to be associated with the use of the drug. As a result, The
British Committee on Safety of Drugs established the 'Yellow Card' system
for physicians to report any suspicion that a prescription drug might have
caused an adverse event. (Throughout this chapter ADE or Adverse Drug
Event refers to adverse events associated with a drug and to drug–drug
interactions that produce adverse events.) The study of adverse drug
events, drug–drug interactions, and untoward drug effects in special populations led to the new term 'drug induced illness'[1]. The study of drug
effects on large, diverse populations led to a new discipline, pharmacoepidemiology[2–4], which can be defined as the assessment of drug
safety through large-scale surveillance of drug usage. The goal of phar-
macoepidemiological studies is to discover and to quantify: rare adverse
reactions, drug–drug interactions, adverse events in special populations,
and adverse effects that occur only after prolonged use.

To increase knowledge of drug safety before marketing, epidemiologists
contribute to expanded Phase III development studies. Traditional efficacy
and safety trials include narrow populations of patients often having no
concomitant disease or other complicating factors. To generate safety
data more quickly and economically during the preapproval stage of development, manufacturers now often conduct large, simple, safety trials
(LST) that include heterogeneous patient populations. Inclusion/exclusion
criteria are relaxed to generate a more representative profile of the patient
population expected to be exposed to the drug after the market launch.

Within the pharmaceutical industry the role of the epidemiologist has
continued to grow. From the inception of clinical programs, epidemiologists help to establish populations at risk of diseases; determine the natural history of diseases; help to define endpoints for therapy in targeted
populations; determine the incidence of diseases (rate in a population)
and the prevalence of diseases (the number of people affected). These
data contribute not only to a better clinical understanding, essential to the
design and conduct of drug development studies, but also provide information used by economists to quantify the economics of drug therapy.

PHARMACOECONOMICS

The health economist's work encompasses a broad scope of study
covering all of medical care. Within the context of drug therapy that
work ranges from determining the cost of illness to the cost of treatment.
Part of the treatment costs can be drug therapy. The cost of drug
therapy includes the cost of the drug, the administration, follow-up,

efficacy or lack of it, the costs of ADEs, and often time lost from work, and other indirect costs. In serving increasingly sophisticated purchasers, economists seek to determine the full costs of employing a given drug therapy. It is important to note that economics comprises more than financial costs and benefits; values that cannot be readily assessed in monetary units, such as the quality of the patient's life, are also measured and used to quantify the value of drugs. To acquire this knowledge pharmacoeconomic studies are often run in parallel with, and at times integrated into, clinical studies. This integration presents challenges to the data management team. These data are critical to decisions made throughout the drug development process, from which drugs to develop, how much to invest, to pricing, and reimbursement schemes. It is the societal emphasis that has given rise to the prominent role of pharmacoeconomics.

Over the past 15 years in most industrialized countries the cost of medical care has risen dramatically. In efforts to control medical costs, governments, insurers and other payers have placed a strong emphasis on cost containment in the purchase of drugs. In Australia manufacturers must provide an economic evaluation of each drug prior to receiving approval on the reimbursement scheme[5], and other countries are considering similar legislation. Most European countries base reimbursement for new drugs, in part, on the results of economic studies. In the United States, market pressures from institutional purchasers and insurers have forced manufacturers to provide economic justification for their products. Faced with a more economically sophisticated and competitive marketplace, drug manufacturers have begun to conduct economic analyses of potential drug candidates much earlier in the drug development process.

Several types of economic analyses are applied to assess the value of drug therapy. Each type of study differs from the others with respect to the study objectives and the outcomes that are measured.

Cost-of-treatment studies include costs for diagnosis and treatment. Cost-of-illness studies determine the wider economic impact of an illness, for example, loss of the patient's productivity, and other indirect costs. In cases in which the clinical outcomes are equal, for example, the control of blood pressure is the same, monetary units might be used to determine the least expensive drug; drug A costs less than drug B for the same clinical result. These are cost-minimization analyses (CMA).

In studies in which single, well-defined clinical outcomes differ in magnitude, monetary units can be weighed against the clinical outcome; therapy A produces a reduction in blood pressure that is worth the cost as compared to the blood pressure reduction produced by drug B and the cost of B. These are cost-effectiveness analyses (CEA). With non-monetary measures such as the patient's quality of life, the patient's quality of life using drug A is compared with that of patients using B. These are cost-utility analyses (CUA). When the clinical outcomes measures differ in kind, the researcher might wish to assess the relative value of spending money on therapy A versus therapy B, that is, one computes a benefit to cost ratio. Using money to purchase a drug for children with leukemia might be a better return on the investment than using the same sum of money to perform cardiac surgery on elderly patients. These are cost-benefit analyses (CBA). Note that the economic difference might not lead to an acceptable societal decision. Cost-benefit analysis is not often used to select therapies because of ethical concerns of placing monetary value on human lives.

SOURCING DATA

When the researcher is able to design a study, recruit the subjects and collect the data, a complete set of data might be available. However, data for epidemiologic and pharmacoeconomic studies come from many sources. Secondary data sets (available from multiple sources; see Table 16.1) do not always provide complete and consistent data. Clinical data from patient records contain unknown biases, and can be incomplete and unreliable. Insurance claims data often lack the outcomes of interest and rarely contain sufficient information on patients' medical histories. Cost data can differ also depending on accounting methods.

Safety data are widely available. The health authorities and manufacturers receive spontaneously reported adverse events, third-party payers (both government agencies and insurers) track adverse events, and in the United States, Health Maintenance Organizations (HMOs), and pharmacy benefit organizations maintain databases of ADEs. The successor to the British Committee on Safety of Drugs, the Committee on Safety of Medicines, continues to compile data of spontaneously reported 'suspicions' of adverse events possibly associated with prescription drug use. With the availability of records from the British National Health Service it is possible to identify patients who have been prescribed a drug and thus to follow prospectively a cohort of users. This approach has been called Prescription-Event-Monitoring (PEM)[6]. In Canada the Adverse Drug Reaction (ADR) reporting program began in 1965. Up to 8000 reports are received annually by the Bureau of Drug Surveillance[7]. Nearly half of the reports come from physicians, pharmacists and hospitals rather than from the manufacturers. The United States Food and Drug Administration (FDA) has maintained a database of reported adverse drug experiences since 1969. There is today an Office of Epidemiology and Biostatistics which maintains a high level of support for post-marketing surveillance of ADEs. In 1993 the FDA received 123 000 adverse drug experience (ADE) reports. The majority of reports came from manufacturers of drugs.

Table 16.1 Examples of computer databases of primary data and sources in the United States

Public sources	• Medicare Enrollment Database (HCFA) • Medicare National Claims History Repository (HCFA) • National Ambulatory Medical Care Survey (NCHS) • National Death Index (NCHS) • National Health Interview Survey: health services use, acute and chronic conditions and other health status, health promotion and disease prevention, etc. (NCHS) • National Health and Nutrition Examination Survey (NHANES): nutritional status, cardiovascular disease, diabetes, overweight, hypertension, etc.; functional status (NCHS) • National Hospital Discharge Survey (NCHS) • National Medical Expenditure Survey (NMES): health services use and expenditures, third party payer coverage, health status, etc. (AHCPR) • National Vital Statistics System: demographic, infant and maternal health, family data, pregnancy outcomes, cause of death (NCHS) • Patient Treatment File: socio-demographic, diagnostic, surgical, episode information for impatient and extended care (Department of Veterans Affairs)
Private sources	• American Hospital Association Tapes: costs, discharges, outpatient visits, hospital characteristics (American Hospital Association) • ARAMIS (Arthritis, Rheumatism, and Aging Medical Information System): disease registry (American Rheumatism Association) • Duke DataBank for Cardiovascular Disease (Duke University Medical Center) • HCIA CHAMP database • APACHE III database • Value Health Sciences compass database • Northern New England Cardiovascular Disease database • HELP System Data Base: clinical records (LDS Hospital, Salt Lake City, Utah) • MEDSTAT Market Scan Data Base (MEDSTAT System)

Reference: The Lewin Group, Fairfax, VA, USA.

Most developed countries have government-sponsored ADE reporting systems. The Council of International Organizations of Medical Science (CIOMS) has been developing guidelines for the reporting of adverse events. The International Conference on Harmonization (ICH), representing the United States, the European Union and Japan, is also working on guidelines and standards for the reporting of adverse events.

Epidemiologic and economic data are sometimes available from the United States government. The government pays medical expenses for many citizens through the Medicare and Medcaid programs that provide state-by-state health care utilization including information on the use of drugs. The US Agency for Health Care Policy and Research (AHCPR) has been collecting patient care data from state governments and private health care data organizations since 1988. The data are used, among other purposes, to develop guidelines on the selection of drug therapies. The billing records can be used by economists to conduct economic research.

Insurers maintain extensive databases on the costs of medical care for their clients. Since the cost of treating adverse drug reactions is an added expense, they not only document reports of adverse reactions, but in some cases may restrict reimbursement for drugs which do not have an acceptable safety profile based on their guidelines.

In the United States HMOs are frequently for-profit companies seeking to provide medical care while controlling costs. They have databases of information on patient care which include drug usage and outcomes of drug therapy, including adverse reactions. Unfortunately access to these data is difficult, time-consuming and expensive. Table 16.1 lists examples of databases from public and private sources in the United States.

Access to epidemiologic and economic data on drug therapy in Europe is more limited. In Europe there are three major commercial databases that can be used for safety and economic data. The IMS MediPlus database contains general practice records continuously collected from 156 computerized practices throughout the UK. There are more than 1.5 million patient records, with comprehensive notes of hospital admission, referrals, and laboratory tests. MediPlus employs Read Codes, used by the UK National Health Service (NHS) as the standard for primary and secondary health care. MediPlus also allows the data to be used in ICD-9 (International Classification of Diseases Version 9) format. There is the GP Research Database (GPRD) from the ERIC group, and IBM has a database available. The Contract Research Organization Quintiles has a database QOST that contains information on costs of medication, laboratory evaluations, diagnostic procedures, hospital tariff charges and medical supplies in France, the UK, Spain, Germany, Belgium and Italy.

When the needed information is not available from existing databases, or the strength of the evidence is insufficient for the intended purpose, comparative prospective studies can provide: the needed data, consistent and common definitions of adverse events, collection of data for all subjects in the target population, an assurance that all investigators are collecting data using common definitions and formats, a duration of exposure to drug that is common to all subjects, and a common format for data capture. When a manufacturer has a potential competitive advantage because of a superior safety profile of its drug, the prospective study can provide strong evidence. However, there are inherent biases with respect to patient selection and to observer bias. The strongest data in comparative clinical efficacy come from controlled studies with patients randomly assigned to therapies, and the observers blind to the treatment received. When a manufacturer wishes to promote the advantage of a drug based on data, the strongest case (and in many countries the only legal case) is proof that is based on a controlled study, blinded if possible. Understanding the strengths of various study designs is key to good data management.

EXPERIMENTAL DESIGNS

The data management team helps assess the quality of the data for each study. The standards for acceptable data quality will depend on the objectives and scientific rigor of the study. Epidemiologic and economic studies are often run in parallel with pivotal clinical studies and follow the same rigorous designs, that is, randomized, controlled trials (RCT). There are, however, epidemiologic and economic studies that differ markedly from the typical clinical study in both objectives and design. When an RCT is either impractical or uneconomical, non-experimental designs may be used. An understanding of the key differences between experimental studies (usually RCTs) and non-experimental studies is essential for the data manager working in these areas. In discussing experimental designs we will generally use pharmacoepidemiologic studies for examples; the principles apply to economic studies as well.

The Experimental Study

The most rigorous design is the *experimental study*, which gives the highest degree of assurance that the data reflect accurately the outcome of therapy in a given population. Experimental studies are based on hypothesis testing, on controls and, most importantly, on the random assignment of patients to pre-selected therapies. Although other types of experimental studies are possible, in the pharmaceutical industry 'experimental' is synonymous with RCT. In the context of safety assessment, experimental studies are prospective, therapeutic interventions designed to test a hypothesis that the incidence and severity of adverse events associated with drug A are the same as those associated with placebo or with drug B. (More complicated designs are possible, but it is not necessary to address them in this context.) Patients are treated in accordance with a strict protocol; all patients in the same treatment arm are to be treated in the same manner. A variety of factors from selection bias to unknown concomitant conditions (confounders) can affect the outcome of treatment. Thus, groups of patients of comparable demographics and medical histories might be recruited and randomly assigned to receive drug A or B, or placebo. The randomization should distribute the confounders equally between the two groups. In the most controlled studies neither the patient nor the treating physician knows which group has received which drug (double-blind study).

The dosing is carefully controlled, and the use of concomitant medications may be restricted. *It is the degree of control in experimental studies that provides the higher degree of certainty that the data reflect the true results of therapy. However, generalizability to other populations and situations is limited.*

Observational Studies

Less rigorous, but of major importance, are non-experimental studies (*observational studies*) in which therapeutic intervention is not pre-selected and controls are less restrictive, for example, the study might not be blinded, or the patients might not be randomly selected to groups (Table 16.2). Charles Anello of the FDA defined observational studies as those not employing randomization of patients to study groups. These naturalistic studies are often preferred to study the economics of the innovation being studied.

In contrast to experimental studies, observational studies are often *not* designed with a predetermined selection of the therapeutic intervention. Either the observational study is retrospective, and all therapeutic intervention is historic, or the study is prospective and learning the type of intervention that is provided to patients is an objective of the study. As described below, an observational study might be used to learn of the existence of adverse effects (descriptive studies), quantify the occurrence of adverse events (surveys to obtain data on the incidence, that is, rate of occurrence of an ADE, or the prevalence, the total number of cases), or to test the hypothesis that those patients exposed to a drug then experience adverse events more frequently or of greater severity than those who do not (case-control and cohort studies).

In *descriptive* studies researchers compile reported instances of adverse events associated with drugs. These observations are used to uncover potentially, drug-related problems. Since descriptive reports are, for the most part, anecdotal, they provide evidence of safety issues that can be studied through more thorough investigations as described in the following paragraphs.

Surveys are designed to ascertain the incidence or prevalence of ADEs in a selected population. Because the universe of patients exposed to the drug cannot always be studied, a sample of the target population is selected using statistical sampling techniques. Of course, not all adverse events are necessarily associated with drug therapy. The underlying disease or condition could be the cause or a contributing factor. To help determine the incidence of ADEs, case-control studies may be used.

Case-control studies look *retrospectively* at two populations that are comparable with respect to demographics and health status: those which have been exposed to the drug (cases) and those which have not (controls).

Table 16.2 Comparison of elements in various types of safety studies

Type of study	Intervention	Hypothesis testing	Retrospective	Prospective	Controlled	Random assignment	Blinding
Experimental	Y	Y	N	Y	Y	Y	Y
Observational (non-experimental)							
Descriptive	N	N	Y	N	N	N	N
Survey	N	N	Y	N	N	N	N
Case-controlled	N	Y/N	Y	N	Y	N	Y/N
Cohort	N	Y/N	Y	Y	Y	N	Y/N

Intervention—researcher has protocol with planned therapeutic intervention for patients
Random Assignment—patients are assigned to treatment group by random selection

The data from each case subject are matched with the data from one or more control patients of the same age, gender, medical history and other potential confounding factors. The use of controls can give a more accurate understanding of what percentage of adverse events is attributable to the drug and not to other factors. The researcher may be testing a hypothesis that the groups differ or may simply be looking for possible differences between the cases and the controls.

In a *Cohort study* the researcher establishes two groups to be studied. The groups are usually designed to be comparable with respect to potential confounders such as gender, age, medical history, and so on, but are not randomly assigned. The two groups may be analyzed through a retrospective analysis of records, or they may be followed over time (prospective study). Usually patients are observed, without any intervention from the researchers; all therapeutic decisions are made independently by the treating physicians.

Retrospective vs. Prospective

While retrospective data searches can provide important information, there are limitations: the desired data might not be available; if the desired data are available, each person or group supplying data might use differing definitions for indications, adverse events, and so on. Other areas of difference: type and amount of data from each source; the duration of exposure to drug; the format in which the data are collected; and in many instances adverse events will not have been noted and recorded. The most important limitation is the relative lack of control. As noted, numerous factors can affect a patient's response to a drug: age, gender, concurrent diseases, other medications, compliance, and so on. In the absence of controls these confounders must be known and accounted for in order to analyze the study results. To acquire more complete and comparable data for two groups being compared, prospective cohort studies are recommended. Prospective safety studies have significant advantages over retrospective studies. Even in the non-experimental cohort study, one has the opportunity to define at the beginning what data are needed, how and by whom they will be collected, the size of the population, the duration of the study, and the analysis to be done. Thus, the collected data are more likely to be complete and to cover the same timespan for all patients studied.

While the *prospective* observational study produces a higher degree of certainty than the *retrospective* observational study, there are still the inherent difficulties associated with non-randomized, non-blinded studies. The absence of randomization means unmeasured confounders could affect the results, and the absence of blinding could allow observer bias. Thus, the prospective study with randomization of subjects to cohorts is the design of choice to demonstrate clinical efficacy and safety. The less controlled, naturalistic designs are useful to establish clinical effectiveness in heterogeneous populations and under varying conditions or, importantly, when randomization might be unethical or blinding impossible. In determining an economic endpoint, a naturalistic design is often preferred to the randomized, blinded trial, particularly when knowledge of the treatment allows variation in medical practice (resource use) to occur. This practice should not be misinterpreted to mean that experimental designs are inappropriate for economic studies, but it does raise the issue of protocol versus non-protocol driven costs and the generalizability of results to routine practice.

The Large Simple Trial

In both the post-marketing and pre-approval phases of drug development, experimental studies (always prospective) are the most rigorous type used to help determine the safety profiles of drugs. Because the controlled, clinical trial is the highest standard for clinical research, it is the most reliable study to determine the safety profile of a drug *if* the patient population studied is large and diverse enough to be representative of the total population that will receive the drug. However, for most clinical development studies the patient population is narrowly defined to help establish the efficacy of the drug under study; too broad a population would generate too many confounding factors and obscure the results. Manufacturers need to ensure that during clinical development the population of patients exposed to drug is representative of the broad population likely to receive the drug once it is marketed. These safety studies must be both practicable and affordable. For this reason, drug firms often conduct large, simple trials in which the inclusion/exclusion criteria are less stringent, the outcomes are more focused on safety and thousands of patients are enrolled. For relatively common ADEs, large, simple studies can uncover potential problems. However, for rarer events, the incidence of the ADE might be so low that tens of thousands of patients must be exposed to the drug before cases are noted. Post-marketing surveillance of thousands of users might detect rarer events associated with drugs.

STUDY VALIDITY, DATA INTEGRITY AND QUALITY

In pharmacoepidemiology and pharmacoeconomics the validity of studies and the integrity and quality of data can differ from the standards in Phase II and Phase III clinical development studies. 'Validity' refers both to study designs and to instruments (equipment and questionnaires). A valid study design together with a valid measure can lead to valid results. 'Integrity' and 'quality' refer to data. Integrity is a measure of the completeness of the data and includes quality. Quality data are accurate in that they correspond to the facts, and precise in that all measures are consistent around a point. For regulatory approvals the validity of studies and study instruments in epidemiologic and pharmacoeconomic studies must be as rigorous as those in pivotal clinical studies.

Data that accurately and precisely reflect the true facts are valid data. Kazdin defines experimental validity as 'the extent to which an experiment rules out alternative explanation[8]. There are numerous factors that can affect the validity of a study. At the highest level is the design of the study and the tools; the questions asked and the tests conducted must be valid. Spilker lists five types of measurement validity[9]:

Construct Validity means how well the measure reflects what it is supposed to measure.
Criterion Validity means how well the measure obtains the same result as an accepted test, scale, or questionnaire.
Discriminant Validity means that the test or measure is able to detect the smallest change that would be considered significant.
Content Validity means the choice and relative importance of each part of a test or questionnaire are appropriate for the intended purpose.
Face Validity means how well the measure correctly measures what it purports to measure.

Clinical scientists and economists are to assure that the measures used in the study are valid. However, even when the study design and the instruments for measuring are valid, it is possible for the data to be incomplete, inaccurate, or false. Thus, there is a question as to the integrity of the data. Spilker defines an *ideal database* as:

1. The population is well defined.
2. Records of all medicines are included.
3. All hospitalizations and diagnoses are included.
4. All deaths are included.
5. All important covariates (potential confounders) are included.

This listing of needed information assumes both that all data are collected and the data have been collected correctly. The perfect data set is an ideal; in nearly every study there is a level of data error. Some sources of error are: not all patients are seen at every scheduled visit; there are unresolved inconsistencies in data; some missing data are unrecoverable;

the data recorded by the observer could be inaccurate or both, spelling and coding might contain errors. How much known or estimated error is acceptable depends on the judgement of the research team.

There are major differences between the level of acceptable data error in prospective clinical trials designed to determine efficacy and safety, and the level of acceptable error in observational studies. In pivotal clinical studies, researchers demand a very high level of confidence in the data. All inconsistencies must be resolved if possible. Errors in data fields must be very low, often less than 0.05%. The number of patients and the completeness of the data is generally designed to allow for analysis to produce confidence levels of 95% with the power of the statistics at 80% or higher. These goals are achievable in many pivotal studies because the study is simple in the sense that a hypothesis is being tested in two, well-defined and controlled populations of subjects. The wider scope of studies conducted by epidemiologists and economists leads to the use of more analytical approaches than those used in interpreting RCTs. Epidemiologists and economists do use study designs amenable to null hypothesis testing. They also often use confidence intervals to interpret how well the data from observational studies reflect the population and in using naturalistic designs and evaluating the relative cost of therapies, economists often strengthen the interpretation of data through sensitivity analyses, the process of varying the estimates to measure their effects on the results.

In observational studies the design might be of necessity less rigorous; the confounders more numerous; the availability of data more limited. There is often far less assurance of the precision of the data. Just as in basic science in which the scientist is working in a new area of research, the confidence in the data is based on logic and completeness. In reporting and analyzing data, the researchers must state the objectives of the study, the limitations of the methods, the assumptions made relative to the population, and so on. It is critical for good reporting of data that the researchers stress the potential errors in their studies. For the data manager these limitations focus on the integrity of the data, that is, the completeness and the quality of the data.

As an example, in a report on the variability of prescription use in patients with AIDS the author noted the bias of omitted variables[10]: 'Removing the bias would require a complementary survey or reconstruction of the records, which would necessitate considerable extra resources.' As a second example, Revicki and co-authors note in their report of medical costs associated with fluoxetine and tricyclic antidepressants[11]: 'Several caveats must be considered when interpreting the results of this study . . . physician charges were missing for 37% of the patients; therefore, estimates of physician-related costs for treating antidepressant over doses may not be as accurate as the hospital cost data.'

THE ROLE OF THE DATA MANAGER

The data manager should be involved in the earliest development of the strategies and tools for data collection. Table 16.3 lists key activities that involve data management prior to the initiation of the study.

Table 16.3 Pre-initiation activities for epidemiologic and pharmacoeconomic studies

---

Design Study: objectives, scope, limitations, comparators (if any), timelines
Develop data collection strategy: patient self-report and/or medical and billing records
Design CRFs
Prepare Guidelines for CRF completion
Design database
Prepare Source document verification plan
Design record log for tracking data collection

In optimal organizations, the data management specialists participate on research teams that include: clinical investigators, statisticians, regulatory personnel, clinical trial managers, CRF designers, epidemiologists or pharmacoeconomists, and the data management specialists. Through participation with the team during the design of the study, the data management specialists gain the necessary understanding of the required data and most importantly the standards expected with respect to data quality. It is also important that members of the data management team understand the source of the data and the form in which the data will be retrieved, especially when data will come from multiple sources, such as: hospital records, insurance and government records, or private physician records. In addition, economic studies may include indirect costs such as time lost from work, requiring diaries, interviews and possibly verification through employer records.

When the study design is complete, and the sources of data have been established, a data collection strategy is required. Because a patient often visits more than one medical care facility, when possible it is imperative to question the patient as to when and where treatment has been received. For prospective studies, patients may be asked to keep a diary or may be interviewed at visits, by telephone or through questionnaires mailed to them. If data are abstracted from medical or insurance records and the patient is not available, it is possible that the owner of the records knows of other care the patient has received.

In the United States obtaining a patient's medical bills for economic studies requires clearance from an Institutional Review Board (IRB). The patient should be identified only by trial number to assure confidentiality of billing as well as of medical records. Billing records are often difficult to obtain in the United States and generally are not available outside the United States. Economists often work with clinical researchers to develop models of treatment regimens and assign costs based on available data from multiple resources. Such models allow individual institutions to input their known costs and calculate results, for example, cost-effectiveness. Cost can be those charged by provider or those reimbursed by insurer.

Measures of quality of life and general well-being are captured with questionnaires. These instruments should be valid for the specific use. There are numerous validated instruments for quality of life and general well-being. However, for the specific study under consideration, it may be necessary to modify an existing questionnaire, or in some cases to design, test, and validate a new questionnaire. When patients are not competent to answer the questionnaire, it is sometimes possible to have family members or other observers complete the forms. Verification of the correctness of patient self-reported data is difficult, if not impossible. With proper randomization of patients to treatment groups being compared, the reporting errors should be randomly distributed to each group.

The design of the CRF should be led by an experienced CRF designer with input from the entire team. The data management specialist has the opportunity to assist in elements of design that contribute to ease of data entry and cross-checking of data from one form to another. Most importantly, the data entry personnel should have a clear understanding of what is meant by each entry. Any potential ambiguity in the CRF must be avoided. In pharmacoepidemiologic studies the concepts and definitions are reasonably standardized. Pharmacoeconomics is a relatively new discipline with a broader scope of inquiry than clinical studies, and new study methods are being developed. For each study, the definition of terms, determining in which fields to enter data, how to handle exceptions, and so forth, requires intensive effort and communication among all members of the research team to assure a meaningful set of data is compiled. All of this information should be incorporated into written guidelines for CRF completion. The use of the CRFs and guidelines should be tested by a pilot use among site personnel and the research staff, especially the data entry and data verification staff.

The establishing of data edits including ranges and cross-checks should be done with the participation of the data management personnel. This is especially important with pharmacoeconomic studies since, as noted above, they are likely to include multiple factors that may be new to the data management personnel.

In the course of the study the data management team should continually audit the data collection and database for completeness and consistency. No study goes exactly as planned, and economic studies with multiple factors new to the data management team are especially likely to generate surprises; corrections in data capture, entry and editing are frequently necessary.

With the rapid growth of pharmacoeconomics and the increasing importance of large safety studies, the data manager needs to be aware of the relevant study designs and become an integral part of each study team. With a thorough understanding of the issues and early participation in the study, the data manager can contribute significantly to a successful study.

SUGGESTED READING

The expansion of pharmaceutical research into epidemiology and economics will continue to demand of data managers an ever broadening knowledge base. Pharmacoeconomics is an especially challenging area because the concepts and terminology are evolving. The following publications are recommended.

An Introduction to Health Economics (1995) M.F. Drummond, Brookwood Medical Publications, Surrey, UK.

British Journal of Medical Economics, Brookwood Medical Publications, Surrey, UK.

Databases for Pharmacovigilance (1995) ed. Stuart R. Walker, Medical Benefits Risk Foundation, London, UK.

Medical Outcomes and Guidelines Sourcebook (1996) Faulkner and Gray, New York, NY.

Peto, R. and Collins, R. Gray (1995) Large-scale randomized evidence: large, simple trials and overviews of trials. *Journal of Clinical Epidemiology*, **48**, 23–40.

PharmacoEconomics published monthly by Adis International, Auckland, New Zealand.

UCSF. *UCSF postgraduate program: outcomes research and clinical epidemiology.* Webside: http:/www.caps.ucsf.edu/epidem/courses/oracle.html

REFERENCES

1. Jick, H. (1977) The discovery of drug induced illness. *N. Engl. J. Med.*, **296**, 481–485.
2. *Lancet* (1979) Controlled trials: Planned deceptions? *Lancet*, **1**, 534–535.
3. Ritter, J.M. (1980) Placebo-controlled, double-blind clinical trials can impede medical progress. *Lancet*, **1**, 1126–1127.

4. Scheiner, L.B. (1979) Clinical trials and the illusion of objectivity. In K.L. Melmon (ed.), *Drug therapeutics—Concepts for Physicians*. Elsevier–North Holland, New York, pp. 167–182.

5. Evans, D., Freund, D., Dittus *et al.* (1990) The use of economic analysis as a basis for inclusion of pharmaceutical products on the pharmaceutical benefits scheme. Canberra, Department of Health, Housing and Community Services.

6. Finney, D.J. (1996) Statistical aspects of pharmacoepidemiology. *Drug Inf. J.*, **30**, 987–990.

7. Appel, W.C. (1996) Postmarketing surveillance in Canada. *Drug Inf. J.*, **30**, 665–669.

8. Kazdin, A.E. (1982) *Single-Case Research Designs. Methods for Clinical and Applied Settings*. Oxford University Press, New York.

9. Spilker, B. (1996) Validation of clinical tests and measures. In *Guide to Clinical Trials*, Lippincott–Raven, Philadelphia–New York, pp. 313–319.

10. Kerleau, M., Le Vaillant, M. and Flori, Y.–A. (1997) Measuring the variability of prescriptions use in patients with HIV infection or AIDS. *PharmacoEconomics*, **11**(3), 246–261.

11. Revicki, D.A., Palmer, C.S., Scott, D.P. *et al.* (1997) Acute medical costs of fluoextine versus tricyclic antidepressants. *PharmacoEconomics*, *11*(1), 48–56.

17 Future Revisited

RUTH LANE

Glaxo Wellcome, Middlesex, UK

INTRODUCTION

Someone once said, 'The future isn't what it used to be'. A few years ago, Clinical Data Management professionals were optimistically predicting the advent of new technologies which would radically increase efficiency by reducing the paper documentation mountains associated with clinical trials and considerably improving the process. The promise has yet to be fulfilled. Although advanced technology has been implemented to enhance various aspects of the data management process, it has not been without difficulty nor has it been developed as rapidly as many had anticipated.

Meanwhile the pressure for a better, quicker and cheaper process has been increasing. The cost of drug development has soared. It is now necessary to demonstrate the economic value of a medicine and not just its safety and efficacy profile. Development costs are rising by almost 10% annually due to an increased number of studies being conducted with more procedures in larger, and more diverse, populations, so there are pressures to be more productive. In Europe, the Economic and Monetary Union's potential effect on pricing strategy could challenge productivity even more. Having a common currency across countries makes for easier comparison and this may keep the price down.

Margins of profit have been reduced through pricing constraints and generic competition. The industry has responded to these increased pressures with corporate mergers and acquisitions. Expenditure on research and development has been affected as profit margins decline and many companies have downsized as a consequence. In North America, for example, the number of people employed by pharmaceutical companies has decreased by nearly 50 000 and R&D spend has declined generally by around 7%. Companies have sought to decrease their fixed costs by reducing headcount and increasing the use of flexible resources such as Contract Research Organisations. There is significant pressure to market a

Clinical Data Management. Second Edition. Edited by R.K. Rondel, S.A. Varley and C.F. Webb.
© 2000 John Wiley & Sons, Ltd

medicine as early in the patent life as possible in order to maximise the period without competition, both to increase total revenue and to shorten the time to peak sales.

The increase in regulatory requirements and competition seen in the 1990s, coupled with reforms in health care services, has therefore created enormous pressure for the pharmaceutical industry. With the aim of meeting these challenges the pharmaceutical companies continue to make a significant investment in technological solutions but have added an additional emphasis on process improvement. The constant challenge is to achieve more with less.

In this environment the effectiveness of the Data Management function is crucial. It is a vital step in obtaining early approval to market a product and in its subsequent, successful marketing. It is often on the critical path and it has been estimated that each day that a medicine is not on the market, up to $1m may be lost, so delays or deficiencies in the Data Management process can be costly. Speed is not enough. There is still the need to strike the right balance between time, cost and quality.

The future shape of Clinical Data Management, as predicted earlier this decade, has not turned out to be what we had anticipated. The future challenges and successes and failures of the past few years need to be understood if a better future is to be assured.

FUTURE CHALLENGES FOR CLINICAL DATA MANAGEMENT

In order to continue to contribute effectively in the next millennium, Clinical Data Management needs to anticipate and prepare for further challenges. The management of clinical trials data must be effective. The differentiator between companies in the future will be the quality of the development decisions they make. Better decisions will be based on rapidly available, good-quality information. Converting good-quality data into high-calibre information is an essential step from which knowledge and wisdom emanate. As the information age matures, the expectations of information users will increase.

Good-quality information will be required throughout the lifetime of a product. The lifetime of the product will almost certainly include mergers/demergers and acquisitions of the parent company along with collaborations and licensing deals.

New areas of discovery and development are emerging. The past few years have seen a blossoming of the application of genetics within the industry, accompanied by tremendous requirements for large databases. Running behind this will be a demand for detailed demographic and phenotypic information from a number of data resources, including the clinical trials arena.

The challenge of costs will continue, with the accompanying need to complete medical development programmes as rapidly as possible.

Technology itself will present challenges as well as opportunities. As investigators and health care technology providers become more sophisticated, electronic data will be available from many sources. These data sources may not conform to the conventional standard approach of many large companies. Technology may also be now reaching the stage of challenging traditional roles within clinical data management.

MEETING THE CHALLENGES

Meeting the challenges of the future for Clinical Data Management requires a holistic approach. Technology clearly has a vital role to play in achieving this but also critical to success are the adoption of relevant working practices and many other factors. In the rest of the chapter we will review and consider a number of these factors under the following headings:

1. *Embracing Technology.* Electronic data capture, Computer Assisted New Drug Applications (CANDA) and Computer Assisted Product Licence Applications were seen to offer the revolution in the past. Progress has been patchy. The future also offers enhanced document management and the exploitation of the Internet.

2. *Enhancing Processes.* The whole Data Management process needs to be challenged. Redundant parts of the process need to be identified and eliminated. Standards are emerging from the regulatory agencies; acceptance and production of guidelines for the electronic age, especially electronic signatures, are offering opportunities to rethink processes.

3. *Embedding Quality.* The acceptable level of quality also needs to be defined. Detection of errors is sometimes overemphasised compared to quality control. Error detection does not in itself control quality but reveals the effectiveness of quality control procedures and may indicate where remedial action is required. Quality standards and data structures provide the basis for dependable and reusable data.

4. *Enforcing Regulations.* Regulation of the pharmaceutical industry is continuing to evolve. The International Committee for Harmonisation has provided a forum for the development of commonality in the USA, Europe and Japan. Data privacy regulations are coming into force in the EU. Data management needs to reappraise systems and assumptions to ensure compliance and to look for opportunities to improve productivity.

5. *Exploiting Databases.* Databases need to be developed so that they continue to be an asset to the pharmaceutical development and marketing organisation. It must be possible to make sense of the data for the lifetime of the drug, irrespective of which system the data are held on. Contexting

information will become more important. Disciplines which generate large numbers of data points are becoming more important in medical development, such as genetics and pharmacoeconomics. The increased use of external information will also offer opportunities and challenges in the future.

6.   *Extending Communication.* Electronic exchange of information has become much more widespread and less complicated. This creates opportunities, both in improved process and in facilitating better two-way communication. However, this does offer some threats to the pharmaceutical developer, such as instant demands for information.

7.   *Expanding Resource.* Increasingly, pharmaceutical companies are able to resource the Data Management function in a number of ways. Contracting in or out, use of technologies and flexible working offer numerous resourcing options. Different skill sets may be required within the pharmaceutical company. Roles may also change as a result of adopting any one of these models.

8.   *Engaging Data Managers.* Opportunities for Data Managers to develop their expertise are plentiful. Different skill sets are emerging. The challenge is to build the skills, recruit and retain good people.

9.   *Evolving Culture.* With the increasing skill set required by Data Management, it is essential that we nurture a culture which attracts the right kind of employees to fulfil this important role if our companies are to overcome the challenges ahead.

10.   *Emerging Markets.* As new regions increase their market share of a pharmaceutical product, we need to be able to work in these to build a relevant clinical information source and to put effective data management structures into place.

Embracing Technology

Since the beginning of the decade, many new technologies have emerged which can be usefully applied to the Data Management component of the clinical development process. The past vision of the future was instant capture of data electronically and more powerful processing systems, both offering significant resource benefits. At the other end of the process electronically compiled submissions were to be commonplace. Where is the revolution?

As an example, in the early 1980s, the industry was beginning to pilot the capture of clinical data remotely, using an electronic tool. Fifteen years later an estimated 95% of clinical trials still use paper CRFs. The reasons for the lack of rapid uptake of this type of technology are many and varied.

Unanticipated difficulties have been encountered when new technology is being introduced. This has occurred especially when there has not been a radical review of how processes and roles need to change to maximise the benefits the technology can offer. Whether you choose to reskill people and train them to use technology to do their job or to change the roles of existing users of technology to include other functions is almost immaterial in some respects. Both approaches require an investment in training, usually in time and money. Expectations of, and from, staff may change and have to be well managed. The skill is to ascertain how to embrace the technology to optimum effect in the operational environment whether it be centralised or decentralised, outsourced or insourced.

The scale-up process has also created difficulties. Piloting a technological application in a small way, in a relatively controlled environment, is often a highly successful exercise. As full-scale implementation gathers pace, both system performance and people performance issues may arise. Both need to be assessed or stress-tested to a degree, to see if they have the capacity to cope with the expected work in terms both of volume and of nature. Support also acquires another dimension as you move from using an application in a simple, single-centre study to a more complex, multicentre, multinational environment. If the technology is designed for investigator use, for example, an electronic Case Report Form, providing 24-hour, multilingual support along with sufficient understanding of the application design and of the communication networks in many countries all over the world is essential if the pharmaceutical company is not to lose credibility. There are a number of strategies for handling this, including the use of contract IT resource to handle the preparation of PCs and local logistics but the key to doing this successfully is to have a well-managed and well-sponsored implementation plan underpinned by a commitment to provide sufficient resources.

No obvious market leader has yet emerged in the world of electronic data capture. Performance and design of the systems have not yet reached the optimal level. Set-up times for studies have been too long and have often required specialist support from the companies that produced the software. These companies have typically been small and there have been difficulties in matching expectations with the large, global pharmaceutical companies. New technologies seem to be changing so fast that they seem to last less time than it takes to conduct the average clinical trial.

Widescale implementation of some of the more sophisticated technologies has also been slower than expected because the industry has been distracted both organisationally and financially by the acquisitions and mergers which have taken place. Introducing yet another way of managing data when two companies combine may prove to be one change too many or too soon, given that both companies usually already have both their own current and legacy systems.

No matter how well the technology and its support are implemented, the benefits of technologies such as electronic data capture will only be obtained by positioning it well in the process and by implementing it well if you want to maximise the benefits for the cost. Attention to this is vital if it is going to be a key means of increasing productivity. If a technological solution is being used, it is important to develop associated working practices to realise the potential benefits. There is little benefit in terms of time saving, for example, if an investigator only completes an electronic CRF some weeks or months after seeing the patient, except that data entry is done at source. In the best situation the working practices should be such that the investigator completes the electronic CRF while seeing the patient. Conversely, the designer needs to be aware of the process within the investigator's office if this is to be feasible or acceptable. Despite the potential benefits to the pharmaceutical company, the investigator, as the end user, needs to be incentivised to use such electronic data capture tools. Failing to offer any benefits to the investigator has also played a part in the lack of uptake.

In an attempt to increase user acceptance of data capture a number of alternatives to the keyboard have been explored. Some parts of CRFs seem to lend themselves more to a particular type of technology than others, for example Optical Mark Reading (OMR) for Quality of Life questionnaires, because of the widespread use of multiple choice questionnaires. Optical Character Recognition (OCR) is still not used extensively in Data Management, predominantly because of variable handwriting recognition rates, particularly where varying types of script are encountered, as in international trials. Other industries, however, have successfully experimented with using three different OCR engines applied to the same data to ensure a higher degree of accuracy for handwriting. The lack of uptake in clinical trials may be related to the variability of the terms that may be used compared to the more limited 'vocabularies' of, for example, finance-based enterprises. The promise offered by pen-based systems seems to have been overtaken by the increasing acceptance of keyboard-based systems for entering data in the investigator's clinic as computer usage amongst the medical profession has increased. Disappointing character recognition and response times of the pen-based systems have also been cited as reasons for their lack of uptake. Neither keyboard nor pen is optimal for real time entry of data if the electronic CRF is not 'portable' either by virtue of networking data capture applications or the actual device used by the investigator and the various other operatives, such as study nurses, who participate in studies.

Acquisition of data in document form has also been explored, from the use of FAX-based systems to simple capture of images of paper CRFs. Many of the predicted benefits of electronic data capture, such as speed of response to the investigator and rapid receipt of data, have been claimed by users of these systems, at a much lower investment cost than PC-based systems. Attempts to convert data from images into a database have had some success but even providing electronic access to copies of paper

CRFs seems to offer some real benefits. Imaging documents, especially CRFs, can mean that local staff and those at headquarters, who may have international responsibilities, can view the data simultaneously with all of the attendant opportunities for improved communication and process.

The Case Report Form is not the only source of data. The increased use of different procedures and facilities during the course of a clinical trial often means that the data generated from one subject are dispersed to many places. The challenge for Data Management is to recombine the data to recreate the subject's profile for reporting from the database. For example, paper-based diary data need to be linked with data entered into the electronic CRF. These, in turn, must be integrated with the results from the haematology and clinical chemistry laboratory analyses and with the time concentration data from the samples taken for pharmacokinetic analysis. ECG data may come via yet another route. As data from each of these different routes become computerised, the data manager has to ensure that each data file contains sufficient identifying information and that the systems are compatible to transfer and recompile the data associated with one patient. One of the key features of capturing or computerising data electronically at source means that the initial quality will be significantly higher if effective validity checks are employed. Care needs to be taken to ensure that these checks are not too intrusive for the user and that data integrity is maintained as the computerised data from different sources are merged. The Data Management role looks likely to become more one of brokers of information rather than processors of it.

So far, most of the discussion has been put into considering how the application of technology can significantly improve the management of clinical trial data. Technology does also offer benefits elsewhere in the clinical development process. The Computer Assisted Product Licence Application (CAPLA) and, more specifically the Computer Assisted New Drug Application (CANDA), have been offering the same promise of process improvement as electronic data capture has held at the front end of the process. The advantages seem clear: it has considerable potential for speeding the review process and to reduce the vast volumes of paperwork that are generated in the process. The orderly construction of a computerised application can also provide a well-structured environment for the compilation and review of the information in-house.

With these potential gains in mind and with considerable pressure on them to increase efficiency and speed up review, the FDA is desirous of moving towards a paperless process for registering drugs. This will mean that both CRFs and the listings can be filed electronically. Despite this the FDA has required three paper copies of each NDA in the past, and computerised versions have been review aids. Recently the agency has changed its policy and regulatory submissions are now permitted with electronic signatures with one paper copy. This is a significant step since the FDA now has the potential to be totally electronic. This offers the benefit to the pharmaceutical company of positioning the CANDA as a submission in its own right, not as a duplicated effort. Paper documents can also be replaced with electronic ones in the archive. At the front end of the process the recognition of the electronic signature will mean that data can also be entered directly into an electronic database so that the initial source data record is electronic, offering gains to the monitoring staff as well as data management. In this regulated environment it is essential that these records are as readable and as accessible as paper ones and indicate authorship. It must be possible to generate a printed copy too. In this electronic environment it is essential, however, to bear in mind that systems can become obsolete and accessing historic electronic records can prove difficult. In Europe, however, progress towards a totally electronic regulatory submission system has been slower. In the UK, you are required to be able to demonstrate that someone posing as the genuine signatory could not have produced the electronic signature, just as you would with a paper-based signature.

In order to respond to the FDA's advance into the electronic age, the pharmaceutical company will need to be able to support access, security, and archiving. Computer-assisted review programs are also being used for submissions. The potential resultant decrease in review time means the pharmaceutical company has to be ready to launch the drug on the market sooner if all goes well. In the UK, the MCA is also working with the industry with respect to electronic submissions, that is, Computer Assisted Product Licence Applications (CAPLAs). These were initially submitted on discs but now CDROMs are favoured.

As the regulatory agencies become increasingly computerised in their work, Clinical Data Management must consider ways to work synergistically in the provision of data to them. One key point to consider when introducing technology generally is how it is going to be used. Simply because a system can perform a particular function, does not necessarily mean it adds value to use it or activate it. Its functionality may enable the user to work in a number of different ways, so, as suppliers of information, data managers need to be cognisant of this in order to ensure that the user of the technology is presented with the right information or message. For example, navigation through a hard copy document may differ in order from in the electronic version so information may be viewed out of context and with different results if care is not taken.

For any stage of the process, implementing technology is a costly business but, if it is done well, the return on investment makes it worthwhile. Data Management needs technological interventions to achieve the necessary productivity levels demanded by the current industry challenges. A system needs to be designed and built so that it can perform the task for which it is intended. Data management, or document management, systems need to ensure that the integrity both of the data and of the associated information is assured. A system must be tested both by the developers and by the user community to ensure it is fit for use. It needs to be reliable and secure in operation as well as being the subject of policies and procedures to ensure its usage is adequately controlled. Disaster recovery plans and virus-vetting procedures can prevent significant loss in future. In addition, it needs to be well documented in terms both of its development and of its use. There should be documented evidence of what the design, testing and scope of usage is intended to be and similarly documented evidence of how this was achieved. Systems, like processes and databases, are auditable so adequate documentation is key. Any failure on the part of Clinical Data Management can be costly to the company.

The Internet is a new phenomenon which is rapidly permeating the world at an unprecedented speed. An estimated one to two million new users are reported to be accessing the Internet for the first time each month. It offers worldwide two-way communication and access to information without needing to understand the systems and applications underlying it.

The pharmaceutical industry seems to be behind others in its usage though there are an increasing number of examples of where it is being applied successfully to aspects of the clinical development process. Other disciplines in the pharmaceutical industry are using web browsers, for example, to access large bioinformatics databases. However, its usage in the industry looks set to surge over the next couple of years and Clinical Data Managers need to be aware of its potential role in the clinical arena.

With so many able to access the Internet from home, it has already been used for recruiting patients into upcoming trials. Recruitment, especially for the larger Phase III trials, is often protracted and increasing the effectiveness of this part of the process could be very valuable. Targeting specific populations via the support groups on the web would be easy. The other area where there is keen interest in the Internet is for computerising and transferring patient data. With the advent of electronic CRFs, investigators may be bombarded by pharmaceutical companies, each with their own hardware to support the running of their clinical trials system. The Internet could do away with the need for different software and hardware on the investigator's desk and is therefore very attractive both to the investigator and to the pharmaceutical industry at large. It could also facilitate communication between the clinics, laboratory, sponsor and so on. A number of studies are reported to have been run using web-based technology for the CRFs.

Internet security is often mentioned as an issue though the encryption technology employed is purported to be more secure than leased telephones and faxes and is now such that, apparently, the US National

Security Agency has not been able to break the code so far. Some also draw comfort from the fact that highly sensitive financial details are already transferred via the Internet seemingly without major concerns. Also, clinical trials are often designed, and the data transferred, in a way that is not easy to understand unless you have information on the treatment code or data structure, which adds another degree of data security. It has been suggested that transferring data via the Internet is not the real challenge but moving away from the paper version is! It is evident that some clinical trials have already been conducted using the Internet and this seems set to increase.

With so much communication between the ever-increasing populations of Internet users, patients in a trial are known to be exchanging information, for example AIDS patients. It is not easy to anticipate how this might affect the progress and outcome of the trial but it is worthy of some consideration. Information may be published easily on the Internet; for example, data output can be converted to HTML quite easily, using SAS. As the Internet lends itself to being both a publishing and a marketing tool, users need to be aware of the consequences of bad practice. To prevent legal action, information published on the Internet must be up-to-date and not be libellous in any way. One advantage to the user is that they do not have to understand the operating system. Clinical Data Management might benefit from seeking out similar opportunities to provide the tools and the operating environment for its customers to interrogate clinical databases. This approach could equally apply to internal customers as well as external ones.

Most would admit that the targeted use of technology in the clinical development process could bring significant benefits. It can mean that data are available on the desktop in real time. This important company asset can be viewed on an ongoing basis. Technology of the future will facilitate access to the data virtually as they are generated. Early decisions can be made on the development of a drug, based on access to study management information such as recruitment and protocol violations, or on safety profiles, for example by accessing laboratory and adverse event data shortly after they are captured. A pharmaceutical company can now access its data on a central laboratory's database or it can receive ready-to-load files within hours of generation from central laboratories and individual sites. As technology has advanced, so have the different data security technologies including encryption, algorithms, closed wide area networks and digitised signatures. Whatever the tool, the Data Manager needs to ensure the integrity of the data whilst providing rapid access to information from clinical trials.

The opportunities to enhance our businesses by embracing technology are endless but the key to success is in the careful positioning of it to optimise its role and minimise any potentially negative impacts its use may bring.

Enhancing Processes

The changes occurring in the pharmaceutical industry have resulted in many companies critically evaluating how they do business. Technology review alone will not guarantee success. There are tremendous gains to be made by process review, either on a large scale, as in full business re-engineering, or at more basic levels within each process. Most pharmaceutical organisations have embarked on such exercises over the past decade. Managing data is a costly part of the R&D process and some have been staggered to learn the true cost to the organisation of each datum collected. It has been viewed as a prime candidate for process review.

Underpinning this review and the continuous monitoring of the businesses are performance metrics. These are seen as an integral measure of the effectiveness of the clinical development process and are the means by which the necessary increase in productivity will be demonstrated.

Over the past 15–20 years the Data Management business has evolved to keep pace with the growing requirements of the clinical development process. Myths and redundant working processes have developed over this time, particularly as guidelines and regulations governing this aspect of clinical development have been open to varied interpretation. Clinical Data Managers sometimes feel compelled to continue to use processes which were implemented for specific historical reasons but may no longer be necessary. For example, certain checks of data on the database versus the CRF may take place when specific problems are experienced but these may continue long after the process causing the problem has changed.

Many process change projects have focused on challenging the current process, eliminating redundant activities, genericising others and standardising the output. If we are to plan for the future now, we need to develop processes which are lean. When defining new ways of working, it is helpful to record the basis for the decision so that as dependencies change, we do not revisit issues unnecessarily and are not caught in the old trap of supporting old assumptions that are no longer valid. Many companies have clinical data stored on more than one database system. Serious adverse event data have proved to be a controversial example in the past where different users of the data have different reporting needs and one system may not have been able to meet both sets of requirements.

Ways in which processes can be enhanced include minimising activities by simplification, readdressing assumptions and automation and the use of standards. Minimising, simplifying and automating the routine, will enable data managers to utilise their skills to better effect. The use of standards in the design of the data capture tool, databases, query resolution and reporting programs is of real benefit to all involved though there is usually some resistance to implementation. This may be overcome by ensuring that there are tangible benefits for those who feel constrained by standards. These might range from agreeing to an earlier delivery date if standards are used through to reinforcing the use of the preferred standards through performance management methods. For example, if time is saved through using the standard, rewards might be given for increased efficiency or enhanced productivity due to increased intellectual input. Finally, since change is becoming a way of life in Clinical Data Management, it is essential to learn how to manage it.

Introducing industry standards for parts of the Data Management process could prove very beneficial. The development of MedDRA, the ICH *Medical Dictionary for Regulatory Activities*, is one step in this direction. This classification system for reporting clinical trial and spontaneous adverse events will enable regulatory authorities to receive information from different companies in a more comparable form. It seems that whilst the FDA intends to mandate its use, other authorities will only recommend that it be used, but especially with electronic submissions. The MedDRA dictionary of terms is to be maintained by an independent international organisation and it will include autoencoding and multilingual functionality.

Whilst technology can undoubtedly be used to good effect to obtain better quality data initially, the process may enhance this too. For example, Data Managers can train both investigators and patients to attain this as well. The process of managing the investigational sites seems to be improving generally to the advantage of Data Management. Recognising the need in this area, facilities are beginning to emerge, such as Site Management Organisations (SMOs), which have the potential to ensure cost and performance efficiencies by increased involvement of the investigator site at the clinical trial conduct level. In the US, during the past five years, the traditional academic-oriented medical centres have been replaced by a new type of investigational centre which typically forms part of a networking enterprise with some level of co-ownership involved. Relevant incentives with good management and information systems mean that there are efficiencies to be gained by conducting a study at one of these centres. This model is also emerging in other countries too, especially in Europe. Care needs to be taken to ensure that there is no conflict of interest, especially by organisations, including CROs, which may, in some respects, be considered to hold a stake in the sites they are scheduled to monitor.

Embedding Quality

When defining processes, it is important to consider the desired quality of the output and then to design and build quality into the process accordingly. This needs to be done irrespective of the tools used. Expressing the quality of the output, whether it is the database or the report, in a meaningful way which conveys confidence to the user of the information is not easy. Perhaps the traditional error rate figures should be replaced by accuracy levels to portray a better sense of the standard of quality achieved rather than the level of inaccuracy.

The quality control steps often present in a paper-based Data Management system are extremely resource intensive and quite a misnomer. They are usually more error detection than quality control. It was not that many years ago that Data Managers seemed to strive for the 100% accurate database that colleagues often expected. In response to the pressures of both the present and the future, the challenge now is how to attain an acceptable level of quality whilst reducing time and cost, that is, how to minimise and manage the risks.

Assuring the integrity of the data on the database is much more than checking that what appears on the CRF, or is first recorded in the electronic data capture tool, is accurately represented in the finalised database. The data need to be traceable from the source to the report with relevant audit trails in place. Detecting falsified data is an activity the Data Manager can assist with by using the data searching tools at their disposal. This may have previously been left for the monitors to detect but Data Management can proactively play a role too. Early detection of fraudulent information may result in its omission from a study analysis. However, late or no detection could result in patients being at risk or, at least, the pharmaceutical company's or CRO's reputation being called into question. Once the genuineness of the data recorded in the clinic is established, the Clinical Data Management function needs to ensure its processes or systems do not introduce further errors which go undetected. Data security is also important. Process-oriented audits, which ensure that procedures are adequate and are being followed, may bring more benefit than output audits in which documents, databases and so on are reviewed. However, there needs to be confidence in the ability of the process to produce the desired result. One future activity that Data Management should consider engaging in is a pre-program dialogue with the regulatory authorities about the acceptable quality standards for the data. Agreeing the philosophy upfront could increase confidence in the data and reduce queries later.

One of the keys to successful drug development and marketing programs is the use which can be made of the information gleaned to date. Integrating data handled on different systems over time and with different working practices is a challenge. However, if defined standards of data quality have been adhered to throughout, this task is much easier.

During the 1990s, the pharmaceutical industry has become increasingly reliant on external resources to raise efficiency. CROs, SMOs and others have been instrumental in this drive but the sponsor must also assure itself that these organisations can deliver the quality of databases, reports and documentation required and to target. Detailed assessments of their capability in the relevant competencies, and especially those of staff assigned to the work, are essential. Ongoing performance review and feedback are also important for a successful collaboration. Clearly the extent to which this is necessary changes as the relationship and confidence become established.

Enforcing Regulations

The pharmaceutical industry is well regulated and it is important that Clinical Data Management keep abreast of new regulations, influencing these as appropriate. It is essential to consider any impact on data collection or handling, database design and so forth, and to ensure compliance.

One key activity over the past few years has been the work of the ICH as representatives from regulatory agencies and the pharmaceutical industry in Europe, the US and Japan have sought to harmonise on drug registration issues. The EU has recently adopted the ICH guidelines for GCP in place of the European ones (which had been effective since 1992) for all clinical trials starting after 1 January 1997 and this seems to have brought increased work for both investigators and sponsors. The US and Japan are planning to adopt these too.

There have been changes to the registration process in Europe. The European Medicines Evaluation Agency was set up in 1995 and the CPMP's summary of the assessment is openly accessible (via the European Public Assessment Report). The EMEA also has a home page on the Internet. Clinical Data Management should maintain an active interest in what the agencies are doing and keep their processes in line with their requirements. For example, there are European guidelines on clinical safety data management and pharmacovigilance. In the US, a policy revision by the National Institute of Health (NIH) in 1994 deemed that women and minorities must be included in all clinical trials. The need for additional subanalyses on different populations highlights the need to ensure that the clinical database can meet changing regulatory needs.

Another EU directive on Data Protection was implemented in October 1998 which restricts the use of confidential patient data. In particular, under the new directive consent will need to be specific and unambiguous and subjects will have the right to access their data. The exporting of data from EU countries to those without adequate data protection legislation without consent will not be permitted. Currently, this would include the USA. Potential consequences could be that unblinding is affected and that regulatory agencies may not be able to exchange information. In addition, the use of data for a subsequent purpose may be prohibited if it is not disclosed and consent obtained. The pharmaceutical industry is working with the European regulatory agencies to find a mutually acceptable and workable solution. Generally regulations in the clinical trials arena are tightening up with ethical guidelines increasingly becoming legal codes of conduct. The data aspects of clinical development are, therefore, coming under increasing control in line with the study conduct component and data managers need to be prepared for these changes.

Exploiting Databases

Increasingly, data from clinical trials are being used to do more than justify that a drug is sufficiently safe and efficacious to market. Clinical databases can increase the rate of acquisition of knowledge within the pharmaceutical organisation if used effectively. The Data Manager can play an influential role in facilitating access to relevant data.

The provision of timely and quality safety data for regulatory reporting, for review by Drug Safety Monitoring Boards or for internal reviews, is key to ensuring that no patients are exposed to unnecessary risks. In addition to this, clinical trial programme databases can assist with managing the drug development programme. They are now being recognised as good sources of information on rates and patterns of recruitment and return of data from the site. Information on the quality of the data that these supply may help with investigator selection and can highlight problems in the data collection process or system. Details of protocol deviations can enhance study design and focus monitoring. Extraction of data from existing databases can obviate the need to conduct a study, for example drug interaction. The uses to which the database can be put are extensive but its depths are still not completely plumbed. Clinical Data Management needs to lead the way in revealing what information is held to minimise collection of duplicate data. Another important role is to feedback on the percentage of data actually used in the final study report or subsequent searches of the database to help minimise data collection in future studies.

Other disciplines that generate large numbers of data points are becoming more tactically important in the medical development process as developers seek to target their drug programmes, and support more effective commercialisation of their products. Large databases of genetic information are being developed. Correlating polymorphisms in candidate genes with disease phenotype is going to be significant in targeting the drug's efficacy and safety in subpopulations. Pharmacoeconomic data are already collected in many trials to ascertain what economic value the medicine might deliver to the market. This information may be important for the pricing and marketing strategy. Data Managers have also had to learn how best to handle pharmacokinetic and pharmacodynamic data for use in models to assist with drug development.

The active management of the drug development process to accelerate, redesign or terminate programs in order to maximise the business benefits, relies heavily on timely and quality data-driven decisions. Rapid access in this environment to individual or summarised data is vital. The data need to be managed throughout the whole of their life cycle to build up this capacity. There is tremendous potential to have more effective development programmes by investing more resource earlier in the process in order to characterise the potential medicine more fully before entering Phases II and III. Use of existing data and techniques such as computer simulation of trials can help to improve study design, reduce numbers of studies and patients and the consequent wastage of resource. Data management can enhance this activity by ensuring that data are available in a form that can be fed back into the system and used in this way.

Data Managers are not restricted to mining data from internal databases. The trawling of multiple external sources can provide data for the company's ever-expanding customer base. Customers include physicians and patients but also governments and those who ultimately pay for the medicines, insurance agencies and Health Management Organisations (HMOs).

The information explosion offers threats and opportunities to the pharmaceutical developer. Data Management needs to be aware of the broader uses of clinical data and information and to consider how it can best use its skills to support medical development. Medical practices are constantly evolving and the effective use of medical data is at the heart of the change. Patient-centred, opinion-based models for treating patients are giving way to evidence-based medicine. Rapid access to factual information and other tools for making biomedical decisions in practice have contributed to this. In the UK, around 90% of GPs now have a computerised surgery but most of them only use it for generating prescriptions at present. The NHS is adopting Internet technology in a highly secure environment to enable patient and health service information to be exchanged. Hopeful patients may demand access to experimental medicines they hear about, for example via the Internet, making it difficult to run a controlled clinical trial. These aspects and the need to differentiate products from one another in a competitive world will change the pharmaceutical company's approach to the drug programme structure.

As technology is advancing, patient information which is already available on health care databases is already being utilised by pharmaceutical companies. Although access is relatively limited at the moment, Clinical Data Management needs to be ready to take advantage of this opportunity as and when it arises. However, care may need to be taken in searching these databases as often they are fairly unstructured.

Extending Communication

Communication methods in the world of clinical trials are on the verge of a revolution. The basis of moving data around the world used to be, and to a large extent still is, by the physical relocation of paper or possibly floppy discs. Electronic file transfer was fraught with difficulty and the need to ensure common standards and systems.

Communication today occurs via a number of different media and how well these are used affects the ability to be effective in business. The information technology revolution has provided global access to networks. Intranets, mini-internets that are accessible only to a defined group of users, usually within the organisation they serve, facilitate the sharing of information to a dispersed workforce and many pharmaceutical companies have taken advantage of this technology during the past 2–3 years. SOPs, project plans, contact telephone numbers can all be made readily available via this type of route. This offers tremendous potential for disseminated workforces with rapid feedback around the organisation worldwide.

The Internet is easy to use and is highly accessible to many people. This is generating a 'pull' for information as well as the more familiar 'push' of information to the consumer. Patients no longer receive health-related information only from their medical practitioner. More than 10% of the searches conducted on the Internet relate to health matters. Geographical separation is no longer a boundary to knowledge. The philosophy that information brings power takes on a new dimension. Patients may have more up-to-date information on medicines and their effects than their physicians or even the pharmaceutical supplier, especially if they communicate with each other on these issues. Instead of receiving the messages someone else deems you need, for example via electronic mail or from your GP, you can search out what you feel you want, probably from the Internet. Expectations of information holders will grow faster than the more regulated and conservative areas of medical development will feel comfortable with.

The pharmaceutical companies need to keep abreast of how these extended communications can impact and enhance business and the Clinical Data Management function is no exception. Some are taking advantage of the many enabling technologies, including PC videoconferencing, scanning and so on, but the regulatory agencies throughout the world are also engaging in closer communication with each other, sharing information. This could have the advantage of driving more common standards between agencies but may also mean that pharmaceutical development organisations will need to be able to meet regulatory queries from different sources more rapidly.

As discussed earlier, the security of sensitive and confidential data transferred electronically needs relevant attention. Although encryption is considered to add a level of security which FAX, for example, may not have, authentication is also important. Information can be sent via the Internet which, seemingly, makes it look as though it has come from a different sender. Firewalls, which prevent outside users accessing secure areas within organisations and systems, and virus checks, also play an important role in the security of electronic data.

Whatever medium is used, it is clear that there is still a need for concise and unambiguous communication, especially in specifications outlining work expected from CROs, central laboratories, and similar establishments. With electronic information usually being accessible to a wider audience than single paper copies, care needs to be taken when considering the target audience, which may mean that contexting data will become even more important.

Expanding Resource

The workload of the Clinical Data Management function in the pharmaceutical company has continued to increase over the last couple of decades. As the volume of data included in a marketing application increases, and as companies have endeavoured to broaden their portfolio of drugs in the pipeline, the demands on Clinical Data Managers have certainly not diminished. One of the key challenges facing this group, therefore, is how to achieve more whilst maintaining headcount or budgets in a steady or declining state. Technology and process changes have offered solutions, but different resourcing strategies are being explored, such as contracting in, contracting out, and homeworking. Each places slightly different demands on the Data Manager.

In particular, there has been a growth in the CRO industry with an estimated 2000 companies now in existence throughout the world. To put this into context, it approximately equals the number of pharmaceutical and biotechnology companies in the world. The quality and timeliness of the output the CROs are able to provide are variable and the quality and nature of the relationship with the pharmaceutical company are of paramount importance. Contracting out the Data Management part of a study or program may be done in order to cope with the peaks in workload. Increasingly, though, this approach seems to be used as a more strategic method of resourcing projects, especially when the CRO can provide support for a range of clinical development activities. Managing the relationships with CRO staff seems to have become a key part of the in-house Data Manager's role over the past 5 years or so. Effective communication and project management skills are essential to both parties to ensure success. Some companies have developed alliances with specific CROs in an effort to help derive mutual benefit from a longer term or higher level of commitment. Staff turnover tends to be higher in CROs than in the pharmaceutical companies though both try to invest in keeping this to an acceptable level. This has to be managed in order not to jeopardise completion of the projects, especially in the CRO environment where resource conflicts may occur between work for different pharmaceutical companies.

Some pharmaceutical companies adopt a different approach and expand their resource by contracting in Data Management staff. Although there are overheads associated with this way of working, some prefer to use their own systems to manage the data and feel they benefit from the degree of control they have over the work in this scenario. Usually the data managers' supervisory and training skills are more in demand in this model.

Pharmaceutical companies probably still manage in the order of half of their work in-house on average. With suitable communication networks and technology now available, some companies utilise flexible working arrangements, including homeworking, to supplement their in-house resource. Telecommuting is possible as access to electronic datafiles and mail complements the more traditional methods of communicating with the office, such as telephone, faxes, post. This type of arrangement is often coupled with more flexible working hours and although this can be advantageous, a homeworker usually needs to be fairly autonomous and self-motivated to make this arrangement work well. Managing the homeworker can require additional effort and be a greater challenge. The range of activities which can be done at home may also prove limiting.

Some organisations thrive on a distributed Data Management function. Many have operations in both the US and Europe and some with other centres in Japan and the rest of the world. Where Data Management is regionalised, strong coordination from the designated centre is necessary. Awareness of cultural differences and effective working in international teams are both necessary attributes for the Data Manager operating in this sort of environment. Technical communications may be problematic and different time zones make direct communication, even by telephone, a challenge, especially if you are trying to link up the US, UK and Japan simultaneously, for example. However, combining data generated in such different cultures where medical practice and data recording philosophies differ, is also a real challenge to the Data Manager if it is to be done meaningfully. If the geographical centres can coordinate effectively, there is considerable potential for a faster feedback loop to local investigators and monitors, faster access to data at the centre and the potential for increasing the effective working day.

One other major impact on resourcing is the use of technology for remote data capture. Generally, the workload peaks and troughs will be at different points compared to the traditional paper method. The intensive data entry and processing component after the study has started reduces significantly for the Data Manager. There may be more effort required, however, in developing and delivering the application to the investigational site and in supporting the use of the technology during the study and possibly at study closure. Start-up times can be slower. Depending on the role which the Data Manager performs in this scenario, they may need to have more advanced technical skills.

The potential for expanding resource in these ways may mean that the role of the in-house data manager becomes more of a coordinating, set-up and progress monitoring role, brokering information. It also gives the opportunity to look at the areas where in-house data management staff could add maximum value and to build on that.

Engaging Data Managers

The challenge facing Clinical Data Management is to decide which strategy, or strategies, best meets their organisational needs. Depending on the roles and responsibilities assigned to the function, some of the skills and competencies for a Data Manager engaged in outsourcing will differ from the one who is employing the advanced technology solution or coordinating an international team. As pharmaceutical companies move into new therapeutic areas or develop an interest in genetics, for example, the Clinical Data Manager needs to understand the implications of the data to ensure they are managed effectively. The approach to database systems is changing too, so an understanding of the relative merits of distributed databases, object-oriented databases and the use of commercial, customised or in-house developed systems is also essential. All require broad Data Management skills but an ability to acquire knowledge and understanding is essential as new areas are explored. Appropriate recruitment, retention and development procedures will be needed to ensure an adequate resource fit. Organisations need to be able to respond to changing needs rapidly so flexibility is important. Search consultants will need to operate globally if suitable Data Managers for this new era are to be found. Opportunities abound in the information-driven world of the future.

In parallel with these opportunities, Data Management is becoming much more business focused. The pressures on the pharmaceutical industry generally are finding their way to areas like the Data Management department because of its high cost to the organisation but also because of the value it brings by handling this increasingly recognised key corporate asset. As the battle is won to reduce the routine elements of Data Management, skill sets will change and the challenge will be to build the skills, recruit and retain good people.

Evolving Culture

In the flattened organisations of the 1990s, empowered teams, networking and effective decision-making based on open sharing of information should be part of the culture if it is to generate a productive environment. Traditionally, Data Management has been perceived to sit somewhere between IT, Statistics and Clinical Research. The boundaries will become more blurred or even redefined depending on the resourcing models adopted. The Data Management role, and that of the Statistician, is also likely to become less well defined. The downsizing of the pharmaceutical industry over recent years to reduce its fixed costs has left many of its employees feeling they no longer have jobs guaranteed for life. As a consequence, many are proactively seeking to acquire skills which are portable to other professions and disciplines or even other industries.

The technical, international project and process management skills of the Clinical Data Manager can profitably be applied to other types of data, even within a pharmaceutical company but also elsewhere. Data Management has the opportunity to play a significant role in the development of the culture of the learning organisation. They have traditionally, if unknowingly, been custodians of institutional knowledge, both in the forms of clinical data but also in their implicit knowledge of the organisation, such as standards, quality of investigators and methodology. With the increasing skill set required by Data Management, it is essential that we nurture a culture which attracts the right kind of employees to fulfil this important role if our companies are to overcome the challenges ahead. Rewards and recognition commensurate with the job are important.

Emerging Markets

As opportunities arise for pharmaceutical companies to enter some of the less well-established markets in various countries around the world, global development and commercialisation will increase. Data Management needs to be ready to respond to the need by increasing its understanding of medical practice in these areas to ensure quality data collection processes are put in place. Similarly, acquaintance with regulatory needs will help obtain a smooth passage through the review process. Recommending how to utilise data collected in some countries for use in others is also an essential role for Clinical Data Management.

CONCLUSION

The pharmaceutical industry is facing, and will continue to face, both internal and external challenges which require a significant increase in productivity. Clinical data is the key corporate asset. The product of the clinical development process, it is compiled to provide evidence of a medicine's efficacy and safety profile and of its potential economic value to the market. Adopting more effective methods for managing the clinical data could enhance the speed with which the drug is developed and commercialised, increasing competitive advantage. The effective use of data capture tools can ensure that high-quality data are available early for review and rapid decision-making. A well-designed and documented database, populated via efficient data feed mechanisms, will ensure regulatory and commercial questions receive rapid responses. As information from the sponsor's clinical database develops into corporate knowledge, the value of the medicine can be realised. Although the regulatory agencies are often considered to be the primary customers of the information supplied by pharmaceutical companies, increasingly the customer-base is broadening. Those who ultimately pay for medicines are economising more and more and want to be convinced of their economic value. Patients are becoming a powerful group of consumers even for prescribed medicines. In a sense, they are voters who want monetary value and quality. They are becoming more educated, seeking out up-to-date medical information, especially from the Internet even though this may prove to be misleading, depending on its origin. There are AIDS activist groups, for example, which are very knowledgeable on what is going on in the industry and also patient advocacy groups. Particularly in the US, many employers could be regarded as consumers of the data and information supplied by the pharmaceutical companies. This is because of their association with Health Management Organisations (HMOs) with respect to their staff. The managed care era which emerged so rapidly in the 1980s, was designed to reduce health care costs often by focusing on preventive measures. All these developments in the pharmaceutical arena demand that Clinical Data Management is at the forefront, leading change, influencing direction.

Data Managers may also need to be longer term in their thinking than their colleagues in Clinical Research. Sustaining an integrated database for initial registration and all subsequent uses, including further claims and so on, is a long process compared to the study report or regulatory submission which may mark the end of involvement for clinical staff in some organisations. In any case, the Data Management function is responsible for building a knowledge base which may need to serve the company for 15–20 years. In order to do this, it needs to employ a broad range of skills. Technical, project management and interpersonal skills all need to be well developed. A concern for compliance is also important in this regulated industry but a willingness to change and proactively seek ways to improve are key to its continued success.

ACKNOWLEDGEMENTS

I would like to thank my secretary, Lisa Lenard, for typing this chapter. In addition, I would like to thank two colleagues for their contribution to the contents. They are Michelle Cotter, who reviewed the first draft, and Lesley Tracey, whose help was invaluable in assisting in structuring it when I had conflicting demands on my time.

Index

Index compiled by Geoffrey C. Jones

Printed in the United States
25993LVS00001B/331-345